Nursing Research and Statistics

Nursing Research Society of India

Pearson

Assistant Editor—Acquisitions: Jigyasa Bhatia
Associate Editor—Production: Vipin Kumar

ISBN: 978-81-317-7570-7

First Impression

Published by Pearson India Education Services Pvt. Ltd, CIN: U72200TN2005PTC057128

Head Office: 1st Floor, Berger Tower, Plot No. C-001A/2, Sector 16B, Noida – 201 301,Uttar Pradesh, India.

Registered Office: Featherlite, 'The Address' 5th Floor, Survey No 203/10B, 200 Ft MMRD Road, Zamin Pallavaram, Chennai - 600044
Website: in.pearson.com; Email:companysecretary.india@pearson.com

Digitally printed in India by Trinity Academy for Corporate Training Ltd, New Delhi in the year of 2025.

Contents

Foreword

It is my great pleasure to write a few lines for the Nursing Research Society of India, which is celebrating 25 years of its existence through this textbook on nursing research. Being associated with NRSI from the very beginning and enjoying most of its conferences organized in different parts of the country, we feel proud at the release of this book.

Our graduates need to find innovative ideas through research in order to bring about effective changes in nursing practice. Nursing research occurs in day-to-day life settings and the demand of the present time is evidence-based practice. Hence, nursing interventions need to be developed depending on evidence-based practice. I hope this book will effectively guide a large number of nursing graduates that India will be producing and who will be contributing to the improvement of nursing practice. I wish that with their earnest effort, they will bring about a substantial change in the country's nursing scenario.

Reena Bose
Ex-President
NRSI
Advisor
Sister Florence College of Nursing

Preface

The Nursing Research Society of India (NRSI) celebrated its silver jubilee in 2012. During the preparations for the celebrations, in one of the executive meetings, the executive members discussed doing something memorable and worthwhile to commemorate this important milestone in the history of NRSI. Publication of a book on research seemed a befitting venture to celebrate this special occasion. Jogindra Vati Gupta, Joint Secretary, NRSI, was unanimously given the responsibility of compiling the book. The authors for writing the chapters were suggested by the executive board.

This book is the product of the thoughts and views of several nurse teachers and nurse scientists who have written chapters on research methodology. There is a widespread notion that evidence-based nursing is largely non-existent in India and most nurses are not oriented toward research. Our purpose of bringing up this book is to promote interest of teachers and nurses in research.

The vision with which this book is being conceived is that the most basic component of a research is 'material and methods'. We in India, until now, have been mostly using methodology based on Western views, whereas our materials (situations) are Indian. While teaching and conducting research, we at times feel uncomfortable and uncertain about how to infuse Western methods with Indian materials. The following question frequently arises: 'Are we doing justice to the research work in hand?' Through this book, this question can be solved to some extent, because it contains many examples from the day-to-day nursing situations in the Indian settings, and our vision of creating a book in Indian perspective will be realized.

Nursing research in India is mostly taken up as an academic exercise for the completion of the master's or bachelor's degree of nursing programs, and research in nursing is rarely done for 'the sake of research'. Through this book, we intend to motivate nurse scientists of India to take up research projects that would truly enrich the body of nursing knowledge and pave the way to conduct research on areas affecting decision-making with an Indian perspective.

We hope this book will provide a comprehensive introduction to nursing research, research methodology, and methods to prepare the papers. The book will be very useful to practising nurses and nursing students at all educational levels. The text is organized into 15 chapters based on research process written by multiple authors. It covers the basics of both qualitative and quantitative approaches to nursing research. The reader can achieve a smooth transition from the theoretical base to actual research situation after going through the contents of this book. The readers are also given directions for developing nursing research proposals and seeking funding and support for conducting research studies and publishing articles in nursing research journals. The chapter on analysing the data focuses exclusively on descriptive and inferential statistics. The examples in the various chapters have been presented from actual clinical nursing research. Thus, this book is a genuine effort in clarifying the basic concepts of nursing research.

We are highly obliged to all the authors for their invaluable inputs whose contributions were extremely helpful in the development of this text. We would also like to recognize the excellent editorial assistance and suggestions given by Jigyasa Bhatia, Pearson Education, from time to time for keeping us on track.

Usha Ukande
Jogindra Vati

About NRSI

NURSING RESEARCH SOCIETY OF INDIA

The Nursing Research Society of India was established in May 1986 to promote research within and around the nursing environment. It is registered under the Societies Act XXI of 1960 with the Registrar of Societies, Delhi Administration (Certificate No. S/18421 dated 2 December 1987).

AIMS AND OBJECTIVES

1. Support the development of nursing research activities in the universities and nursing health care institutions to provide nursing care standards.
2. Provide a platform to nurse scientists to exchange views on nursing research.
3. Promote and sponsor scientific meets, seminars, and conferences to advance nursing research.
4. Create public interest in the contribution of nursing in promotive, preventive, and restorative activities contributing to health and family welfare.
5. Establish Nursing Journal of India to communicate knowledge pertaining to innovations in nursing.

About the Contributors

T. M. Assuma Beevi is Principal of MIMS College of Nursing. She is a Joint Director of MIMS Academy.

R. Sreevani is Professor at Shri Devraj URS College of Nursing, Tamaka, Karnataka.

Sister Tessy Sebastian is Professor at the Department of Psychiatric Nursing and Dean of Faculty of Nursing, Smt. Radhikabai Meghe Memorial College of Nursing, Sawangi (Meghe), Maharashtra.

Sneha Pitre is Vice Principal and Head of the Department of Bharati Vidyapeeth College of Nursing, Katraj-Dhankawadi, Pune, Maharashtra.

Jogindra Vati is Professor and Principal of SGHS College of Nursing, Mohali.

Raj Rani is Principal of College of Nursing, Baba Farid University of Health Sciences, Faridkot, Punjab.

Bandana Bhattacharya is Former Professor and Vice Principal(Retd), Adesh College of Nursing, Muktsar, Punjab.

Pity Koul is Professor at Nursing School of Health Sciences, IGNOU, New Delhi. She is also the Secretary of NRSI.

Manju Chhugani is Principal of Rufaida College of Nursing, Jamia Hamdard University, New Delhi.

Usha Ukande is Principal of Choithram College of Nursing, Indore. She is also the President of NRSI.

Ratna Prakash is Professor and Principal of Himalayan College of Nursing, HIHT, Dehradun.

H. C. Rawat is Vice Principal of College of Nursing, Baba Farid University of Health Sciences, Faridkot, Punjab.

A. V. Raman is Director of Nursing Research and Education, Westfort College of Nursing, Thrissur, Kerala.

K. Lalitha is Professor at National Institute of Mental Health and Neurosciences (NIMHANS), Bengaluru.

Santosh Yadav is Officer on Special Duty at Rufaida College of Nursing, New Delhi.

Ghansham Sharma is Lecturer at the Department of Community Medicine, Guru Gobind Singh Medical College, Baba Farid University of Health Sciences, Faridkot, Punjab.

chapter 1

Introduction to Nursing Research

OBJECTIVES

Upon completion of this chapter the learner will be able to:

- Identify the types of knowledge used by nurses in their practice
- Discuss the historical developments of nursing research
- Explain the meaning and definition of research
- Differentiate between research in nursing and nursing research
- Differentiate between problem-solving, scientific method, and research
- Explain basic and applied research
- Identify the characteristics of nursing research and researcher
- Discuss the significance of nursing research
- Explain research utilization
- Differentiate between research utilization and evidence-based practice
- Discuss various aspects of evidence-based practice
- Define evidence-based research

NURSING RESEARCH: A PERSPECTIVE

Managing clinical responsibility is a challenge for nurses and nursing profession. Nurses require extraordinary range of knowledge, skills, and talents to provide quality care to their patients. Historically, nurses' practices were based on certain types of knowledge. The mechanisms that nurses usually used to provide patient care were as follows: traditions and customs, common sense, authority, experience, intuition, logical reasoning, and assembled knowledge. Carper stated that there are four types of knowledge that nurses use to base their practice, namely empirics, aesthetics, ethics, and personal knowledge. Park had described three types of knowledge. They are *representational knowledge* (to describe, explain or understand a phenomenon), *relational knowledge* (knowing a person both affectively and cognitively), and *reflective knowledge* (bringing changes by reflecting on agreeing to the values, which inform the world in which we live). Whatever may be the type of knowledge, it gets outdated quickly in today's scientific world. The half-life of scientific knowledge is getting shorter than before. Nurses must access and evaluate extensive clinical information and incorporate it into their clinical decision-making to provide quality care in a compassionate manner. This is possible only through the efficient use of research findings. This can be achieved by purposeful reading of research reports and research summaries in the practice area and by conducting or participating in research studies to develop new knowledge. Nursing research generates new knowledge that boosts scientific practices and is the only valid knowledge that nurses can rely upon in their practice. So, nurses need to be cognizant and proficient in the research process.

HISTORICAL DEVELOPMENT OF NURSING RESEARCH

The need of research was emphasized in modern nursing practice from its inception. Florence Nightingale established her system of nursing and nursing education over a hundred years ago. However, she envisioned the development of nursing as a scholarly human and scientific discipline. She used the research process and records to formulate ideas for improving nursing and health care. This incidence directs the need of observation and documentation in the practice of nursing. This may be the reason why she is still remembered by the statisticians as a pioneer in statistics. Florence Nightingale focused on the importance of a healthy environment for patients. She used aspects of research such as ventilation, cleanliness, purity of water, and healthy diet. She began her research during the Crimean War (1853–1856) and collected data based on her observations. She used statistics and graphs to present results. She had based her nursing care on research findings. Her most important findings were that mortality rate decreased from 42 per cent to 2 per cent for wounded or ill soldiers after the environment was cleaned. Although Florence Nightingale paved way for scientific basis for nursing practice, nurse's education was mainly based on apprenticeship training model in early period. During this period, the primary emphasis was on the availability of student's services in patient care rather than on developing knowledge base for the nursing profession.

Nursing Research Development in USA

The historical background on the development of nursing research in the USA shows that from 1900 to 1950 most leaders in nursing had advanced preparation in the field of education. As a result, many research studies focused on education rather than practice and that improved the educational system of nursing. During 1900–1950s, many articles on nursing care of patients with communicable diseases, hygiene, sanitation, asepsis, infant mortality, and maternal mortality were seen in nursing literature. This shows nurses' awareness towards research. The *American Journal of Nursing* was first published in 1900. In 1920, the journal published its first case study, which was used as a teaching tool for students at that time. Even now, case studies are found to be one of the best teaching tools for nursing. In 1920s, the first graduate programme in nursing was started in the USA. The 1930s witnessed the evaluation of the effectiveness of nursing procedures and distinguished nursing orders from medical orders. During 1930–1940s, nursing leaders conducted studies on the status of nursing students and the findings helped to relieve excess nursing duties from students to fully benefit from educational programmes. After World War II, a broader concept of nursing care related to public health nursing was developed. The importance of including social sciences and humanities into nursing education was emphasized during this period. Social sciences and humanities helped nurses to have a broader concept of family-centred care. This promoted nurses with research background to conduct studies on the sociological and psychological aspects of illness. The research resulted in the fundamental paradigm shift of nursing care from patient-centred care to family-centred care. In 1950, graduate-level programmes were started in nursing. The aim was to prepare nurses for leadership positions, advance practice and research. In 1950, the American Nurses Association (ANA) initiated a five-year study on nursing functions and activities. 1952 was a landmark year in the history of nursing research with the publication of the *Nursing Research Journal*. This helped to communicate the growing body of knowledge to professionals in nursing. In 1953, the Institute for Research and Service in Nursing Education was established by Teacher's College, Columbia. In 1955, the ANA established the American Nurses Foundation to support and promote research activities. In 1956, the articles that appeared in journals show reflections on the ideas about conceptual development of nursing as a science and a profession.

During 1955–1965, researchers focused their work on the characteristics of students for selection, retention, and educational processes. Articles focusing on quality of patient care, chronic heart diseases, cancer, stroke, and so on were also published at that time. Hospitals began to report experiences with intensive care unit and automation. In 1963, the publication of *International Journal of Nursing Studies* was started. Sigma Theta Tau first published *Image* (now *The Journal of Nursing Scholarship*) in 1967.

Prior to 1970, the *Nursing Research Journal* was the only major publication. However, by 1970, the number of publications increased, which included *Western Journal of Nursing Research*, *Advances in Nursing Sciences*, *Nursing Science Quarterly* and *Scholarly inquiry for Nursing Practice*. In 1970, the ANA funded the formulation of a national commission for the study of nursing and nursing education. During this period, some private sources also published independent investigations of the quality of nursing in USA. Five hundred US nurses earned doctoral degrees in the 1970s, which is considered as a landmark achievement in the development of nursing research. In 1970, the Commission on Nursing Research was formulated in the USA to advance research activities. In 1972, the Council of Nurse Researchers was established. In 1973, the National Commission for Nurses in the USA concluded that nursing is a science and an art. *Advances in Nursing Science* and *Research in Nursing* were first published in that year, followed by *Western Journal of Nursing Research* (1979). During 1977–1986, 720 journal articles related to nursing research were published with 95 per cent nurses as first authors. During 1976–1981 and in 1985, the ANA developed the statement of priority on nursing research. In 1986, the National Center for Nursing Research was established in the USA with Dr Ada Sue Hinshaw as the first director. In 1993, the National Center for Nursing Research became the National Institute for Nursing Research. The current work of this institution is related to expansion in clinical practice, ethical practice and protection of human subjects. Another area of concern is the use and evaluation of nursing theories. The *Qualitative Research Journal* was first published in 1994. 1997 witnessed the foundation of Canadian Health Services. In 2004, world view on *Evidence Based Nursing Journal* was started.

History of Nursing Research in Europe

In Europe, especially in the UK, the United Kingdom Central Council for Nursing (UKCC) and the National Institutes of Health (NIH) also took up nursing research as a main agenda for nursing fraternity to improve evidence-based nursing practice. In the 1950s, sociologists and psychologists were more involved in researching nursing and nurses. Marjorie Simpson started a self-help group for nurse researchers in 1959 called the Research Discussion Group. This later became the Research Society of the Royal College of Nursing. By 1980s, nurses in the UK obtained doctoral degrees from various universities. They obtained research qualification even after a baccalaureate programme. Tierney identified the UK, Finland and Denmark as having developed in a similar way over 30 years, with Estonia, Lithuania, and Slovenia developing their research activities only in the past 10 years.

Nursing Research in India

The first attempt at nursing research in India dates back to Florence Nightingale's report on unsanitary conditions in Indian military men's living areas. In 1946, the Bhore Committee in its report recommended improvement in various aspects of nursing, including the need for higher education. Following these recommendations, nurses from India were sent to Columbia University to acquire research qualifications. Ms Edith Buchanan of Rajkumari Amrit Kaur College of Nursing (RAKCON) was the first nurse in India to obtain a doctoral degree in education with the sponsorship of the World Health Organization (WHO). In 1955, Ms Margaretta Craig attended the International Council of Nurses meet and presented a paper on the need for nursing research in India.

From 1960 onwards, postgraduate nursing students started progressively involving themselves in research at RAKCON, Delhi, and College of Nursing, Christian Medical College, Vellore. In 1963, the Indian Nursing Council (INC) conducted a study on the health services of India to revise General Nursing and Midwifery (GNM) syllabus. Dr Marie Ferguson of RAKCON along with other nurse leaders conducted an activity study to define nursing and non-nursing functions of nurses in selected health institutes of India. The Trained Nurses Association of India conducted a study on nurses' time utilization with the assistance of Ms Anna Gupta, under the guidance of Dr Sulochana Krishnan. Ms Margaretta Craig was the chairperson. Dr Aparna Bhaduri and Dr Marie Farrel had authored *Health Research: A Community Based Approach*, which was published by WHO. They conducted a series of seminars in various parts of the country to create awareness about nursing research among nursing educators. The first nursing research conference was organized at College of Nursing, Bengaluru, in 1982. The title of the conference was 'Nursing Research in India: Prospect and Retrospect'. This conference had made the following recommendations:

1. Each nursing college should have a research cell.
2. The faculty at a nursing college should encourage students and provide time for conducting research.
3. The college of nursing should foster research attitude among nursing students.
4. The central and state governments and private institutions should include budget for nursing research.
5. Opportunity should be provided for faculty to visit foreign countries on short-term basis to learn about nursing research.
6. Efforts should be taken to establish collaborative areas of research and scholastic interactions with nursing colleges in other countries.

In 1984, the University Grants Commission sponsored a conference at Bengaluru titled 'Teaching Nursing Research to Nursing College Teachers' for all teachers of nursing colleges in India.

The first M. Phil. programme for nurses started at RAK in 1986 followed by MAHE, Manipal, in 1992; doctoral programmes are now offered by many universities in India for nurses as well as other disciplines such as psychology, education and other humanities. The INC now offers Doctor of Philosophy in Nursing (PhD) programme in collaboration with WHO at Rajiv Gandhi University, Bengaluru. Other prestigious universities that offer PhD programme in India are MAHE, Manipal; JNU, New Delhi; SNDT, Mumbai; University of Kerala; University of Calicut; MG University; Kottayam; The Tamilnadu Dr MGR Medical University, Chennai and Devi Ahilya Vishwavidyalaya Indore and many other universities, Indore. As far as research articles are concerned, the *Nursing Journal of India* (NJI) gives preference for research articles. From 1978 to 1980, Dr Aparna Badhuri and Dr Marie Farrel wrote on nursing research in a series of articles in NJI. Many Indian nurses were sponsored by the Rockefeller Foundation to achieve their doctoral degree from Columbia University during 1950–1970s. In 1998, the National Institute of Mental Health and Neurosciences Bangalore (NIMHANS) organized a nursing research interest section. In 2002, INC revised the GNM syllabus and included nursing research in the curriculum. Another landmark achievement in nursing research in India was the establishment of the Nursing Research Society of India (NRSI) in 1986, with Dr Inderjit Walia as the founder president and Mrs Uma Handa as the first secretary. The work of NRSI has helped in creating awareness on research among nurses. Every year, the society organizes conferences for nurses on current issues in the nursing field pertinent to nursing in the country. NRSI now has zone-wise activities, as India is a vast country and it may not be able to cater to the needs of all nurses in this diversified country.

NRSI has provided a portal for the dissertations conducted in the country as a curricular requirement by postgraduate students (www.nrsi.org). Now, there are many indexed journals that are published for dissemination of nursing research articles; examples of such journals are *Nursing and Midwifery Research Journal, Nightingale's Nursing Times, Journal of Nursing and Midwifery, Journal of Nursing Research Society of India, Indian Journal of Nursing Studies, Journal of Nursing Education*, and *Kerala Nurses' Forum.*

PhD Consortium and Its Role in Research Development

The INC in collaboration with Rajiv Gandhi University of Health Sciences and WHO has initiated a doctoral programme in nursing under the Faculty of Nursing to promote doctoral education in various fields of nursing (www.indiannursingcouncil.org). Currently, there are six study centres (College of Nursing, NIMHANS, Bengaluru; R.A.K. College of Nursing, New Delhi; C.M.C. College of Nursing, Vellore; C.M.C. College of Nursing, Ludhiana; Government College of Nursing, Thiruvananthapuram and Government College of Nursing, Hyderabad). These centres are connected by video conferencing facilities. Currently, the seventh batch of students is doing the doctoral research under the PhD consortium. The consortium can be contacted at phd@indiannursingcouncil.org.

Indira Gandhi National Open University had also started PhD in nursing in the year 2010. The current enrolment is fixed for postgraduate nurses who have completed five years of experience after postgraduate qualification.

DEFINITION AND MEANING

In today's world, nurses must be lifelong learners capable of evaluating and modifying their clinical practice based on new knowledge. Nurses are increasingly expected to become producers of new knowledge through nursing research. The term research in Latin means 'to know'. The word 'research' is derived from the French language and its literal meaning is 'investigate thoroughly'. It is a new way of experiencing reality. Research is to search again or to examine carefully. It is the process of collecting, analysing and interpreting data to understand a phenomenon. Specifically, research is diligent, systematic enquiry, or investigation to validate and refine existing knowledge and generate new knowledge. Research in its broadest sense is an attempt to gain solutions to problems; more precisely, it is the collection of data in a rigorously controlled situation for the purpose of prediction or explanation. ANA defines nursing research as the development of knowledge about health and the promotion of health over the full life span, care of persons with health problems and disabilities, and nursing actions to enhance the ability of individuals to respond effectively to actual or potential health problems. According to ANA, nurses use research to provide evidence-based care that promotes quality health outcomes for individuals, families, communities, and health care systems. Nursing research is a systematic approach to examine the phenomena that are important to nursing and nurses. Nursing research is the systematic enquiry designed to develop trustworthy evidence about issues of importance to the nursing profession, including nursing practice, education, administration, and informatics.

NURSING RESEARCH VERSUS RESEARCH IN NURSING

Nursing research focuses on the practice of nursing. Research in nursing studies the nursing profession and the characteristics of the nurse. Nursing research is mainly concerned with clinical problems. Research in nursing is the broader study of the nursing profession and includes historical, ethical and political studies. Nursing research includes all studies concerning nursing practice, education, and administration. Studies concerning nurses themselves also can be included in nursing research. It provides objective and reliable nursing knowledge to improve the quality of nursing practice. It is important for every nurse to know that studies related to patient care or promoting wellness are usually termed 'clinical nursing research'.

SCIENTIFIC METHOD AND RESEARCH PROCESS

Scientific method is the basis of scientific investigation. It involves experiments on samples or specimens. In scientific method, the scientist poses a question and formulates hypotheses. The hypothesis stays as the potential explanation or answer to the question. Here, the researcher with empirical evidence and rigorous control attempts to answer the question under consideration. So, it is a process that starts with a question. It is a systematic and objective method of enquiry. Scientific method helps a researcher to develop new knowledge, expand and validate existing knowledge, and reaffirm previous knowledge. The rigorous control is the core of scientific method. Hence a specific problem is studied in a systematic and objective way by keeping rigorous control and holding conditions constant which permit only variation to phenomena comes under study. It also focuses on the structure and control to establish cause and effect relationship between variables by supporting or rejecting the hypothesis. The scientific problem-solving helps in theory testing and not theory developing. This method helps to test fractions of theory rather than a whole theory. That is, a fraction of the theory can be tested while specific problems are investigated because it is structured. Theory generation is possible only when a loosely structured research method is used, as it helps to depict the totality or wholeness of the human experience under study.

Research process covers all branches of research with a whole lot of methodology and not only the scientific method of experimentation. Research uses non-experimental observations for gathering information. In a historical research, the researcher may collect data on experiences of people in a retrospective perspective. However, in scientific the method, the researcher performs the observation as a by-product of some intervention. Research process refers to the actual gathering of information. This can be observation, interview or even gathering information on the Internet. In the scientific method, rules and answers are derived through several steps and it ends with a conclusion as proving or disproving, or accepting or rejecting, the hypothesis posed. Research is a step in the knowledge quest. Research today has a wide spectrum from researching a book and writing a review to locating best evidence from different sources to answer a burning clinical question in the context of nursing research. When research is used in the context of science, it is a step of scientific method. Scientific method is specific and often uses the following steps:

1. State a hypothesis—a tentative prediction of relationship between variables.
2. Design an experimental procedure to test the hypothesis and construct equipment and tools necessary for testing.
3. Conduct experiment.
4. Analyse data collected from experiment.
5. Refine or correct hypothesis and continue the experiment if necessary.

The scientific method has many limitations compared with other research methods in nursing. Because nursing uses human beings as subjects, it poses moral and ethical issues. The complexity of human behaviour will not allow rigorous control, and the measurement of behaviour poses difficulty due to influence of external variables. Keeping conditions constant is a difficult task.

NURSING RESEARCH AND PROBLEM-SOLVING

A problem is a situation that can be quantitative or qualitative, confronts an individual or a group of individuals, and requires resolution. Problem-solving is a powerful human activity. It is a process, an activity, whereby the best value is determined for an unknown, subject to a specific set of conditions. It is a means by which an individual uses previously acquired knowledge, skills, and understanding to satisfy the demands of an unfamiliar situation. It is impossible to teach specific facts that will always lead to a solution. The ability to solve a problem comes from doing it. Many things must pull together to solve a problem. Problem-solving is a skill necessitating a combination of experience, knowledge, process, and art. The problem-solving process is a series of logical steps, which when followed produce an optimal solution, given time, and resources as two constraints. There are different steps involved in problem-solving and different experts give several types of steps. However, all these experts agree on the following steps:

1. **Specify the Problem:** This involves evaluating the present state and determining how it differs from the stated goals.
2. **Analyse the Problem:** Analysing the problem involves learning as much as you can about it.
3. **Formulate Possible Solutions:** Identify a wide range of possible solutions.
4. **Evaluate Possible Solutions:** Weigh the advantages and disadvantages of each solution.
5. **Choose a Solution:** Consider three factors: compatibility with your priorities, amount of risk, and practicality.
6. Implement the solution.
7. Evaluate and revise if necessary.

Both nursing research and problem-solving use abstract critical thinking and complex reasoning to identify new information. However, research process needs to be distinguished from problem-solving. Problem-solving targets a single problem of a patient or an organization, for example, a patient complaining that a particular nurse behaves absent-mindedly while providing care. This may be a problem related to that particular nurse; the reasons for such behaviour need to be analysed and solutions are to be determined to change the behaviour of that particular nurse. Research process, on the other hand, contributes to the profession of nursing by validating, predicting, explaining, and controlling phenomena of interest to nursing with the help of statistics. For example, a study can be conducted to find the level of satisfaction among patients receiving chemotherapy in the day care centre. The knowledge derived from this study can be used to change the practice. The study can be replicated in another place for further validation of findings. A solution derived for a problem cannot be replicated as the problem may not be the same for another situation or place. Research involves an explicit process of informed consent for subjects of the study, which is not customary in a problem-solving scenario. In the example of the absent-minded nurse, she can be called and questioned about the reasons of absent mindedness, whereas the patients participating in the study on the level of satisfaction need to give informed consent expressing their willingness of participation. Research is subjected to external and peer review and replication to ascertain validity and ethical principles. A problem of absent mindedness of a particular nurse is an isolated problem and a solution is necessitated for that situation. However, the level of satisfaction of patients is related to multiple factors that are not only related to the nurse's behaviour. It needs a thorough exploration of the structure, process and output in the health care organization. The factors may be similar in different organizations and need

TABLE 1.1 *Differences between Research and Problem-solving*

S. No.	Research	Problem-solving
1.	Start with selection of a research topic.	Target a single problem.
2.	Perform the rigorous process of collecting and analysing data using statistical methods.	No statistical analysis is used.
3.	Control the extraneous and confounding variables.	No control is imposed.
4.	Informed consent of participants is necessary.	No informed consent is needed.
5.	Findings of the research study can be generalized.	No generalization is needed.
6.	Replication of the study is possible.	No replication is possible and is situation based.

replication to identify best evidence. Table 1.1 summarizes the differences between research and problem-solving:

NEED AND IMPORTANCE OF NURSING RESEARCH

The most important purpose of nursing research is to develop a scientific knowledge base for nursing practice. Practitioners of human care and treatment throughout history have been viewed with respect, and their services were unquestioned compared with those in other professions. However, these differences are diminishing. Now, nurses must account for what they do, why they do, what they produce and how much it costs. So, nursing is accountable to society for providing cost-effective state-of-the-art quality care, and nurses are accountable to their patients. A solid research base will provide evidence of the nursing action that is effective in promoting positive patient outcomes in terms of positive aspects of health including survival rates, states of physiological, physical and emotional health, and satisfaction with health care services. The classic definition of outcome of medical treatment of death, disease, disability, discomfort, and dissatisfaction (5 Ds) need not be the outcome of nursing research. So, the care given must be routinely assessed and remedial measures must be taken to decide the outcome of nursing practice. Nurses need to seek ways to improve nursing care through research. Research results create a strong scientific base for nursing practice, especially when deliberately and carefully evaluated for application to specific clinical topics. During the career of a nurse, many practice issues and clinical questions will be raised, which require research to answer such queries confidently. Pursuing research in such areas will help nurses to acquire valid and reliable information that would enable them to provide quality care. Findings of nursing research not only aim at affecting the direct provision of nursing and health care to recipients of nursing care but also need to generate knowledge in areas that affect nursing care processes indirectly. Burns and Groove stated that research within the realms of nursing education, nursing administration, health services, characteristics of nurses and nursing roles provides evidence for effectively changing these supporting areas of nursing knowledge.

Validates Nursing as a Profession

Nursing like other professions has educational standards, autonomy, socialization, an established knowledge base, licensure, formal entry examinations, code of ethics, technical expertise, professional standards, altruistic service, and public trust. These are the main characteristics of a profession. The knowledge base of nursing is updated through the same rigorous process of research similar to other scientific professions. Nursing practice activities are substantiated to produce reliable outcomes by a number of researches.

Critics assert that nursing is a borrowed knowledge, and hence, there is a challenge for nurses to identify those elements that are unique to nursing and build scientific knowledge base unique to nursing. Nursing practice activities can be substantiated as predicting valid and reliable outcomes for patients only after a body of knowledge has been established and confirmed by substantial amount of research.

The total body of knowledge called nursing is composed of many facts, concepts, principles, and theories. Much of this knowledge is borrowed from the medical, biological, and social sciences. So, it is imperative for nurses to develop their own body of knowledge in nursing that describes and explains nursing problems and nursing care. Thus, research is essential to develop scientific principles and theories specific to nursing. Researchers in nursing are now conducting research that applies scientific principles from general sciences to nursing care problems to aid in developing scientific base for the profession. Nursing research confirms and expands the body of knowledge to validate the profession with its own knowledge base. For example, if a study on patient comfort suggests that a relationship exists between high level of stress and noise level in patient care unit, the nurse can very well adopt a practice of keeping a lower level of noise in the unit, promoting comfort. These findings can be incorporated into practice and can be suggested as a scientific base for validating nursing interventions related to stress reduction strategies. There it forms a part of nursing knowledge base. New knowledge obtained through research needs to be tested in practice. Nursing care should also generate new areas for research. Thus, research helps in validating the profession.

The highest goal of nursing research is the establishment of nursing theories and principles to provide sound bases for practice that validate the profession. While providing nursing care, the choice of nursing intervention is determined from the body of nursing knowledge and factual information about the patient. So, certain standard principles of practice appropriate to particular situation are selected from the body of knowledge. A time should come when it can be said that the scientific base for a particular nursing intervention has arrived from a knowledge base from nursing itself. This will be possible only by developing scientific basis for the profession through research.

Refines Existing Knowledge on Nursing Practice

Research helps in the discovery of new knowledge and refines existing knowledge. The knowledge generated can be used to improve clinical practice, nursing education, nursing administration, and different nursing roles. For example, diagnosis of type 2 diabetes was made previously with fasting blood sugar 160 mg/dl and GTT (Glucose Tolerance Test) as criteria. The new criteria are FBS (Fasting Blood Sugar) $\geq$ 126 mg/dl—two separate occasions, symptoms, and positive 2-hour GTT—and HbA1C > 6.5. This is an example of refining existing knowledge. Researches in the area of care of newborns have identified that keeping infants in the supine position is better than the prone (face down) position to prevent sudden infant death syndrome (SIDS). Previously, newborns and infants were kept face down to drain secretions; this resulted in the suffocation of infants, leading to SIDS. For example, a child sleeping face down may move his or her face into such a position that the nose and mouth are completely obstructed. This may alter the levels of oxygen or carbon dioxide in the infant's blood. Protective responses to stressful stimuli may be defective in infants who are vulnerable to SIDS. Furthermore, it is identified that items in a baby's crib and his or her sleeping position can combine with a baby's physical problems to increase the risk of SIDS. Babies who are placed on their stomachs or sides to sleep may have more difficulty breathing than those placed on their backs. Lying face down on a fluffy comforter or a waterbed can block an infant's airway. Draping a blanket over a baby's head is also risky. This is not the only reason for SIDS, but these findings definitely helped nurses to refine existing knowledge on care of infants to reduce the incidence of SIDS.

Provides Scientific Basis and Demonstrates Accountability to Profession

The scientific knowledge of nursing is derived from the focus or unique perspective of the discipline and provides an organizing framework for nursing practice. The knowledge obtained through research helps nurses to substantiate and justify their actions by referring to research findings. Research results create a strong scientific base for nursing practice, especially when deliberately and carefully evaluated for application to specific clinical topics. In this era of accountability, nurses are accepting the challenge to document outcomes of care. Nursing research had progressed to account for nursing practices and potential effects and document their worth to hospital administration and policy-makers. Thus, nurses can prove the benefit of their appointment over others for providing cost-effective quality care, especially in the current scenario of economic crisis. Research is essential to validate nursing actions, which in turn provide justification for the cost of nurses versus unlicensed assistive workers. Through research, the scientific basis for our actions is being challenged constantly. Nursing research equips the nurses for description, explanation, prediction, and control of nursing phenomena in their clinical practice.

Description is done through identifying and understanding the nature and attributes of nursing phenomena and sometimes the relationships among these phenomena. Through research, nurses are able to do the following:

1. Describe what exists in nursing practice
2. Discover new information
3. Promote understanding of situation
4. Classify information for use in the discipline

A study conducted to find out the stressors of leukaemic children and their coping mechanisms towards hospitalization provided an insight into the common stressors and described the same in terms of children and their parents. The factors identified as most stressful by parents were not even considered stressful by nurses and doctors. This provided new information regarding different perspective on stressors. Hence, research that concentrates on description is an essential groundwork for studies that will provide explanation, prediction, and control of nursing phenomena.

Explanation, according to Burns and Groove, is concerned with the clarification of relationship among and between phenomena. This helps to identify the reasons why certain events occur. Explanation helps to the organization of concepts and derivation of concepts and principles. Quite often description follows explanation. When enough facts exist, explanation of relation between such facts is necessary. The explanation of phenomena helps to predict the occurrence of certain events. Through research, *prediction* on the chance of occurrence of certain events can be estimated and precautionary measures can be taken. The probability of occurrence of certain events can be possible only through scientific research using inferential statistics. For example, the Meteorological Survey of India gives prediction on climate or weather changes for each day and gives red alert to fishermen to take precautions by not going to sea on certain days when there is a possibility of a hurricane or heavy tides. These weather reports are obtained through research and monitoring. Here, the people can take precautions, as there is an anticipated risk of turbulent sea. In a similar manner, in nursing, the use of Norton's scale for bedsore risk assessment help nurses to predict the anticipated risk of developing bedsore in certain hospitalized patients. This example explains that the probability of developing certain conditions or complications is there if certain situations or risk factors are present. Hence, nursing research helps nurses to promote wellness through preventing the occurrence of risk factors. As mentioned earlier, once the outcome of phenomena is predicted through research, the *control* can be exercised through manipulation of the situation or risk factors. Wiedenbach described control as the ability to write a prescription to produce the desired results. For example, if a patient is found to be prone to develop bedsore, the nurse can very well prescribe to the patient a water mattress, which would control the occurrence of pressure ulcer in that patient. Estimating and anticipating the outcome in a particular situation is thus possible through research.

In a nut shell, nursing research does the following for nursing as a profession:

1. Validates nursing as a profession (by providing distinguishing criteria to consider nursing as a profession, a service, occupation)
2. Provides scientific basis for practice by explaining, describing, predicting, and controlling phenomena important to nursing and nurses
3. Helps in formulating theories
4. Helps in formulating models and frameworks for practice
5. Helps in testing the proposed theory
6. Helps in testing models for practice
7. Helps in developing cost-effective quality nursing interventions

CHARACTERISTICS OF A GOOD RESEARCH

1. Research is a systematic process that identifies variables and tests the relationship between them.
2. It is logical and so it can be duplicated by others.
3. It has clearly defined purposes.
4. It exerts control over situations or extraneous variables and the variables under study.
5. It is reductive, as it investigates a small sample and findings can be generalized to a larger population.
6. It creates empirical evidences as decisions are based on the data collected.
7. It produces reliable results that can be replicated as others may find the same results.
8. It produces valid findings that are reproducible.
9. It maintains accuracy in all steps.
10. It maintains originality.
11. It meets ethical principles.
12. The informed consent is obtained from the participants.
13. It tests a whole theory or the parts of a theory.
14. It develops theory.
15. It uses logical reasoning in generation of knowledge both deductively and inductively.
16. The findings can be used for description, prediction, and explanation of phenomenon of interest

Attributes of a Researcher

A researcher should have certain characteristics to effectively conduct the research. They are as follows:

1. A researcher should be a subject expert; they should have qualities such as endurance, commitment and a sensitive mind and should be purpose oriented.
2. The researcher should also have scientific temper with a spirit of enquiry and rational approach.
3. The researcher must be objective and avoid sentiments and emotional interpretations of facts.

TYPES OF RESEARCH

Nursing research activities may be classified into two types.

Purpose

Basic Research

It is the fundamental or pure research for establishing new knowledge with the development and refinement of theories. The findings are not immediately applicable to practical problems, but they provide scope for further research to expand the body of knowledge. In basic research, a specific purpose is not delineated by the researcher like that of applied research, but it stimulates new ways of thinking about divergence that have the potential to change and improve how practitioners deal with a problem.

Major aims of basic research are as follows:

1. Gather and generate information.
2. Expand the body of knowledge of the particular discipline in which the study is conducted.
3. Refute or support theories.
4. Refine existing knowledge or theories and principles.

Example: A researcher conducts a study on adolescents' attitude towards hero worship. Here, the researcher observes that the adolescents believe in positive role modelling rather than hero worship. So, a theory can be evolved on the benefits of role modelling in developing positive attitude among adolescents.

Applied Research

This type of research also helps in generating new knowledge but can be applied to practical setting without undue delay. It has functional purposes and practical use. Applied research is done to find a solution to a problem that requires an impending solution. It is action oriented and involves collection and analysis of data to arrive at a solution for existing problems in any organization or practice area. So, applied research attempts to solve problems in the organization, make decision, evaluate programmes, and develop new strategies for pursuing change in existing practice.

Example: A researcher might have seen that there is a wide variation in oxygen saturation of patients receiving different modes of oxygen delivery after giving the same amount of oxygen. So, the researcher may conduct a study to identify the reasons and the best method of oxygen delivery to improve saturation within a prescribed period of oxygen delivery.

Table 1.2 provides a comparison of the basic and applied researches.

TABLE 1.2 *Comparison of Basic and Applied Research*

S. No.	Basic Research	Applied Research
1.	Basic research is the pure or fundamental research.	It is used in the field of practice to solve a problem.
2.	It is done to study a general phenomenon, a process.	It is targeted at solving a specific problem for a utilitarian purpose.
3.	It is abstract or theoretical.	A theory or part of the theory is tested to find the utility.
4.	It is knowledge for the sake of knowledge and is believed as a starting point in knowledge expansion.	It is useful in creating evidences.

Approach to Research

The following are the various approaches to research:

1. Descriptive research:
   (a) Classified as surveys
   (b) Qualitative strategies
2. Experimental research:
   (a) Purely experimental
   (b) Quasi-experimental
3. Historical (documentary)

In the historical approach, the researcher does the systematic collection and critical evaluation of data related to past occurrences. It examines what has already occurred. The investigator has no control over manipulating the independent variables. Experimental approach is future oriented and predicts what will occur. In this approach, the investigator has control in the manipulations of the independent variables in the experimental settings, and the subjects are randomly arranged (each individual is assigned a place in a group based on chance alone) to the treatment (experiment) condition specified in the study. Quasi-experimental research refers to modification of the experimental approach. The investigator may have control in manipulating the independent variables, although the subjects are not randomly arranged to the treatment condition.

The type of research used by a researcher depends on the objectives and framework of the study, kind of data and nature of problems to be solved. The researcher's skills, background and academic preparation, and areas of competence will influence the selection of the type of research that they do. Difference between research approaches is determined by their time orientation and the extent to which the investigator has control over manipulating the independent variables and the type of philosophy a researcher holds. The philosophy of the researcher influences what type of research they perform. A person holding positivist philosophy may propagate quantitative experimental studies to develop empirical evidences. Naturalistic philosophical perspective advocates qualitative researches. They hold the view that whatever be the control exercised by the researcher, there will be a researcher influence in any experiment. A person believing in critical social theory may propagate yet another approach or mixed methodology.

RESEARCH UTILIZATION

Research utilization (RU) is the use of research findings in practice to improve the quality of care provided to patients. It is the use of findings of a particular study and is different from evidence-based practice (EBP). RU involves critical analysis and evaluation of research findings and then determines how they fit into clinical practice. Incorporating the findings into practice helps to close the gap between research and practice. More recently, RU efforts in nursing have been replaced by EBP.

EVIDENCE-BASED PRACTICE

Though RU and EBP are used synonymously by many people, there are differences between these two. RU uses the available research findings to guide the nursing practice and the efforts of the nurses to improve patient outcomes, whereas EBP is the conscientious use of current best evidence in making decisions about patient care. EBP is a problem-solving approach to clinical practice that integrates a systematic search for and critical appraisal of the most relevant evidence to answer a burning clinical question. This includes patient data and research data, one's own clinical practice and patient preferences, and values. 'EBP de-emphasizes ritual, isolated and clinical experiences, ungrounded opinion and tradition as a basis for nursing practices—and stresses instead the use of research findings and, as appropriate, quality improvement data, other operational and evaluation data, the consensus of recognized experts, and affirmed experience to substantiate practice.'

Table 1.3 lists the differences between RU and EBP.

TABLE 1.3 *Differences between Research Utilization and Evidence-based Practice*

Research Utilization (RU)	Evidence-based Practice (EBP)
RU is the use of knowledge typically based on a single study.	EBP takes into consideration the findings based on a series of studies and the expertise of the practitioner as well as the patient preferences and values.
In RU, we use the results of studies often conveniently selected as supported for nursing care.	EBP is far more rigorous: • Here the nurse selects all research that has been done in an area. • Then the research results are analysed together and synthesized, coming up with a through integrative review. • The results are then put into the context of clinical expertise and the value system of the patient and particular protocols of the best practices that are developed. EBP encompasses multiple types of evidence such as research findings, research reviews and evidence-based theory and the integration of that evidence with clinical expertise, and patient preferences and values.
Findings are usually applied at the organization level.	Findings are usually applied in the bedside and are tailored to individual patient care needs.
It follows the steps of RU.	It synthesizes all the evidences and integrates with expert opinion, patient preferences and values.

EBP is positioned to become a major driving force in the disciplinary life of clinicians, students, educators, administrators, and policy-makers.

Extensive work is being done on the best ways to translate research into practice, generating a new area of health care science called *translation science*. Eventually, the promise of translation science is to provide evidence on the best ways to incorporate best evidence into health care, including nursing practice.

Importance of Evidence-based Practice in Nursing

Nursing is a practice profession; it is important that clinical practice be based on scientific knowledge. Evidence generated by nursing research provides support for the quality and cost-effectiveness of nursing interventions. It has been observed that EBP improves patient care. A meta-analysis of 84 studies conducted showed that 72 per cent of patients receiving EBP had 28 per cent better outcomes than the control group. The Committee on Quality of Health Care in America, Institute of Medicine, named EBP as Rule 5 of the 10 Rules for Health Care in Crossing the Quality Chasm as a means of quality improvement. It has been seen that only a small percentage (21%) of health care providers are incorporating research findings into patient care decisions. The use of EBP in practice may improve use of research findings. Balas and Boren identified that it takes approximately 17 years to translate research findings into practice. EBP improves nurses and other health care professional's job satisfaction and reduces employee turnover. It has seen that hospitals that had incorporated EBP in nursing practice had less turnover compared with other hospitals. Hospitals with magnet accreditation used EBP in nursing and witnessed fewer turnovers among nurses. This is attributed to job satisfaction among nurses who use EBP. Without current best evidence, practice rapidly gets outdated. Health care providers need to judiciously find the best evidence to make informed care decisions as there are now innumerable amount of information on drugs, health care products, emerging information on risks and benefits of products, alternative medicine approaches, and so on. EBP is a problem-solving approach to clinical practice that incorporates the best evidence from well-designed studies, patient values, and patient preferences.

In EBP, questions are generated in a different manner from research questions. The widely used model is the *PICO* acronym. PICO stands for the following:

P: Patient population
I: Intervention of interest
C: Comparison intervention or status
O: Outcome of interest

The following example illustrates the use of PICO format for a clinically burning question. With hypertensive patients (BP 150/80), what is the effect of giving patients choice versus no choice in the selection of their food items on their weight maintenance or blood pressure?

P: Patient population (patients with BP 150/80)
I: Intervention (choice—patient selects his own food)
C: Comparison intervention (no choice group)
O: Outcome (maintenance of weight or BP)

Patient Population—Questions to Ask: On what patient group is the information required. Starting with your patient, ask how you would describe a group of patients similar to yours.

Intervention (Exposure): This is the second part of the question. It can be an action to make a change in a situation or a nursing care on which you want to study the effect. On what medical or nursing intervention do you want to study the effect? What is key intervention that you want to consider?

Comparison: Here the comparison of usual intervention to another mode of intervention to find the effect. In the given example, the patients' choice of food selection rather than a prescribed food menu is compared. What is it compared with? Is it better or worse than no intervention at all or than another intervention? What is the main alternative to compare with the intervention?

Outcome: It is the fourth component of PICO. What do we anticipate as an outcome? Until now, we have learned how to formulate a burning question for finding evidence; patient population or patient condition needs to be carefully delineated so that the search for evidence provides relevant information. In the same way, intervention of interest requires similar delineation. The comparison of interest can be a comparison with another intervention similar to the one stated in the given example or the standard of care. The outcome of interest is the desired accomplishment, measurement, or improvement as a result of selected intervention. After formulating a burning clinical question for finding evidence, it is very important to locate the answer to the clinical question formulated. It requires understanding of the information sources. There are many resources available. If the first source is not of help, go for the next, then again the next, and so on. Research studies and clinical trials published in the journal literature form the foundation of scientific evidence. However, not all research meets the highest standards of quality. So, those who practice EBP should do systematic reviews or meta-analysis.

Determining Best Evidence

The most accepted way of finding evidence is through a *systematic review*. 'A systematic review is a summary of evidences on a particular topic, typically by an expert or expert panel that uses a rigorous process for identifying, appraising, and synthesizing studies to answer a specific clinical question.' Conclusions are drawn about the data gathered through this process. Many systematic reviews summarize results from multiple studies. They are called *meta-analysis*. Systematic reviews or meta-analysis and evidence-based clinical practice guidelines are regarded as the strongest level of evidence on which practice decisions are based. If one research study or clinical trial provides good evidence, several studies with similar findings give even stronger evidence or negate previous findings. This logic is applied by researchers to systematically identify, appraise, and synthesize evidence from individual studies on a particular topic. Here comes the use of meta-analysis of several studies with statistical analyses. These processes translate into the literature as systematic reviews and summaries of evidence.

The key to knowing whether the significant and relevant evidence have been found is through further evaluation of the selected studies from a successfully executed search. This evaluation method is called the *critical appraisal of the evidence*.

After completing searches in the appropriate information resources, critically analyse the retrieved documents for validity, reliability, and applicability to the following factors:

1. A defined clinical situation
2. The original clinical question
3. The individual patient needs
4. Do the findings apply to this clinical setting and patient population?
5. Is the evidence strong enough to warrant a change in practice

Apply: Once the evidence has been gathered, it is time to apply. Before applying, evaluate whether the intervention should be accepted, rejected, or modified for clinical practice. Think about your own clinical expertise and patients' preferences and values.

Educate the Staff About Its Importance: Solicit staff input so that they will more readily get into the recommended practice. Determine who should be involved in the approval process for the practice change. If costs are likely to increase as a result of the practice change, provide rationale or decide how to handle it. Conduct a trial implementation by focusing on one area where practice change can be carried out easily.

Critical Appraising Knowledge for Clinical Decision-Making: Each clinical decision made or action taken is based on the nurse's knowledge, as described earlier in this chapter. Knowledge is derived from a variety of sources: experience, tradition, trial and error, authority, logical thinking, research, and theories.

Grading the strength of the evidence should incorporate the following three domains:

1. Quality
2. Quantity
3. Consistency

Integrating the Evidence

Evidences that had been critically appraised may be integrated into practice. The common evidences the nurse integrate into clinical practice in order are as follows:

1. Evidence from the literature search
2. Health care provider's expertise
3. Clinical assessment of the patient
4. Available health care resources
5. Patient preferences and values

Evaluating the Effectiveness

The effectiveness of the evidence-based intervention is evaluated in terms of how the treatment worked or how effective the clinical decision was with a particular patient or practice setting. This type of evaluation is essential in determining whether the change based on evidence resulted in the expected outcome. If the treatment did not produce the expected effect or the outcome, the analysis should include the formulation of all possible alternative explanations for the findings. A short list of broad strategies that apply regardless of the setting is as follows:

1. Assessment of barriers to EBP
2. Correction of misperceptions about EBP goals and processes
3. Questioning of current clinical practices

Evidence-based research is used to describe a type of research where the researcher is aware of certain evidence before exploring the subject. Precisely, the researcher does not enter the project unbiased. They are aware of a theory derived from the evidence and use research to test its validity.

KEY POINTS

- Traditionally, nurses use different ways of knowledge in their practice.
- Assembled knowledge is obtained through thought process and scientific way.
- The four types of knowledge used by nurses are empirics, aesthetics, ethics, and personal knowledge.
- Nurses also use representational knowledge, relational knowledge, and reflective knowledge.
- Research in nursing studies the nursing profession and the characteristics of the professional, whereas nursing research is concerned with practice issues.
- The main goal of nursing research is to create and maintain scientific basis for professional practice and validate nursing as a profession.
- Nursing research helps nurses in describing, explaining, predicting and controlling the nursing phenomenon of interest.
- The two major types of research are basic and applied research.
- Nurses need to know the historical development of nursing research to appreciate the previous works and present development to move further.
- Much of the nursing research is based on positivism, naturalism, or social critical theory.
- Research process and problem-solving use abstract critical thinking and complex reasoning to identify new information, but both are distinct in the characteristics of bringing new information.

- The scientific method has many limitations compared with nursing research process. The complexity of human behaviour will not allow rigorous control. Research process covers all branches of research with different approaches, contrary to the scientific method of experimentation.
- RU in nursing is the use of knowledge typically based on a single study, whereas EBP uses findings of many studies, expertise of practices, patient preferences and values.
- EBP includes many steps, with formulating a clinical question as the first step. PICO is a tip for nurses to formulate a burning clinical question.
- The evidences derived need to be critically analysed before being applied in practice.

QUESTIONS

I. Essay-type Question

1. How will you substantiate the importance of nursing research to nursing profession?

II. Short Notes

1. What are the types of knowledge nurses use in their professional practice?
2. How will you differentiate nursing research from research in nursing?
3. How will you differentiate scientific method from research process?
4. How will you differentiate problem-solving from research process?
5. What are characteristics of a nursing research?
6. What is EBP?
7. How will you differentiate RU from EBP?
8. Why it is important for nurses to use EBP in nursing?

III. Multiple-choice Questions

Circle the alphabet before the correct answer

1. A problem-solving method that uses experience, intellectual faculties and thought process with both inductive and deductive reasoning is
   (a) logical reasoning
   (b) scientific thinking
   (c) experiential knowledge
   (d) positivist thoughts
2. The scientific knowledge derived through testing theories by objective approach is
   (a) intuition (b) empirics
   (c) aesthetics (d) ethics
3. The chance of occurrence of certain events estimated is called
   (a) description (b) explanation
   (c) prediction (d) recapitulation
4. A positivist philosophy in research proposes is
   (a) qualitative study
   (b) quantitative study
   (c) mixed methodology
   (d) experiential research
5. The use of a research finding in practice to improve the quality of care provided to patients is
   (a) EBP
   (b) RU
   (c) translation science
   (d) experiential knowledge

6. A new area of health science that translates research findings to practice is
   (a) EBP
   (b) RU
   (c) reflective knowledge
   (d) translational science
7. Ms Smitha would like to conduct a study on the professional aspects of nursing. You will categorize her study into
   (a) research in nursing
   (b) nursing research
   (c) clinical research
   (d) qualitative research
8. If a research finding helps nurses to change existing practices for better patient care outcome, it is
   (a) validating practice
   (b) providing scientific basis for practice
   (c) refining existing practice
   (d) testing theory
9. Fundamental or pure research is called
   (a) basic research
   (b) applied research
   (c) interventional research
   (d) quantitative research
10. Which of the following is the central core of scientific method?
    (a) objectivity (b) control
    (c) systematic (d) replicable
11. NRSI was established in the year
    (a) 1976 (b) 1986
    (c) 1996 (d) 2006

Answer Keys

1. (b) 2. (b) 3. (c) 4. (b) 5. (b) 6. (d) 7. (a) 8. (c)
9. (a) 10. (b) 11. (b)

FURTHER READING

Balas, E. A., Boren, S. A. 2000. 'Managing Clinical Knowledge of Healthcare Improvements'. In V. Schattauer (ed.), *Yearbook of Medical Informatics* (pp. 65–70). Stuttgart, Germany: Schattauer.

Burns, N., Grove, S. 2005. *The Practice of Nursing Research: Conduct, Critique and Utilisation*. Fifth edition. St Louis, MO: Elsevier Saunders.

Carper, Barbara A. 1978. 'Fundamental Patterns of Knowing in Nursing', *Advances in Nursing Science*, 1(1): 13–24.

Centre for Reviews and Dissemination. 2001. *Undertaking Systematic Reviews of Research on Effectiveness.* Second edition. York, UK: CRD, University of York.

Chinn, P. L., Karmer, M. K. 1999. *Theory and Nursing: Integrated Knowledge Development*. Fifth edition. St. Louis: Mosby.

Chulay, M. 1997. 'Bridging the Research-Practice Gap', *Critical Care Nurse*, 17: 80–85.

Estabrooks, C. A. 1999. 'The Conceptual Structure of Research Utilization', *Research in Nursing and Health*, 22: 203–216.

http://www.indiannursingcouncil.org/

http://www.nrsi.org/

http://www.nursingworld.org /

Joseph, M. 2001. *Stressors of Parents of Leukaemic Children*. Unpublished Master's thesis, Submitted to the University of Calicut as a requirement for partial fulfilment of Master's Degree in Nursing.

Melnyk, B., Fineout-Overholt, E. 2005. *Evidence-Based Practice in Nursing and Healthcare.* Philadelphia: Lippincott Williams & Wilkins.

Melnyk, B. M., Fineout-Overholt, E., Stone. P., Ackerman. M. 2000. 'Evidence-Based Practice: The Past, the Present and Recommendations for the New Millennium', *Pediatric Nursing*, 26(1): 77–80.
Nightingale, F. 1969. *Notes on Nursing: What it Is Not*. New York: Dover Publication.
Park, P. 2001. *Knowledge and Participatory Research in Handbook of Action Research*. London: Sage Publication.
Polit, D., Beck, C. 2008. *Nursing Research: Generating and Assessing Evidence for Nursing Practice*. Eighth edition. Philadelphia: Lippincott Williams & Wilkins.
Sackett, D. L., Strauss, S. E. 1998. 'Finding and Applying Evidence during Clinical Rounds: The Evidence Cart', *JAMA*, 280: 1336–1338.
Sackett, D. L., Strauss, S., Richardson, W. S., Rosenburg, W., Hayness, R. B. 2000. *Evidence-Based Medicine: How to Practice NS Teach EBM*. Second edition. London: Churchill Livingstone.
Stetler, C. et al. 1998. 'Evidence-Based Practice and the Role of Nursing Leadership', *JONA*, 28(7/8): 45–53.
Talbot, A. L. 1995. *Principles and Practice of Nursing Research*. St. Louis: Mosby.
The statistic observed with regards to infection rate.
Tierney, A. 1998. 'Nursing Research in Europe', *International Nursing Review*, 45(1): 15–19.
Treece, E W., Treece, J. W. 1986. *Elements of Research in Nursing*. Fourth edition. St. Louis: Mosby.
Wiedenbach, E. 1968. 'The Nurse's Role in Family Planning: A Conceptual Base for Practice', *Nursing Clinics of North America*, 3(2): 355–365.

chapter

2 Research Process

OBJECTIVES

Upon completion of this chapter the learner will be able to:

- Define research process
- Explain the steps in quantitative and qualitative research process
- Identify the research process of ethnographic, phenomenological, grounded theory, and historical methods

INTRODUCTION

Nurses are the largest professional group among healthcare workers endowed with the challenge of making quick yet critical informed decisions relating to a variety of patient problems occurring within the context of a complex and rapidly evolving health care system. During the interventions, as they directly interact with the patients and their caregivers, they have a direct bearing on their well-being. It, therefore, makes sense that the nursing practice should be based on sound research evidence. According to the American Nurses Association, research based practice is essential if the nursing profession is to meet its mandate to society. Nursing research refers to the use of systematic, controlled, empirical, and critical investigation in attempting to discover or confirm facts that relate to a specific problem or question about the practice of nursing.

Research Process

Research process is a systematic logical and orderly way to obtain scientific knowledge through careful collection and scientific examination of data and empirical testing of hypothesis. The process follows a set of sequential steps and each step consists of a general flow of research activities.

Phases and Steps in Quantitative Research

The research process involves conceptualizing a research study, planning and implementing that study, and communicating the findings. The scientific research process proceeds in an orderly fashion and involves a logical flow as each step builds on the previous steps. Nearly every author refers to the formulation of the research problem as the first step and the communication of research findings or the utilization of research findings as the final step in scientific quantitative research. The scientific research process consists of following phases (Table 2.1).

TABLE 2.1 *Phases of Quantitative Research*

Phases	Description	Steps
1. Conceptual phase	In the conceptual phase, activities include reading, conceptualizing, theorizing, re-conceptualizing, and reviewing ideas with colleagues or advisers. During this stage, researchers call on such skills as creativity, deductive reasoning, insight, and a firm grounding in previous research on the topic of interest.	• Identify the problem. • Determine the purpose of the study. • Review the literature. • Develop a theoretical or conceptual framework. • Identify the study assumptions. • Acknowledge the limitations of the study. • Formulate the hypothesis. • Define study variables.
2. Design and planning phase	In design and planning phase, the researcher makes decision about the methods and procedures to be used to address the research questions, and plan for actual data collection.	• Select the research design. • Identify the population. • Select the sample. • Specify methods to measure the research variables. • Develop methods for safeguarding human rights. • Conduct a pilot study.
3. Empirical phase	The empirical phase, one of the most time consuming parts of the research process, involves collecting data and preparing data for analysis.	• Collect the data. • Organize the data for analysis.
4. Analytic phase	During the fourth phase, analysis and interpretation of findings takes place and it provides answers to the questions posed in the first phase of the research process.	• Analyse the data. • Interpret the findings.
5. Dissemination phase	In this final phase, the research report can be shared with others.	• Communicate the findings. • Utilize the findings.

1. **Identify the Problem:** The first step, and one of the most important steps, in the research process is to identify clearly the problem that will be studied. In general, a broad topic area is selected, and then it is narrowed down to a specific one-sentence statement of the problem. This step of the research process may be the most difficult of all and may take a great deal of time. Martin contended that a 'good' problem statement helps the researcher to move through the steps of the research process. Study problems can be identified from personal experiences, from literature sources, from previous research, or through the testing of theories. The problem should be of interest to the researcher and be significant to nursing. The problem statement should specify the sample and the variables that are being studied. A variable is a specific characteristic or attribute that differs among the persons, objects, events, and so forth, that is being studied (like age or blood type). Here is an example of a problem statement: Effectiveness of body–mind–spirit intervention on the well-being of depressive patients.

2. **Determine the Purpose of the Study:** The problem statement addresses what will be studied; the purpose furnishes why the study is being done. There must be clear justification for every research project. If the purpose of a study is clearly presented and justified, the researcher will be much more likely to receive approval for the study and also will be more likely to obtain subjects for the study. Consider the problem statement concerning the effectiveness of body–mind–spirit intervention on the well-being of depressive patients. A study to examine these variables might have the following purpose: explore the well-being of depressive patients and to develop and evaluate the effectiveness of a psychosocial group intervention based on the integrated body-mind-spirit approach.
3. **Review the Literature:** Quantitative research should build on previous knowledge. Before beginning a quantitative study, it is important to determine the information that already exists about the topic. There are many routes to access published literature. They can be located through library card catalogues, indexes, abstracts, and computer-assisted searches. Besides determining the extent of the existing knowledge related to the study topic, the review of the literature also helps to develop a theoretical or conceptual framework for the study. Finally, the review of the literature can help the researcher plan study methods and identify tools that can be used to measure the study variables. The review should be continued during the course of the investigation until the time of data collection. This ensures the researcher that he or she has as much information as possible and the most up-to-date information on the study topic.
4. **Develop a Theoretical or Conceptual Framework:** The goal of research is to develop scientific knowledge. Research and theory are intertwined. Research can test theories as well as help develop and refine theories. Thus theoretical frameworks are a valuable part of scientific research. The theoretical or conceptual framework assists in the selection of the study variables and in defining them. The framework also directs to formulate hypotheses and the interpretation of the findings.

   A purely descriptive research may not require a theoretical framework. Most nursing studies can profit, however, from the identification of a framework for the study. Research conducted within the context of a theoretical framework, compared to research that is not theory based, is more valuable in providing understanding and knowledge that can be used in the future. Research without a theory provides a set of isolated facts.
5. **Identify the Study Assumptions:** Assumptions are beliefs that are held to be true but have not necessarily been proven. Every scientific investigation is based on assumptions. These assumptions should be stated explicitly. Study assumptions influence the questions that are asked, the data that are gathered, the methods used to gather the data, and the interpretation of the data.

   Assumptions are of three types: universal, theoretical and research based assumptions, Universal assumptions are beliefs that are assumed to be true by a large percentage of society. Here's an example: 'Man is bio-psycho-social being'. Assumptions also may be derived from theory or previous research. If a'-study is based on a certain theory, the assumptions of that theory become the assumptions of the study based on that particular theory. In addition, the results of previous studies can form the basis for assumptions in the present research investigation. For example if an investigator conducting a study to evaluate the effectiveness of body-mind-spirit intervention among depressive patients, the universal assumption might be that depressive patients will have bodily problems, mind problems and spiritual problems. The theoretical assumption may be based on body-mind-spirit model, that is, mind, body and spirit are interrelated. An assumption based on research might be holistic intervention is effective for depressive patients.
6. **Acknowledge the Limitations of the Study:** Limitations are uncontrolled variables that may affect the study results and limit the ability to generalize the findings. Generalization is the

extension of the implication of the research findings from the sample to a larger population. For example, the findings from studying adult female survivors of child abuse might be extended from this sample studied to all women who have survived child abuse. There are two types of limitations, namely theoretical and methodological limitations. In nearly every nursing study, there are variables over which the researcher either has no control or chooses not to exercise control. These variables are called *extraneous variables.* For example, the educational level of subjects would be a study limitation if the researcher could not control this variable and thought that it might influence the study results. In experimental studies, uncontrolled variables are referred to as threats to internal and external validity.

The researcher should try to identify study limitations or weaknesses and openly acknowledge the limitations of a study, as much as possible, before data is collected. Other limitations may occur while the study is in progress, for example, malfunctions of equipment or subject dropout. The limitations must be taken into consideration when the conclusions of a study are formulated and when recommendations are made for future research.

7. **Formulate the Hypothesis or Research Question:** A researcher's expectation about the results of a study is expressed in a hypothesis. A hypothesis predicts the relationship between two or more variables. Whereas the problem statement asks a question, the hypothesis furnishes the predicted answer to the question. The hypothesis contains the population and a variable, just as the problem statement does. In addition, the hypothesis proposes the relationship between the independent and the dependent variables. In experimental studies, the *independent* variable is the 'cause' or the variable thought to influence the dependent variable. The *dependent* variable is the 'effect' or the variable influenced by the researcher's manipulation. A hypothesis must be testable or verifiable empirically, which means that it must be capable of being tested in the real world by observations gathered through the senses.

   Consider the problem statement: Is there a correlation between well-being and depressive symptoms among depressive patients? After the review of the literature on the topic, a theory might be discovered that predicts a negative relationship between well-being and depressive symptoms. The following hypothesis might then be formulated: the more the patients experience depressive symptoms, the less their level of well-being. This type of hypothesis is referred to as *a directional research hypothesis.* It contains the direction of the researcher's expectations for the study results.

   Although the null hypothesis (which predicts that no relationship exists between variables) is tested statistically, the directional research hypothesis is the preferred type for nursing studies. This type of hypothesis is derived from the theoretical/conceptual framework for the study, and should, therefore, indicate the expected relationship between variables.

   Experimental, comparative, and correlational studies call for hypotheses. In qualitative studies and some descriptive studies, a hypothesis is not needed. In such studies the research is guided by research questions. For example, the problem statement might be as follows: 'What are the adjustment behaviours of family members when the husband/father is suffering with schizophrenia?' The research questions might be any of the following: 'Do family members become closer or more distant in their interpersonal relationships with each other?' 'What is the greatest adjustment difficulty reported by family members?' 'Do different families report similar adjustment problems?'

8. **Define Study Variables:** The variables and terms contained in the study hypotheses or research questions need to be defined so that their meaning is clear to the researcher and to the reader of a research report. The definitions are usually dictionary definitions or theoretical definitions obtained from literature sources. In addition to a dictionary or theoretical definition, a variable should be operationally defined. An *operational definition* indicates how a variable will be

observed or measured. Operational definitions frequently include the instrument that will be used to measure the variables. If depression is being measured, the theoretical definition might be taken from a certain theorist's description of depression. The operational definition would then be indicated by the identification of the tool or behaviour that would be used to measure depression.

The operational definition allows replication of a study. If a researcher would like to replicate a study, using another group of subjects or another setting, it would be necessary to know exactly how the variables were measured in the previous study.

Besides defining the variables in a hypothesis or research question, the population for the study should be limited or narrowed down to the specific group that will be studied. If the population in the hypothesis is identified as depressive patients, this group could be further defined as women between the ages of 20 and 40 years who have experienced a first episode and who are attending outpatient department in a district hospital.

9. **Select the Research Design:** A research design refers to the researcher's overall plan for obtaining answers to the research questions and testifies the research hypothesis. It is concerned with the type of data that will be collected and the means used to obtain these data. For example, the researcher must decide if the study will examine cause-and-effect relationships or will only describe existing situations. The researcher chooses the design that is most appropriate to test the study hypotheses or answer the research question(s).

   Research designs can be categorized as quantitative or qualitative. They also can be categorized as experimental or non-experimental. Experimental designs can be further divided into true experimental, quasi-experimental, and pre-experimental designs. Non-experimental designs include descriptive, correlational, and comparative studies.

   In experimental research, the investigator plays an active role and has more control over the research situation than in a non-experimental study. More control can be exercised over the extraneous variables that might influence research results. In experimental nursing studies, a nursing intervention is usually introduced. The nurse researcher manipulates this variable by deciding who will and will not receive an intervention. Frequently, one group receives the usual intervention while another group receives some new intervention that is hoped to be more effective. In non-experimental research, the investigator collects data without actively manipulating any variable.

10. **Identify the Population:** The *population* is the complete set of individuals or objects that possess some common characteristic of interest to the researcher. The researcher must specify the broad population or group (target population) of interest as well as the actual population (accessible population) that is available for the study.

    The *target population*, also called the *universe*, is made up of the group of people or objects to which the researcher wishes to generalize the findings of a study. The *accessible population* is the group that is actually available for study by the researcher.

    By identifying the population, the researcher makes clear the group to which the study results can be applied. Scientific research is concerned with generalizing research results to other subjects and other settings. Although the researcher would like to assert that the study results apply to a wide target population, this population must be similar to the accessible population for such an assertion to be made. For example, the accessible population might be depressive patients in one hospital. These patients are 20 to 40 years, with first episode. The target population would be 20- to 40-year-old first episode depressive patients.

11. **Select the Sample:** Sample is a subset of the population that is selected for a study. The sample is chosen to represent the population and is used to make generalizations about the population. Obtaining data from an entire population is costly and time consuming, and it may even be

impossible, at times, to contact or locate every member of a given population. If the sample is carefully selected, the researcher can make claims about the population with a certain degree of confidence. The method of selecting the sample determines how representative the sample is of the population.

Probability samples are those chosen by a random selection process in which each member of the population has a chance of being in the sample, if non-probability sampling is used; the researcher has less confidence that the sample is representative of the population. The investigator cannot estimate the probability that each element of the population has a chance of being selected for the sample, and the possibility of a biased sample is great. The researcher must make the determination of which sampling method to use, after considering the advantages and disadvantages of the various types of probability and non-probability sampling methods.

12. **Specify Methods to Measure the Research Variable:** Quantitative researchers must develop methods to measure the research variables as accurately as possible. The common quantitative data collection approaches are bio-physiological measurements, self-reports, observation methods. Before finalizing the data collection plan, researchers must carefully evaluate whether the chosen methods capture key concepts accurately.
13. **Developing Methods for Safeguarding Human Rights:** The investigator must seek, by every means at his disposal, to ensure that the rights of subjects are rigorously protected through all phases of the investigation, and need to develop procedures to ensure that the study adheres to ethical principles. Each aspect of the study plan needs to be reviewed to determine whether the rights of subjects have been adequately protected. Often that review involves a formal presentation to an external committee.

    As nursing research is generally conducted with human beings, subjects' rights must be considered and the proper permissions secured before subjects are approached to participate in a study. All research with humans must involve voluntary participation of the subjects.
14. **Conduct a Pilot Study:** A pilot study involves a miniature trial version of the planned study. It is advisable to conduct a pilot study before the study subjects are approached and the actual study is carried out. People selected for the pilot study are similar in characteristics to the sample that will be used for the actual study.

    A pilot study could be called the building blocks to larger studies. It is also called primary prevention since a pilot study could prevent the researcher from conducting a large-scale study that might be an expensive disaster (Box 2.1).

Box 2.1 *Purposes for Conducting a Pilot Study*

Purposes for conducting pilot study:

1. To examine issues related to the design, sample size, data collection procedures, and data analysis approaches
2. To test a new instrument or to evaluate an existing instrument that has been altered
3. To evaluate the study procedures and, in general, help to get the bugs out before the actual study is conducted
4. Factors can be examined, such as how long it will take to conduct the data collection and how subjects can be expected to respond to the data collection methods

After the pilot study is conducted, necessary revisions should be made. It may be advisable to carry out another pilot study if changes have been made in the instrument(s) or in the research procedures.

15. **Collect the Data:** The pieces of information or facts that are collected in scientific investigations is called the *data*. Through the data collection procedures, the variable or variables in a study must be measured. Data collection should be a systematic process. These questions must be answered: What data will be collected? How will the data be collected? Who will collect the data? Where will the data be collected? When will the data be collected?

    A multitude of data collection methods are available to nurse researchers. The choice of methods is determined by the study hypotheses or the research question(s), the design of the study, and the amount of knowledge available about the study topic.

16. **Organize the Data for Analysis:** After the data is collected, it is necessary to organize the data for tabulation and evaluation. If questionnaires have been used, it will be necessary to determine if they have been completed correctly. Decisions will have to be made about missing data. If interviews have been recorded, the tapes will have to be analysed and data then placed in some kind of written form.

    A statistician should be consulted in the early phase of the research process, as well as in the data analysis phase of the study. Just as plans for organizing the data should be made before data collection begins, plans for analysing the data also should be made before obtaining the data. The statistician can help determine the type of data needed for a study and what statistical procedures will be appropriate to analyse the data.

17. **Analyse the Data:** Analysis of data consists of putting all of the individual observations, scores, measures, interview data and so forth into some manageable form. Quantitative information is usually analysed through statistical procedures. Data should be analysed in terms of the stated problem. If questions were posed, findings should answer those questions. If hypotheses were stated, findings should support or not support them. Tables, graphs, and line drawings are helpful to summarize data from which relationships between data can be seen.

18. **Interpret the Findings:** After the data is analysed, the findings should be interpreted in light of the study hypotheses or research question(s). If a hypothesis was tested, a determination is made as to whether the data support the research hypothesis. Also, the framework for the study is discussed in light of the findings. If the data support the research hypothesis, then the theoretical or conceptual framework is also supported. Conversely, if the research hypothesis is not supported, the framework for the study is also not supported. Of course, the researcher should discuss any problems incurred in the course of the study or any limitations of the design that may have influenced the study results.

    The results of the present study are compared with those of previous studies that investigated the same or similar variables; the researcher, thus, is able to contribute to the existing body of knowledge on the study topic. After the findings are interpreted, the researcher should indicate the implications for nursing. Considerations are made for changes that might be called for in nursing practice, nursing education, or nursing administration as a result of the study findings. Finally, recommendations for future research are proposed.

19. **Communicate the Findings:** This step of the research process may be the most important one for nursing. No matter how significant the findings may be, they are of little value to the rest of the nursing profession if the researcher fails to disseminate these results to other colleagues.

    Research findings can be communicated through many different mediums, through publication in research journals, present research results in person to colleagues at national, regional, state, and local gatherings of nurses, and through poster sessions.

20. **Utilize the Findings:** The concluding step of a high quality study is to plan for its utilization in practical settings. The researcher may not actually implement the findings, but he or she can make recommendations about how the findings could be integrated into nursing practice. For example, the researcher could act as a consultant to nurses in health care agencies who want to use the study findings. They can also contribute to the process by including, in their research reports, recommendations regarding how the evidence from the study could be incorporated into the practice of nursing and by vigorously pursuing opportunities to disseminate the findings to practicing nurses.

QUALITATIVE RESEARCH

Steps in Qualitative Research

Quantitative research involves a fairly linear progression of tasks; researcher plan in advance the steps to be taken to maximize study integrity and then follow those steps as truly as possible. In qualitative studies, by contrast, the progression is closer to a circle than straight line—qualitative researchers are continually examining and interpreting data and making decisions about how to proceed based on what has already been discovered. The flow of activities varies from one study to another. The following are some of the major activities in qualitative research.

1. **Conceptualizing and Planning Phase:** This involves the following
   (a) **Identifying the research problem:** Qualitative researcher usually focuses on an aspect of a topic that is poorly understood and about which little is known. Therefore, they do not develop hypothesis. Researcher may proceed with a fairly broad research question that allows the focus to be sharpened and delineated once the study is underway.
   (b) **Doing literature review:** According to qualitative study, the phenomena should be elucidated based on participant's viewpoints rather than on any prior information. Some researchers do a literature review at the end of the study. Some researchers conduct preliminary upfront literature review to obtain some guidance.
   (c) **Selecting and gaining entry into research site:** In qualitative research, gaining entry is likely to be an ongoing process of establishing relationships and rapport with gatekeepers and others at the site including prospective informants.
   (d) **Developing research design:** Research design emerges during the course of the data collection (emergent design).
   (e) **Developing methods to safeguard participants:** Ethical issues are special concerns in qualitative studies because of the more intimate nature of the relationship that typically develops between researchers and study participants.
2. **Developing Data Collection Strategies:** In this phase the researcher decides what type of data needs to be collected and how to collect it. Researcher also decides how to enhance trust worthiness.
3. **Conducting Study:** Qualitative researchers begin by talking with or observing a few people who have first-hand experience with the phenomenon under study. The discussions and observations are loosely structured, allowing for the expression of full range of beliefs, feelings, and behaviours. In contrast to using valid instruments for data collection, in qualitative research the researcher takes steps to demonstrate the trustworthiness of the data while in the field.

The researcher confirms that the findings accurately reflect the experiences and viewpoints of participants rather than perceptions of the researchers.

4. **Data Analysis:** The actual process of data analysis involves clustering together related types of narrative information into a coherent scheme. Researcher begins to identify themes and categories which are used to build a rich description or theory of the phenomenon. The sample size is guided by the data collected. Many researchers use data saturation, which occurs when themes and categories in the data become repetitive and redundant, such that no new information can be gleaned by further data collection. Qualitative reports are usually filled with rich verbatim passages directly from participants. Qualitative findings are used as the basis for the formulation of hypothesis, later tested by quantitative research.
5. **Disseminating Findings:** During this phase researcher communicates the findings of the study. The researcher's responsibilities are not completed until the study results are disseminated (Fig. 2.1).

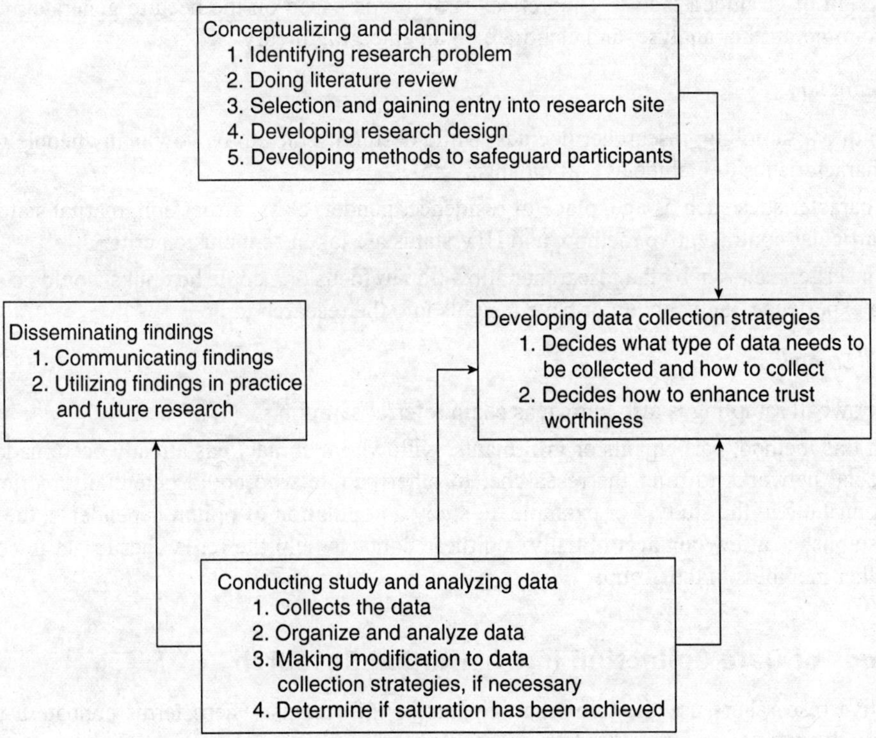

Figure 2.1 *Flow Diagram Showing the Steps of Qualitative Research Method*

Sampling in Qualitative Research

1. The goal of sampling is to develop a rich, thick description of the phenomenon being studied.
2. The sampling principles are not based on number of interviews, participant observations or ability to generalize data, but rather on how accurately the data represents the full context of the phenomenon under study.

3. Participants are recruited based on their personal knowledge of experience with the culture or phenomenon of study.
4. Sample sizes depend on the resources and time available, as well as the study's objectives.

Sampling Methods Used in Qualitative Research

1. Purposive sampling
2. Quota sampling
3. Snowball sampling

Purposive Sampling

1. Sampling purposefully selected by the researcher according to preselected criteria relevant to a particular research question.
2. Theoretical sampling is a form of purposive sampling that is used primarily in the qualitative design of grounded theory. Theoretical sampling is based on the need to generate more data to examine, further analyse, and elaborate on an emerging theory.

Quota Sampling

1. In quota sampling, researcher decides, while designing the study, how many people with which characteristics to include as participants.
2. Characteristics such as age, place of residence, gender, class, profession, marital status, use of a particular contraceptive method, and HIV status are taken as inclusion criteria.
3. The criteria chosen by the researcher allow him to focus on people he thinks would be most likely to experience, know about, or have insights into the research topic.

Snowball Sampling

1. Snowball sampling is also known as chain referral sampling.
2. In this method, participants or informants, with whom contact has already been made, use their social networks to refer the researcher to other people who could potentially participate in or contribute to the study. For example, to study a population of opium dependents, the researcher establishes a few contacts initially and these contacts help the researcher to get in contact with other members in the group.

Methods of Data Collection in Qualitative Research

Qualitative researchers use the terms participants or informants. These terms connate a position of active involvement or a partnership between participants and researchers.

Obtrusive Methods

1. Semi-structured interviews
2. In-depth interviews
3. Focus group discussions
4. Narrative and life history
5. Participant observation

Unobtrusive Methods

1. Simple observation
2. Document analysis (written records)
3. Audio–visual

Visual Records: Photographs, films, and videos provide visual records of daily and life events of the phenomenon under study. Visual methods can document cultural and life events, ceremonies, and behaviours in a natural setting.

Artefacts, archival, and written records can contain rich data that is useful in creating and enriching an understanding of the phenomenon or culture of interest. The data can be in the form of any communication materials such as newspapers, books, letters, emails, speeches, photographs, work of art, music, or household goods.

Interview: Interviews can be unstructured, open-ended, or semi-structured.

1. Unstructured interviews are appropriate when little is known about a phenomenon. This type of interview usually begins with open ended questions and allows the participant unlimited opportunity to elaborate on the phenomena of interest.
2. In semi-structured interviews the researcher exerts more control over the interview and commonly has a set of questions prepared to guide the interview. The questions may not be strictly followed to allow latitude in the participant's responses. The interviewer may also guide the discussion by asking specific questions.
3. A focus group is a type of group interview in which specific people assemble to give their opinion or impressions about the phenomenon of interest. The groups can be convened for various reasons such as evaluating a new product, sharing feelings about an upcoming policy, or discussing experiences with a particular form of treatment. The focus groups generally range in size from 5 to 10 people who have been selected because they share similar qualities. Group discussions can generate data that may not be elicited from a single guided interview. Creative thinking and collective responses stimulated by a focus group can lead to improvement of whatever is evaluated, marketed or discussed.

Observation: The most common method of observation is participant observation, in which the researcher become immersed in the field and observes the activities of the participants. The researcher uses all his senses to generate data about the observations. Involvement in the natural setting of the participants allows the researcher to experience first-hand the phenomenon under study. Detailed, descriptive, and systematic recordings of the observation are kept as field notes.

Different approaches to participant observation are as follows:

1. **Complete Observer:** Complete observer in which the researcher fully observes but has no direct social interactions with the participant or the setting.
2. **Observer as Participant:** In observer as participant, the researcher may minimally participate in activities or do some interviewing but the majority of the time is spent observing.
3. **Participant as Observer:** In the participant as observer, the researcher becomes part of the group, that is, he can be a worker in the setting as well as the researcher. Role discard and conflict with primary responsibilities may occur in this type of observation role.
4. **Complete Participant:** In complete participant, the researcher participates in the setting as a member of the group and the researcher's identity and purpose are concealed. This approach, sometimes referred to as 'going native', is difficult to justify and is considered unethical by current standards.

Recording the Data in Qualitative Research

Most researchers record or document their data through the use of field notes or tape records. Field notes document the researcher's observations and interviews. Data from interviews or focus groups can be recorded as hand written, field notes, or tape-recorded.

Errors in Data Collection and Data Analysis in Qualitative Research

In qualitative research errors can be introduced into a study in two major ways: Problems can occur with the processes of data collection or analysis, or both. To avoid errors, qualitative researchers ensure the rigor of both processes. Rigor is a strict process of data collection and analysis. It is reflected in the consistency of the data analysis and interpretation, the trustworthiness of the data collected, the transferability of the themes, and the credibility of the data (Table 2.2).

TABLE 2.2 *Aspects of Rigor in Qualitative Research*

Aspect	Definition	Methods
Trustworthiness	The honesty of the data collected from and about the participants	Establishment of ongoing or meaningful interactions. Use of a protocol.
Conformability	The consistent, repeatable nature of the data collection and analysis	Use of computer software to organize and analyse data. Audit trails.
Transferability	The extent to which findings relate to other settings or groups	External checks, seeking disconfirming cases, or outliers
Credibility	The confidence in the truth of the findings	Triangulation, Member checks

Analyzing Data in Qualitative Research

The philosophy underlying a research study directs the interpretation of results and therefore it is inextricably linked with data analysis.

Analysis of data involves examining words, descriptions, and processes. Data is analysed using a non-statistical approach that is consistent with the research philosophy, question, and design. Multiple methods of data collection and analysis may be used simultaneously, such as re-reading and coding of transcript while watching a video tape to enhance the appreciation of non-verbal communication.

Steps for Analyzing Data

1. Organize and prepare the data for analysis
2. Read all data, get a sense of the whole
3. Begin detailed analysis with coding process
4. Generate a description of the setting or people as well as categories or themes for analysis
5. Identify themes (writing, visual, etc.)
6. Interpret and make meaning out of data

Qualitative studies use transcribed text that is systematically analysed through a process of coding. Codes are generally one to four word descriptions that capture the broad meaning of paragraphs of data.

The researcher organizes the data into these preliminary abstractions (coding). Then the researcher begins to see common elements among the participant's remarks. The researcher finally takes the leap from looking at discrete individual experiences of the phenomenon to understanding the commonalities of the experience for a given group of informants. At this magical moment themes begin to emerge from the data.

Themes are groups of codes that unify into more abstract common denominators and the researcher moves from analysis to synthesis of the data. As the identification of the themes begins, the researcher writes and rewrites ideas of how the data fall together.

Data is more easily managed with the use of software programs such as Computer Assisted Qualitative Analysis Software (CAQAS). This software is helpful for quickly coding data and schematically drawing representations of how codes might form themes.

Ensuring Validity of Information in Qualitative Research

Throughout data collection and analysis researchers typically record personal reflections, observations, questions, ideas, hunches, and feelings. These vital steps help to judge and interpret data and ultimately to construct meanings.

The commonly used methods to ensure validity of information are reflectivity, bracketing, and member checking (Box 2.2).

Box 2.2 *Commonly Used Methods to Ensure Validity of Information*

1. **Reflectivity/reflective thought/reflective critique** is an interactive process that the researcher goes through to uncover underlying factors that may influence the study's findings. The researcher explores the dynamic interaction between the self and the data, and integrates this added insight and understanding into the study. Researchers are encouraged to keep a record of their feelings, thoughts, reactions, and biases to determine how their personal views may have influenced their interpretation of findings. This introspective process requires critical thinking and self-awareness. Researcher's reflectivity is important because in qualitative research, the researcher becomes part of the research and may influence the study during data generation and analysis.
2. **Bracketing** refers to setting aside personal beliefs, expectations, and what is known about the phenomenon.
3. **In member checking** the researcher goes back to the participants during data analysis to determine whether the participants recognize the experience as their own. This mechanism helps to preserve the integrity of participants' statements.

Evaluation of Results of Qualitative Research

When the outcomes of qualitative studies are interpreted, a different set of questions need to be asked. First, the trustworthiness of the study needs to be established. To be judged trustworthy, four objectives must be attained.

1. **Credibility:** It is similar to validity and means that the investigator has developed, believable interpretations, and conclusions based on the data analysis. It can be established by comparing the data with data obtained from other sources (triangulation); having colleagues explore and clarify the investigator's interpretations to reveal potential biases; searching for disconfirming evidence; and returning to the study participants to validate and verify the investigator's conclusions and interpretations.

2. **Transferability:** It refers to judgment by a non-involved investigator that the findings are applicable to another setting or context.
3. **Dependability:** It means that a non-involved investigator can logically follow the processes and procedures used in the study.
4. **Conformability:** It means the findings, conclusions, and recommendations are supported by the data and that there is internal agreement between the interpretations and the actual evidence.

Ethical Principles of Qualitative Research

1. Respect for persons
2. Beneficence
3. Justice
4. Respect for communities

Types of Qualitative Research

Ethnography

The word ethnographic means portrait of people. Ethnography is a description and interpretation of a cultural or social group or system. The research examines the group's observable and learned patterns of behaviour, customs, and ways of life, focuses on culture, and how people interact with each other. An underlying assumption of the ethnographer is that every human group eventually evolves a culture that guides the members' view of the world and the way they structure their experience. The product of ethnographic research usually is a rich and holistic description of the culture under study. Among health care researchers, ethnography provides access to health beliefs and health practices of the culture, helps to facilitate understanding of behaviour affecting health and illness. The ethnographer is the primary research instrument; the researcher spends one year or more in the field long enough to see a full cycle of activity. The goal of ethnographer is to understand the natives' view of their world or the emic view. 'Emic'—insiders views about their culture and 'etic' perspectives—outsiders view about experiences of that culture. Data collection methods used in ethnography are direct observation, participant observation, unstructured in-depth interviews, records, and physical evidences like diaries, letters, and photographs. For example, wittig conducted an ethno-nursing study focusing on organ donation beliefs of Afro-American women living in rural area. Wittig made numerous visits to the site and conducted in-depth interviews with 10 Afro-American women.

Three broad types of information are usually sought by ethnographers:

1. Cultural behaviour (what people will do)
2. Cultural artefacts (what members of the culture make use of)
3. Cultural speech (what people say)

Phenomenology

Phenomenology describes the subjective reality of an event, as perceived by the study population; it is the study of a phenomenon. Nursing phenomenological studies have contributed greatly to our knowledge about human experiences in health and illness, healing and dying (for example the loss of an unborn child or recurrence of cancer), and the meaning of these experiences to the patients. For example, Rungreangkulkij and Chesla conducted a phenomenological study of Thai mothers' experiences caring for a child with schizophrenia. In-depth interviews were conducted with 12 Thai mothers who had adult schizophrenic children.

Sampling in phenomenology is always a convenience sample. In-depth interviews are conducted to describe experiences as they are lived. As data is collected the researcher uses the process of intuiting, analysing, and describing to discover essential themes in the experience of the phenomenon. Researcher often starts by identifying his perceptions or expectations about the phenomenon to be studied and then attempts to consciously bracket them—hold them separate—so that they will not colour either the data collection or the analysis process.

Grounded Theory

Grounded theorists study social processes in everyday human life and interactions. For nurse researchers, the grounded theory approach facilitates the development of mid-range theory grounded in the life and language of people living with illness conditions. The goal is generating or discovering a theory.

It uses a variety of data sources, including quantitative data, review of records, interviews, observation, and surveys. Example of a grounded theory study—Knobf sought to develop a substantive theory to explain women's responses to chemotherapy induced premature menopause within the context of breast cancer.

Historical Research

Historical research is the systematic collection, critical evaluation and interpretation of historical evidence. Historical research answers questions about causes, effects, or trends relating to past events that may shed light on present behaviour or practices. Many nurse researchers have undertaken biographical histories—the experiences or contributions of individuals, social histories—that focus on a particular period in attempts to understand prevailing values and beliefs that may have helped to shape subsequent developments; and for intellectual histories, historical ideas, or ways of thinking are scrutinized. Data sources in historical research are records, video tapes, photographs and interviews, and review of published reports.

Lusk analysed images of nurses in advertisements from 1930 to 1950. She hypothesized that nurses' relative status in advertisements would be higher in 1940 (when women were encouraged to enter nursing as a patriotic duty) than in 1930 or 1950.

Qualitative research must be systematic, rigorous, and planned to make it credible and dependable. It involves critical self-scrutiny (active reflexivity) to produce explanations. Such investigations produce social explanations which are somewhat generalizable.

SELECTING QUANTITATIVE VS QUALITATIVE RESEARCH

1. If it is found that little is known about phenomena, and the researcher wanted to get a more holistic sense of their experiences, select qualitative study.
2. If substantial knowledge already exists choose a quantitative design.
3. If the purpose is to gain an in-depth understanding of the overall phenomena, use a qualitative design.
4. If you are interested in learning cultural patterns, use ethnographic method.
5. If you are interested in understanding human experience, use phenomenological method.
6. If you are interested in uncovering social processes, use grounded theory method.
7. If you are interested in capturing unique stories, use case study method.

8. The purpose of the study is to describe the relationship between specific variables use a descriptive design.
9. To test an intervention (manipulating the independent variable), use experimental design.
10. Some elements of control are missing, use quasi-experimental design.

KEY POINTS

- Research is needed to evaluate the effectiveness of nursing intervention modalities to determine the impact of nursing care on the health of the patients.
- Research is analytical, empirical, and logical, and directed toward the solution of problems.
- Research may be classified as basic, applied, experimental, non-experimental, retrospective, prospective, qualitative, and quantitative.
- The researcher chooses the method based on the research question and current level of knowledge about the phenomenon and the problem to be studied.
- Basic research generates theory or knowledge that is validated in practice through applied research.
- In experimental research, researcher actively intervenes or introduces a treatment, in non-experimental research; researcher makes observations of existing situations and characteristics without intervening.
- In retrospective research, phenomenon existing in the present is linked to phenomenon that occurred in the past. Prospective research starts with a presumed cause and then goes forward in time to the presumed effect.
- Quantitative research is inductive in nature. It is a formal, objective, and a systematic process in which numerical data is used and centres on hypothesis testing. Qualitative research is deductive in nature and a systematic approach to explore phenomena.
- A few important steps in quantitative research process are identifying the problem, review the literature, develop a theoretical or conceptual framework, formulate the hypothesis, select the research design, identify the population, collect the data, analyse the data, interpret the findings, and communicate, and utilize the findings.
- Quantitative research methods can be classified into descriptive, correlational, quasi-experimental, and experimental.
- A few important steps in qualitative research process are identifying the research problem, doing literature review, selecting and gaining entry into research site, developing research design, developing methods to safeguard participants, developing data collection strategies, conducting qualitative study, data analysis, and disseminating findings.
- Purposive, quota, and snowball sampling methods are commonly used in qualitative research.
- Commonly used data collection methods in qualitative research are semi-structured, in-depth interviews, focus group discussions, participant observation, photographs, films, and videos.
- Trustworthiness, conformability, transferability, and credibility are criteria for judging the scientific rigor for qualitative research study.
- In qualitative research, data are analysed using a non-statistical approach that is consistent with the research question.
- Phenomenological methods provide an in-depth data about a particular life experience and therefore are particularly useful in answering descriptive questions, especially when very little is known about the topic of interest.

- Ethnographic methods provide immersion and active participation in a particular culture or subculture, and assist in answering descriptive and linkage and connection questions.
- Grounded theory methods provide data about social interactions, which can be built into a theory based on reality. These methods are particularly useful in answering questions about interactions or links among social processes.
- Historical methods provide data about past processes to gain insight about the present and future. They answer questions about links and connections.
- The key difference between quantitative and qualitative methods is their flexibility.
- In qualitative methods, the relationship between the researcher and the participant is often less formal than in quantitative research.
- Both qualitative and quantitative researches are used in nursing studies. Qualitative research is concerned with complete and detailed descriptions of events, whereas quantitative research creates statistical models to explain events.

QUESTIONS

I. Essay-type Questions

1. Define nursing research and describe in detail the steps involved in quantitative research process.
2. Describe the steps involved in qualitative research process.
3. Define research and explain various types of research with suitable reference to nursing.

II. Short Notes

1. Define research process
2. Pilot study
3. Ethical aspects of qualitative research
4. Analysis of data in qualitative research
5. Types of quantitative research methods with suitable example
6. Types of qualitative research methods with suitable example
7. Analysis of data in quantitative research

III. Multiple-choice Questions

Circle the alphabet before the best answer

1. Which of the following is *not* a method of quantitative research?
   (a) Grounded theory research
   (b) Correlational research
   (c) Quasi-experimental research
   (d) Experimental research
2. Deductive reasoning is applied in:
   (a) Qualitative research
   (b) Quantitative research
   (c) Action research
   (d) Applied research
3. Which of the following is a qualitative research design where live experiences of individuals are examined in their 'life-world'?
   (a) Ethnography
   (b) Ethology
   (c) Phenomenology
   (d) Grounded theory

4. Which of the following is a characteristic of qualitative research?
   (a) Deductive process
   (b) Control over the context
   (c) Fixed research design
   (d) Inductive process

5. Qualitative research design involves
   (a) Emergent design
   (b) Correlative design
   (c) Experimental design
   (d) Cohort design

Answer Keys

1. (a) 2. (b) 3. (c) 4. (d) 5. (a)

FURTHER READING

Burns, N., Grove, S. K. 1999. *Understanding Nursing Research*. Second edition. Philadelphia: W.B. Saunders Company.

Knobf, M. T. 2002. 'Carrying On: The Experience of Premature Menopause in Women With Early Stage Breast Cancer', *Nursing Research*, 51:9–17.

Lusk, B. 2000. 'Pretty and Powerless: Nurses in Advertisements, 1930-1950', *Research in Nursing and Health*, 23:229–236.

Martin, P.A., 1994. 'The Utility of the Research Problem Statement'. *Applied Nursing Research*, 7:47–49

Polit, D. F., Beck C. T., Hungler, B. P. 2001. *Essentials of Nursing Research: Methods, Appraisal, and Utilization*. Fifth edition. Philadelphia: Lippincott.

Polit D. F., Hungler B. P. 1999. *Nursing Research: Principles and Methods,* Sixth edition. Philadelphia: Lippincott.

Rungreangkulkij S., Chesla C. 2001. 'Smooth A Heart with Water: Thai Mothers Care for a Child with Schizophrenia', *Archives of Psychiatric Nursing*, 15:120–127.

Schotfetdt R. M. 1977. 'Nursing Research: Reflection of Values', *Nursing Research*, 26(1):4–8.

Wittig D. R. 2001. 'Organ Donation Beliefs of Afro-American Women Residing in Small Southern Community', *Journal of Transcultural Nursing*, 12:203–10.

chapter

3 Research Problem

OBJECTIVES

Upon completion of this chapter the learner will be able to:

- Define research problem
- Discuss the criteria for the selection of a research problem
- Identify a research problem
- Enlist the steps of formulating the research problem
- Define research objectives
- Describe the need for research objectives
- List down methods of writing research objectives
- Define variables
- Enumerate the types of variables
- Define hypothesis
- Describe the types of hypotheses
- Formulate research hypothesis
- Define limitations
- Define delimitations
- Define assumptions
- Differentiate between assumptions and hypotheses

INTRODUCTION

The word 'problem' originates from the Greek word *proballein*, meaning 'to throw forward', 'a question proposed for solution' or 'a matter stated for examination'.

A research problem is a question that a researcher wants to answer or a problem that a researcher wants to solve. Identification and formulation of a research problem is the first step of the research process. However, it is considered as one of the most challenging and difficult phases of any research project. It is believed that the selection of a good research problem is a discovery in itself.

RESEARCH PROBLEM

Definitions of Problem

According to Kerlinger, a problem 'is an interrogative sentence or statement that asks: What relation exists between two or more variables?'.

R. S. Woodworth defines problem as 'a situation for which we have no ready and successful response by instinct or by previously acquired habit'.

Whitney states, 'To define a problem means to put a fence around it to separate it by careful distinctions from like questions, found in related situation or need.'

Why Define the Research Problem?

Defining the research problem is similar to defining the destination before beginning a journey; it determines the following:

1. What you will do?
2. Will it withstand scientific scrutiny?
3. How you will do it?
4. What you may achieve?

Selection of a Research Problem: Criteria

Selection of a research problem depends on several factors such as the researcher's knowledge, skills, interest, expertise, motivation, and creativity with respect to the subject of enquiry. In addition, a researcher needs to ensure that the selected problem has high significance and implication for his/her profession and that it is a suitable, feasible, testable, and solvable research problem.

No rules have been established for making a final selection of a research problem. Some criteria, however, should be kept in mind in the decision process. The four most important considerations are the significance of the problem, its researchability, the feasibility of the problem, and the interest of the researcher.

Significance of the Problem

A crucial factor in selecting a problem to be studied is its significance to nursing. The research question should have the potential of contributing to the body of knowledge in nursing in a meaningful way.

Researchability of the Problem

Not all questions are amenable to study through scientific investigation. Problems or issues of a moral or ethical nature, although provocative, are incapable of being researched. An example of a philosophically oriented question is whether nurses should join unions. The answer to such a question is ultimately based on a person's values. There is no right or wrong answer, only points of view. The question as stated is more suitable to a debate than to scientific research. However, it is possible to modify the question so that the aspects of the issue could be researched. For instance, each of the following questions could be investigated in a research project.

What are nurses' attitudes towards unionization?

Do younger nurses hold more favourable opinions of unions than older nurses?

Does a person's role (nurse versus nursing administrator versus hospital administrator) affect his/her perceptions of the consequences of unions on the delivery of health care?

Is opposition to unionization for nurses based primarily on perceived outcomes to patients and clients or on outcomes to the nursing profession?

The findings from these hypothetical projects would have no bearing, of course, on the answer to the original question of whether or not nurses should join union, but the information could be useful in developing a comprehensive understanding of the issues and in facilitating decision-making.

In general, researchable problems are those that involve variables capable of being precisely defined and measured. For example, suppose the researcher was trying to determine what effect early discharge had on the general well-being of patients. General well-being is too broad and fuzzy a concept to measure.

Hence, the researcher would have to establish the criteria against which the patient's progress towards well-being could be assessed.

When a new area of enquiry is being pursued, however, it may not be possible to define the concepts of interest in precise terms. In such cases, it may be appropriate to address the problem using in-depth qualitative research. The problem may then be stated in fairly broad terms to permit full exploration of the concept of interest.

Feasibility of the Problem

A problem that is both significant and worth researching may still be inappropriate if it is not feasible. The issue of feasibility encompasses a variety of considerations. Not all of the following factors are relevant for every problem, but most of them should be kept in mind in making a final decision.

Time and Timing: Most studies have deadlines or at least informal goals for their completion. Therefore, a problem must be one that can be adequately studied within the time allotted. This means the scope of the problem should be sufficiently restricted that enough time will be available for carrying out the various steps required. It is usually better to be generous in allocating time to the various tasks because research activities often require more time to accomplish than one anticipates. A related consideration is the timing of the project. Some of the research steps—especially data collection—are more readily performed at certain times of the day, week or year than at other times.

For example, if the problem focused on patients with peptic ulcers, the research might be more easily conducted in the fall and spring because of the increase in the number of patients with peptic ulcers during these seasons than in the summer or winter months. When the timing requirement of the task does not match the periods available for their performance, the feasibility of the project may be jeopardized.

Availability of the Subject: In any study involving humans, the researcher needs to consider weather individuals with the desired characteristic will be available and willing to cooperate. Securing people's cooperation may in some cases be easy, but other situations may pose more difficulties for the researcher. Some people may not have the time while some may have no interest in a particular study that has little personal benefits. Some others may not feel well enough to participate. Fortunately, people are usually willing to cooperate with a researcher if the demands on their time and comfort are minimal. If the research is time consuming, additional effort, and the payment of a monetary incentive may be necessary to obtain a sufficiently large sample of subjects. An additional problem may be that of identifying and locating subjects with the needed characteristics.

Cooperation of Others: Often it is insufficient to obtain the cooperation of prospective subjects alone. If the sample includes children, mentally incompetent people or senile individuals, it is almost always necessary to secure the permission of the parents or guardians. In institutional settings, such as hospitals, clinics, public schools or industrial firms, access to the personal records of clients or staff members usually requires administrative approval. Many health care facilities require that any project be presented to a panel of reviewers for approval before permitting the study to be conducted.

Facilities and Equipment: All research projects have some resources requirement, although in some cases the needs may be modest. It is prudent to consider what facilities and equipment will be needed and whether or not they will be available before embarking on a project so that disappointment and frustration can be prevented.

Money: Monetary requirement for research projects vary widely ranging from \$10 to \$20 for small student projects to hundreds of thousands of dollars for large-scale federally sponsored research. The following are some of the costs associated with research:

1. **Literature Costs:** index cards, reproduction of articles from books and journals, and computerized literature search service charges
2. **Personnel Cost:** payments to individuals hired to help with data collection, coding, data entry typing, and so on
3. **Subject Cost:** payment to subject as an incentive for their cooperation
4. **Supplies:** paper, envelopes, computer disks, postage, and so on
5. **Printing Cost:** payment to printers for printing forms, questionnaires subject recruitment notices, and so on
6. **Equipment:** laboratory apparatus, calculators, and so on
7. Computer services charges
8. Laboratory fees for the analysis of biophysiological data
9. Other services charges, such as the cost of duplicating materials
10. Transportation costs

Experience of the Researcher: The problem should be chosen from a field about which the investigator has some prior knowledge or experience. The researcher will have a difficult time in adequately developing a study project on a topic that is totally new and unfamiliar. In addition to substantive knowledge, the issue of technical expertise should not be overlooked. A beginning researcher usually has limited methodological skill and therefore should avoid a research problem that might require the development of sophisticated measuring instruments or involve complex statistical analyses.

Ethical Consideration: A research problem may not be feasible if the investigation of the problem would pose unfair or unethical demands on the participants. The ethical responsibilities of researchers should not be taken lightly; people engaged in research activities should be thoroughly knowledgeable about the rights of human or animal subjects.

Interest of the Researcher

Even if the tentative problem passes the tests of researchability, significance and feasibility, there is still one more criterion for its selection, which is the researcher's own interest in the problem. Genuine interest in and curiosity about the chosen research problem are important prerequisites to a successful study. A great deal of time and energy are expended in any scientific investigation and interest and enthusiasm ebb and flow throughout the time required for the completion of the project. The problem selected should extend the researcher's personal knowledge as well as the base of knowledge for others.

Personal interest in a research problem is least likely to be high when the topic has been suggested or assigned to the researcher by others. Beginning research students often seek out suggestions and may be grateful for assistance in selecting a topic area; often such assistance can be helpful in getting started. Nevertheless, it is rarely wise to be talked into a research topic towards which you are not personally inclined. If you do not find a problem attractive or stimulating during the beginning phases of a study—when the opportunity for creativity and intellectual reasoning is at its highest—then you are bound to regret your choice later in the project.

Characteristics of Good Topics

The following are the important characteristics of a good research topic:

1. Interesting—keeps the researcher interested in it throughout the research process
2. Researchable—can be investigated through the collection and analysis of data
3. Significant—contributes to the improvement and understanding of nursing theory and practice
4. Manageable—fits the researcher's level of research skills, needed resources and time restrictions
5. Ethical—does not embarrass or harm participants

Defining Terms in a Problem Statement

Sometimes, definitions and classification of concepts can be inserted into the statement of the problem itself. However, this usually makes the statement inordinately complex and clumsy.

Dictionary definitions of terms and concepts are almost always inadequate for research purposes. The definition provided by the researcher must imply or specify a method of operationalizing the variables. Let us take the following problem statement as an example: Is early discharge of mastectomy patients related to postoperative problems? In this example, early discharge might be defined as 'discharged prior to the fourth postoperative day', and postoperative problems might be defined in part as 'the patient's inability to comb her hair'. If adequate definitions are appended to a well-formulated problem statement, there should be little confusion about what is being studied.

Identification and Formulation of Research Problem

Where Do You See Problems That Can Ignite Your Mind to Think About Research?

The common sources from which a researcher may find ideas to identify and formulate research problems include the following:

1. Classroom
2. School
3. Community
4. Own teaching experience
5. Classroom lectures
6. Class discussions
7. Seminars/workshop/paper presentation
8. Internet
9. Out of class exchange of ideas with fellow students and professors
10. Reading assignments
11. Textbooks
12. Special assignments
13. Research reports
14. Consultation with
    (a) Course instructor
    (b) Advisor
    (c) Faculty member

Formulation of Research Problem

The formulation of a research problem involves the following steps:

1. **Selection of a Research Area:** Formulation of a research problem begins with the selection of a broad research topic from personal experience, literature, previous research and theories in which the researcher is interested, and which has significance for the nursing profession.
   For example, a researcher gets an idea to conduct a study on female foeticide. Therefore, he/she initially begins with such a broad research topic.
2. **Reviewing Literature and Theories:** After getting a broad idea for research, he/she needs to review the nursing literature and theories. Literature is reviewed to know what had already expanded the existing body of knowledge in the respective area of research. Review of nursing theories provides an opportunity for the nurse researcher to plan a research problem to contribute towards either testing or development of a theory or a conceptual model.
3. **Delimiting the Research Topic:** In this step, the researcher proceeds from a general research area of interest to a more specific topic of research to conduct a study.
   For example, initially a researcher decides to conduct a study on female foeticide; later, in this stage, the researcher limits it to a specific research topic: 'A study on the perception of women about causes and prevention of female foeticide in selected rural communities of district Shimoga'. At this stage, the researcher clearly identifies the variables, population and setting of research study. Furthermore, the researcher is also quite clear about the phenomenon to be studied, where and on whom.
4. **Evaluating the Research Problem:** Once the researcher is clear about the specific research problem, the research problem must be carefully evaluated for its significance, researchability, and feasibility. Feasibility of the research problem should be evaluated for time, cost, availability of subjects and resources, administrative and peer support, ethical consideration, and researcher's competence and interest.
5. **Formulating Final Statement of Research Problem:** After establishing the significance, researchability and feasibility, the researcher formulates a final statement of the research problem.

Thus, it is preferable that the formulation of a research problem fulfils the features given in Fig. 3.1.

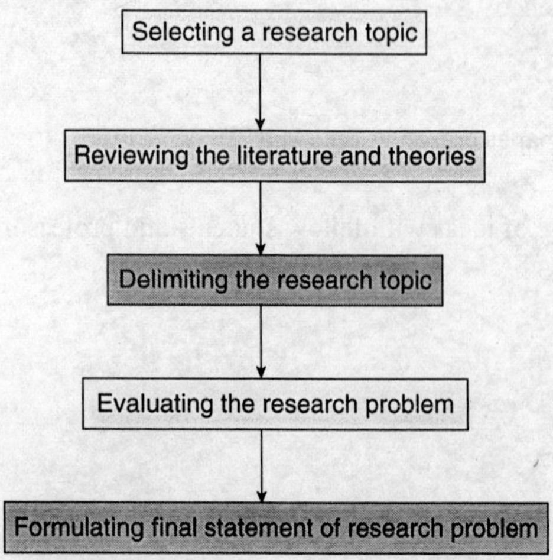

FIGURE 3.1 *Formulation of Research Problem*

RESEARCH QUESTION

Questions emerge from the researcher's topic of interest plus information gathered during the literature review.

RESEARCH OBJECTIVES

The objectives of a research project summarize what is to be achieved by the study.

Types of Research Objectives

General Objectives: These are the outcomes of the researcher's expectation at the end of the study.

Specific Objectives: The specific objectives include the factors influencing various aspects of the statement of the problem.

Characteristics of Research Objectives

The following are the essential characteristics of a research objective:

1. It is a concrete statement describing what the researcher is trying to achieve.
2. It should be relevant, feasible, logical, observable, unequivocal, and measurable.
3. It is a purpose that can be reasonably achieved within the expected timeframe and with the available resources.
4. It is the specific accomplishment the researcher hopes to achieve by the study.
5. It includes obtaining answers to research questions or testing the research hypotheses.

Need for Research Objectives

The formulation of research objectives will help the researcher to perform the following:

1. **Focus:** With clearly defined objective, the researchers can focus on the study.
2. **Avoid:** It helps the researcher to avoid the collection of data that is not necessary for understanding and solving the problem that he/she had defined.
3. **Organize:** It helps to organize the study in clearly defined parts or phases.
4. **Direct:** Properly formulated specific objectives will facilitate the development of research methodology and will help to orient the collection, analysis, interpretation, and utilization of data.

Methods of Stating Objectives

While stating the objectives of the study, the following guidelines must be taken care of:

1. The objectives should be presented briefly and concisely.
2. They should cover different aspects of the problem and its contributing factors in a coherent way and in a logical sequence.
3. The objectives should be clearly phrased in operational terms, specifying exactly what the researcher is going to do, where, and for what purpose.
4. They should be realistic and consider the local conditions.
5. They should use action verbs that are specific enough to be evaluated.

VARIABLES

Variables are qualities, properties or characteristics of persons, things or situations that change or vary.

Chin and Kramer stated, 'Variables are concepts at different level of abstraction that are concisely defined to promote their measurement or manipulation within study; variables are classified based on their nature, actions and effects on the variables'.

Types of Variables

The main types of variables are as follows:

1. **Independent and Dependent Variables:** These two variables are interrelated and are mainly observed in correlational, interventional, pre-experimental, quasi-experimental, and experimental research studies.
2. **An Independent Variable:** It is a stimulus or activity that is manipulated or varied by the researcher to determine the effect on the dependent variable.
3. **A Dependent Variable:** It is the variable that the researcher wants to predict or explain and is the outcome or response due to the effect of the independent variable.
4. **Research Variables:** In descriptive, exploratory, comparative, and qualitative research studies, variables are observed or measured in natural setting as they exist, without manipulating or imposing the effect of intervention or treatment. Here, no independent variable is manipulated and no cause–effect relationship is examined; these variables are considered as research variables. Therefore, research variables can be defined as qualities, attributed properties or characteristics that are observed or measured in a natural setting.
5. **Demographic Variables:** Common demographic variables are age, gender, educational status, religion, social class, marital status, habitat, occupation, income, and medical diagnosis. These characteristics and attributes of the subject under study are considered as demographic variables. In addition, sometimes researchers even try to establish a relation of the demographic variables with their research variables.
6. **Extraneous Variables:** Extraneous variables are the factors that are not the part of the study but may affect the measurement of the study variables. These variables are usually recognized and controlled by researchers in quasi-experimental and experimental studies. However, in other research studies too, the researcher may do so wherever it is possible. In general, specific research design and sample inclusion and exclusion criteria are used to control the influence of extraneous variables.

Dependent Versus Independent Variables

An important distinction can be made between two types of variables in a research study, and it is a distinction that needs to be mastered before proceeding to later reading. It is the distinction between the independent and the dependent variable. Many research studies are aimed at unraveling and understanding the causes underlying a phenomenon. Does a drug cause improvement of a medical problem? Does a nursing intervention cause more rapid recovery? Does smoking cause lung cancer? The presumed cause is referred to as the independent variable and the presumed effect is referred to as the dependent variable.

Variability in the dependent variable is presumed to depend on the variability in the independent variable. For example, the research may investigate the extent to which lung cancer depends on smoking or an investigator may be concerned with the extent to which a patient's perception of pain depends on the different types of nursing approaches.

The terms independent variable and dependent variable are frequently used to indicate the direction of influence rather than a causal connection. For example, let us say that a researcher is studying the attitude of nurses towards abortion and finds that often senior nurses hold less favourable opinion about abortion than younger nurses. The researcher might be unwilling to infer that the nurses' attitude was caused by their age. Yet the direction of influence clearly runs from age to attitudes. That is, it would make little sense to suggest that the attitudes caused or influenced age. Even though in this example the researcher does not infer a causal relationship between age and attitude, it is appropriate to conceptualize attitude towards abortion as the dependent variable and age as the independent variable.

The dependent variable usually is the variable the researcher is interested in understanding, explaining or predicting. In lung cancer research, it is carcinoma that is of real interest to the research scientist, not the smoking behaviour per se. In studies of the effectiveness of therapeutic treatment for alcoholics, it is the drinking behaviour of the subjects that is the dependent variable. Although a great deal of time, effort and resources may be devoted to designing new therapies, the primary interest of all these therapies are related to improvement in drinking behavior and overall functioning of alcoholics.

Many of the dependent variables that are studied by researchers have a multiplicity of causes or antecedents. If we are interested in studying the factors that influence people's weight, for example, we might consider their age, height, physical activity, and eating habits as the independent variables. It has to be noted that some of these independent variables are attribute variables, and others can be influenced by the investigator's manipulation. Just as a study may examine more than one independent variable, two or more dependent variables may be of interest to the researcher. For example, an investigator may be concerned with comparing the effectiveness of two methods of nursing care delivery for children with cystic fibrosis. Several dependent variables could be designated as measures of treatment effectiveness, such as length of stay in the hospital, number of recurrent respiratory infections, presence of cough, dyspnoea on exertion, and so on. In short, it is common to design studies with multiple independent and dependent variables.

The reader should not get the impression that variables are inherently dependent or independent. A variable that is classified as dependent in one study may be considered an independent variable in another study; for example a researcher may find that the religious background of a nurse has an effect on the nurse's attitude towards death and dying. Another study, however, may analyse the extent to which the attitudes of nurses towards death and dying affect their job performance. To illustrate this point with another example, consider a study that examines the relationship between contraception counseling and unwanted pregnancies. Yet another research project could study the effect of unwanted pregnancies on the incidence for child abuse. In short, the designation of a variable as independent or dependent is a function of the role the variable plays in a particular investigation. Some researchers use the term criterion variable rather than dependent variable. In studies that analyse the consequences of a treatment, therapy or some other type of intervention, it is usually necessary to establish the criteria against which the success of the intervention can be assessed; hence, the origin of the expression criterion variable. The term dependent variable, however, is broader, and more general in its implication and applicability. Therefore, we use the term dependent variable more frequently than criterion variable although in many situations the two are equivalent and interchangeable.

HYPOTHESIS

Wording the Research Hypothesis

A workable hypothesis states a relationship between two variables and is capable of empirical testing. This section takes a look at how the hypothesis should be stated and provides examples of various kinds of hypothesis.

A good hypothesis is worded in simple, clear and concise language and provides a definition of the variable in concrete, operational terms. These two requirements may be in conflict if the operational definition needs extensive explanation, in which case the variable should be operationally defined separately. The hypothesis should, however, be specific enough so that the reader understands what the variables are and whom the researcher will be studying. A hypothesis denotes a conjecture or proposition about the solution to the problem, the relationship of two or more variables, or the nature of some phenomenon.

Sources of Hypothesis

Hypothesis in research studies cannot be developed merely with wild guesses or assumptions, but they are generated from a variety of sources such as theoretical or conceptual frameworks, previous research findings, real life experiences, and academic literature (see Fig. 3.2).

1. **Theoretical or Conceptual Frameworks:** The most important sources of hypotheses are theoretical or conceptual frameworks developed for the study. Through a deductive approach, these hypotheses are drawn from theoretical or conceptual frameworks for testing them.

   For example, Roy's Adaptation Model is used in a research study where a hypothesis can be drawn from a concept of the theoretical model that 'patients' adaptation to a chronic illness depends on the availability of social support for them'.

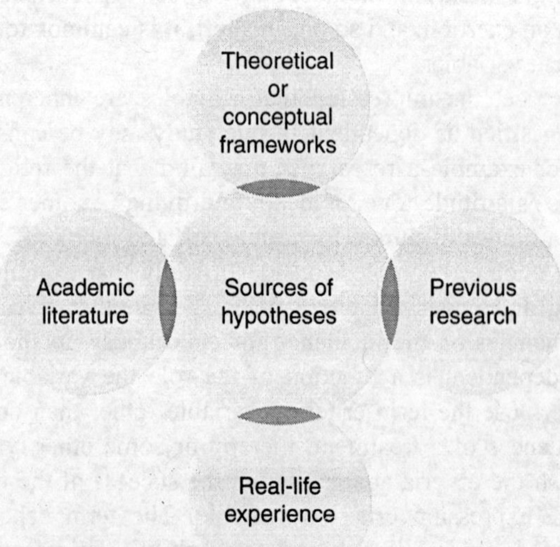

FIGURE 3.2 *Sources of Hypotheses*

2. **Previous Research:** Findings of the previous studies may be used for framing the hypotheses for another study.

   For example, in a small sample descriptive study, a researcher found that a number of patients admitted with coronary artery disease had increased body mass index. In another research study, a researcher may use this finding to formulate a hypothesis as 'obese patients have increased risk for development of coronary artery disease'.
3. **Real-life Experience:** Real-life experience also contributes in the formulation of hypothesis for research studies. For example, Newton had a life-changing experience of the falling of apple and formulated a hypothesis that earth attracts all the mass towards its centre, though several researches were conducted before generating the law of central gravity.
4. **Academic Literature:** Academic literature is based on formal theories, empirical evidences, experiences, observations and conceptualizations of academicians. This may serve as a good source for formulating hypotheses for the research studies.

Characteristics of a Good Hypothesis

A good hypothesis should have the following characteristics:

1. Be simple and clear
2. Be able to provide a definition of the variables
3. Be able to show the relationship between two or more variables
4. Be specific enough and able to test in a meaningful manner

Types and Forms of Hypotheses

The following are the various types of hypotheses:

1. **Simple Hypothesis:** It is a statement that reflects the relationship between two variables.
2. **Complex Hypothesis:** It is a statement that reflects the relationship between more than two variables.
3. **Associative Hypothesis:** It reflects a relationship between variables that occur or exist in a natural setting without manipulation.
4. **Causal Hypothesis:** It predicts the cause and effect relationship between two or more dependent and independent variables in experimental or interventional studies, where the independent variable is manipulated by researcher to examine the effect on the dependent variable.
5. **Directional Hypothesis:** It specifies not only the existence but also the expected direction of the relationship between variables. Here, to express the direction the directional terms such as positive, negative, less, more, lower–higher; lesser–greater are also used.
6. **Non-directional Hypothesis:** It reflects the relationship between two or more variables, but it does not specify the anticipated direction and nature of relationship such as positive or negative.
7. **Null Hypothesis (H0):** It is also known as statistical hypothesis and is used for statistical testing and interpretation of statistical outcome. It states that there exists no relationship between the dependent and independent variables.
8. **Research Hypothesis (H1):** It states the existence of relationship between two or more variables.

Formulation of a Research Hypothesis

A researcher starts the formulation of a research hypothesis with a research question and then generates operational definitions for all variables. When the researcher formulates the research hypothesis need to keep in mind the following:

1. Expected relationship or differences of variables.
2. Operational definitions.

Tips on Developing Research Problems and Hypotheses

The following are a few tips on developing research problems and hypotheses for those planning to conduct a study.

1. As noted earlier in this chapter, your personal experiences as a nurse or nursing student are a provocative source for research topics. Here are some hints on how to proceed.
2. Watch for recurring problems and see if you can discern a pattern in the situation that led to the problem.

   For example, why do many patients complain of being tired after being transferred from a coronary care unit to a progressive care unit?
3. Think about the aspect of your work that is irksome, frustrating or do not result in the intended outcome; then try to identify the factors contributing to the problem that could be changed.

   For example, why is supper time so frustrating in a nursing home?
4. Critically examine some of the decisions you make in the performance of your actions. Are these decisions based on tradition or are they based on scientific evidence that supports their efficacy? Many practices in nursing that have become customs might be challenged.

   For example, what would happen if the visiting hours in the intensive care unit were changed from 10 minutes every hour to the regularly scheduled hours existing in the rest of the hospital?
5. As an alternative to identifying problematic situations, identify the aspects of nursing that you most enjoy or in which you have the greatest interest. For example, think about what coursework has been most interesting to you, what rotation you most enjoyed or what part of your job you liked the best. Then do some reading in the research literature on this general area to see if a topic suggests itself.
6. If needed, do not hesitate to replicate a study that is reported in the research literature. Replications provide a valuable learning experience and have the potential to make valuable contributions because they can corroborate earlier findings.
7. If you are wording your problem statement as a statement of purpose, be careful in your choice of verbs because the verbs communicate information about the nature of your research design and possibly about your level of expertise. Among the verb choices are the following: describe, explore, examine, investigate, address, understand, compare, evaluate test, assess, explain and predict.
8. In wording your research questions or statement of purpose, it may be useful to look at published research reports for models. However, you may find that some reports fail to state unambiguously the problem under investigation. Thus, in some studies, you may have to infer the research

problem from several sources, such as the title of the report. In other reports, the problem is clearly stated but may be difficult to locate. Researchers most often state their research problem at the end of the introductory section of the report.

9. In designing a study of your own, do not be afraid to make a prediction, that is, to state a hypothesis; being wrong is part of the learning process.
10. If you formulate a hypothesis, avoid stating them in null form. When statistical tests are performed, the underlying null hypothesis is usually assumed without being explicitly stated.

Research Problem

While formulating a research problem, the following need to be ensured:

1. The research problem is clearly, precisely and concisely articulated.
2. It clearly states the variables, population and research setting under study.
3. The variables are expressed in measurable terms.
4. The type of study also may be included in the statement of a research problem.

LIMITATIONS

Limitations are restrictions of the study due to theoretical or methodological reasons, which may decrease the credibility and generalizability of the research findings.

Usually, there are two types of limitations in research studies.

Theoretical Limitations

Theoretical limitations restrict the ability of the research findings to generalize due to the use of specific theoretical concept in study or limit the study of variables through operational definitions.

Methodological Limitations

Methodological limitations usually result from some of the methodological factors such as un-representative sample, weak design, single setting, limited control over extraneous variables, poor implementation of treatment protocol, research tools with limited reliability and validity, poor data collection procedure and ineffective use of statistical analysis. Every study, no matter how well it is conducted, has some limitations. This is why it does not seem reasonable to use the words *prove* and *disapprove* with respect to research findings. It is always possible that future research may cast doubt on the validity of any hypothesis or the conclusions from a study.

Limitations in Case Studies: The case study includes the behaviour of a person. The behaviour of an individual is unique and a causal conclusion cannot be made from case studies.

Limitations in Co-relational Studies: In co-relational study as well, conclusion cannot be made because the alternative explanations of the variables are not easily available. Because of the lack of possibility of getting the explanations of variables in a meaningful way, the limitations of such studies will be more.

Limitations in Randomized Experiments: In randomized experimental studies, the variables will mostly be manipulated; the manipulated variables are always confused, and a causal conclusion is not possible in the confused situation. The limitations are beyond the control of researcher.

DELIMITATIONS

Delimitations are the boundaries of the study for the researcher. It aids the researcher as a guide. It also shows the path, horizontal and vertical, in the study. The common parameters of delimitation include sample size and the settings of the study.

ASSUMPTIONS

An assumption is a realistic expectation, that is, something that we believe to be true. However, no adequate evidence exists to support this belief. In other words, an assumption is an act of faith that does not have empirical evidences to support it. Assumption provides a basis to develop theories and research instrument and therefore influence the development and implementation of research process.

Assumption is defined as the 'statements that are taken for granted or are considered true, even though they have not been scientifically tested'.

'Assumptions are principles those are accepted as being true based on logic or reason, but without proof or verification.'

Assumptions Versus Hypotheses

The differences between assumptions and hypotheses are listed in Table 3.1.

TABLE 3.1 *Differences between Assumptions and Hypotheses*

Assumptions	Hypotheses
Basically beliefs and ideas that we hold to be true.	Predictions.
Often with little or no evidence and are not statistically tested in research.	Can be statistically tested and may be accepted or rejected.
Beliefs about the variables.	Predictions about the relationship of two or more variables.
The researcher attempts to discover a correlation based on the beliefs.	The researcher predicts a relation between variables statistically tests it to conclude the study.

Uses of Assumptions in Research

The following are the various uses of assumptions in research:

1. Research is built upon assumptions; since a foundation is needed to move forward, one must assume something to discover something.
2. Assumptions listed in a research paper may be good sources of research topics.
3. Assumptions provide the basis to the conduct of the research study.
4. Tested assumptions through research studies expand the professional body of knowledge.

Types of Assumptions

Figure 3.3 shows the various types of assumption:

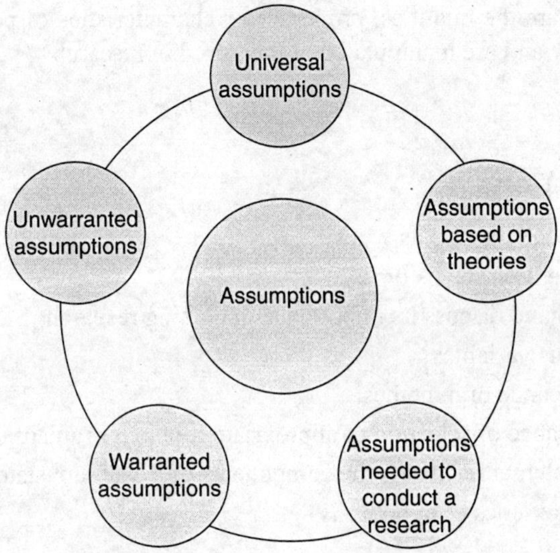

FIGURE 3.3 *Types of Assumptions*

Universal Assumptions: These are beliefs that are assumed to be true by a large part of society but testing such assumption is not always possible.

Assumptions Based on Theories: Assumptions may also be drawn from theories; if a research study is based on a theory, the assumption of the particular theory may become the assumption of that particular research study.

Assumptions Needed to Conduct a Research: Some of the common sense assumptions may be developed to conduct a particular study.

Warranted Assumptions: These are stated along with evidence to support.

Unwarranted Assumptions: These are stated without any supportive evidence. For example, the statement 'Almighty God exists everywhere in this universe'.

KEY POINTS

- **Research Problem:** This is an area of concern in which there is a gap in the knowledge base needed for nursing practice. Research is conducted to generate essential knowledge to address the practice concern, with the ultimate goal of providing evidence-based practice.
- **Assumptions:** These are statements taken for granted or considered true, even though they have not been scientifically tested.
- **Demographic Variables:** These are the characteristics or attributes of subjects that are collected to describe the sample for example, dependent groups' subjects or observations selected for data collection that are in some way related to the selection of other subjects or observations.

- **Hypothesis:** This is a formal statement of the expected relationship between two or more variables in a specified population.
- **Independent (Treatment or Experimental) Variables:** This is the treatment or experimental activity that is manipulated by the researcher to study its effect on dependent variable.
- **Variables:** These are the qualities, properties or characteristics of persons, things or situations that change or vary and are manipulated or measured in research.

QUESTIONS

I. Essay-type Questions

1. Define hypothesis and discuss its types.
2. Define variable and describe its types.
3. Define assumption and discuss its importance in nursing research.
4. What are extraneous variables?
5. Discuss the significance of hypothesis.
6. Discuss the importance of selection of appropriate research problem in nursing research.
7. Define problem statement. Discuss the components of a problem statement.
8. Explain the characteristics of hypothesis.

II. Short Notes

1. Characteristics of research objectives
2. Methods of stating objectives
3. Types of variables
4. Characteristics of good research topics
5. Sources of hypotheses
6. Importance of research in nursing

III. Multiple-choice Questions

Circle the alphabet before the best answer

1. A statement that asks what relation exists between two or more variables is a
   (a) problem (b) situation
   (c) question (d) habit
2. A situation for which we have a known and successful response by instincts is a
   (a) questions (b) research
   (c) problem (d) formula
3. The existence of relationship between two or more variables is
   (a) operational definition
   (b) differences
   (c) inductive hypothesis
   (d) research hypothesis
4. In a research project, 'what is to be achieved by the study' is the
   (a) variable
   (b) research objective
   (c) problem
   (d) population
5. Restrictions of the study due to theoretical or methodological reasons are
   (a) directions (b) objectives
   (c) limitations (d) methods

6. The boundaries of the study for the researcher are
   (a) hypothesis
   (b) demography
   (c) de-limitations
   (d) variables
7. The factors that are not the part of the study but may affect the measurement are
   (a) research variables
   (b) independent variables
   (c) dependent variables
   (d) extraneous variables
8. The activity that is carried out to create the effect on the dependent variable is
   (a) hypothesis
   (b) research problem
   (c) dependent variable
   (d) manipulation
9. To know what had already been done to expand the existing body of knowledge in respective area of research is
   (a) review of literature
   (b) delimitation
   (c) limitation
   (d) formulation
10. The existence of no relationship between the dependent and independent variable is
    (a) hypothesis
    (b) complex hypothesis
    (c) research hypothesis
    (d) null hypothesis

Answer Keys

1. (c) 2. (d) 3. (d) 4. (b) 5. (c) 6. (c) 7. (d) 8. (d)
9. (a) 10. (d)

FURTHER READING

Bhaskara Raj, Elakkuvana D. 2010. *Nursing Research and Biostatistics*. Rajaji Nagar, Bengaluru: EMMESS Medical publishers.

Couchman, W., Dawson, J. 1996. *Nursing and Health Care Research: A Practical Guide*. London: Bailliere Tindall.

DeVault, M. 1990. 'Social Problems: Talking and Listening from Women's Standpoint: Feminist Strategies for Interviewing and Analysis', *Social Problems*, 37(1): 96–116.

Fontana, A., Frey, J. 2000. 'The Interview: From Structured Questions to Negotiated Text'. In N. K. Denzin and Y. S. Lincoln (Eds), *Handbook of Qualitative Research*. CA: Sage Publications.

Grady, K. A., Wallston, B. S. 1988. *Research in Health Care Setting: Applied Social Research Method Series*. Vol. 14. New Delhi: Sage Publications.

Korb, M. 1994. 'Anorexia as Symbolic Expression of a Woman's Rejection of Her Mother's Life', *Western Journal of Nursing Research*, 16(1): 69–80.

Notter, L. E., Hott, J. R. 1988. *Essentials of Nursing Research.* Fourth edition. New York: Springer Publishing Company.

Polit, Denise F., Hungler, Bernadette P. 1995. *Nursing Research Principles and Methods*. Fifth edition. Philadelphia, PA: J. B. Lippincott Company.

Sharma, Suresh K. 2011. *Nursing Research and Statistics*. New Delhi: Elsevier Publication, p. 65.

Sharma, Suresh K. 2011. *Nursing Research and Statistics*. New Delhi: Elsevier Publication, pp. 46–47, 51.

Woods, N. F., Catanzaro, M. 1988. *Nursing Research Theory and Practice*. St Louis: C. V. Mosby Company.

chapter

4 Review of Literature

OBJECTIVES

Upon completion of this chapter the learner will be able to:

- Define literature review
- Recognize the importance of literature review in research
- Determine the purposes of literature review
- Recognize the relationship between literature review and research process
- Appreciate the various skills required for literature review
- Identify various sources for literature review
- Discuss the process of literature review
- Critique the literature review section of research articles
- Follow ethical considerations for literature review

INTRODUCTION

The quest for quality and cost effective health care has brought nursing research into the forefront. Research-based practice is considered as a hallmark of professional nursing. Nowadays, research has become an integral part of all nursing programs. It is required to undertake a literature review at some point, either as part of a course of study, as a key step in the research process, or as part of clinical practice development or policy. For student nurses and novice researchers, it is often seen as a difficult task. It demands a complex range of skills, such as learning how to identify topics for exploration, acquiring skills of literature searching and retrieval, developing the ability to analyse and synthesize data, and becoming skilful in writing and reporting, often within a limited timescale. The purpose of this chapter is to present a step-by-step guide to facilitate understanding the critical elements of the literature review process in research.

MEANING

Literature review means a 're' view or 'look again' at what has already been written about the topic. It is not a literary review, which usually is a brief critical discussion about the merits and weaknesses of a literary work such as a play, novel, or a book of poems. Literature review compiles various research projects published by recognized scholars and researchers. It is not just a descriptive list of the material available or a set of summaries; it provides the background for the problem the researcher is interested in, or helps to put the problem into historical perspective and, at times, shows how others have addressed similar problems in the past.

DEFINITIONS

Scholars have defined literature review in different ways, some of which are as follows:

A literature review is an objective, thorough summary and critical analysis of the relevant available research and non-research literature on the topic being studied.

Review of literature in a research report is a summary of current knowledge about a particular practice or problem, and includes what is known and unknown about the problem.

A literature review is an evaluative report of information found in the literature related to your selected area of study.

The review should describe, summarize, evaluate, and clarify the literature. It should give a theoretical base for the research and help you (the author) determine the nature of your research. Works that are irrelevant should be discarded and those that are peripheral should be looked at critically.

From these definitions, one can understand that literature review serves many purposes and entails a wide variety of activities such as summarizing, synthesizing, and analysing the work done by different scholars related to the topic. It is also done to update the knowledge related to a selected research problem.

However as a researcher, one must keep it in mind that, *review literature is not any of the following*:

1. **An Annotated Bibliography:** An annotated bibliography is a list of citations to books, articles, and documents. Each citation is followed by a brief (usually about 150 words) descriptive and evaluative paragraph, the annotation. The purpose of the annotation is to inform the reader of the relevance, accuracy, and quality of the sources cited.
2. **Literary Review:** A literary review is a brief critical discussion about the merits and weaknesses of a literary work such as a play, novel, or a book of poems.
3. **A Book Review:** It is a form of literary criticism in which a book is analysed based on the content, style, and merit. These reviews are reviewed by scholars and are published in scholarly journals.
4. **A Description of Studies Previously Done:** It is not a study-by-study or article-by-article description of studies previously done, a restatement of the studies previously done, or a brief overview of articles.

GOALS OF LITERATURE REVIEW

Literature review is a goal-driven activity. According to Neuman, the main goals of literature review are as follows:

1. To demonstrate a familiarity with a body of knowledge and establish credibility. A review tells a reader that the researcher knows the research done in that area and the major issues. A good review increases the reader's confidence in the researcher's professional competence, ability, and background.
2. To show the path of prior research and how a current project is linked to it. It outlines the direction of research in question and shows the development of knowledge. A good review places a research project in context and demonstrates its relevance by making connections to a body of knowledge.
3. To integrate and summarize what is known in an area. It pulls together and synthesizes different results. It points out areas where prior studies agree, where they disagree, and where major questions remain. It collects what is known up to a point in time and indicates the direction for future research.

4. To learn from others and stimulate new ideas. A review tells what others have found so that a researcher can benefit from the efforts of others. A good review identifies blind alleys and suggests hypotheses for replication. It divulges procedures, techniques, and research designs worth copying so that a researcher can better focus hypotheses and gain new insights.

IMPORTANCE OF LITERATURE REVIEW

Research is done in order to inform people about new knowledge or discovery, but one cannot expect that people will believe whatever is presented in the research project unless it is supported by other researches on the same topic. It also proves that the researcher is not writing about any random subject, but many others have also communicated and given valuable input about the same topic. Review plays an important role in this aspect.

1. Literature review is important for establishing a link between the researches that have been done already and their relationship with the proposed study. It informs the reader about the aspects of the topic that have been explored by other researchers and that need to be studied further.
2. A good researcher usually does extensive literature review, which helps avoid duplication of work; in case of replication, it provides an option for modifying the research problem with new perspective in terms of setting, sampling technique, population, research design, and so forth, thus making it more valuable.
3. When literature review is performed sincerely and honestly, it yields a lot of information but it may not be possible to include everything in the study. Some information may be directly relevant to the study and some may give clues about the issues of interest.
4. Another importance of literature review is to trace the intellectual progression or the recent advances related to the topic. Depending on the situation, literature review also helps to evaluate the sources and advise the reader on the most pertinent or relevant sources.
5. Literature review seeks to summarize the available literature on any one topic with different perspectives. It helps the reader to gain knowledge without reviewing individual studies. This is very important as there is a tremendous amount of literature available, and it is not feasible for every health care professional to read and assimilate all information.
6. Usually by the end of a literature review, the researcher can identify the gaps related to the topic and the significance of undertaking the study. For example, if someone wants to assess the perception of children towards chronic illness and about death, there may be very few studies and almost none in the Indian scenario.
7. Lastly, review of literature plays an important role in identifying the difference of opinions and the contradictory findings and explanations given by various researchers related to the topic. For example, if anyone is interested in evaluating the effect of traditional medicines on blood sugar level among patients with *diabetes mellitus*, a researcher may get the information from various sources that may reveal similar or exactly opposite findings. In such situations, a review will provide a guideline for selecting appropriate medicines that can be used in the proposed study.

PURPOSES OF REVIEW OF LITERATURE

The overall purpose of a literature review is to critically appraise and synthesize the current state of knowledge relating to the topic under investigation, as a means of identifying the gaps in the knowledge that a new study would seek to address. Hart proposes that a literature review is fundamental to the success of any academic research in that it ensures the feasibility of researching the chosen topic before the study actually commences.

Literature Review for Research Purposes

1. To explore the area of interest in view of narrowing down the topic
2. To summarize and assess the state of existing knowledge. In this, the researcher is interested to find out answers to many questions such as the following:
   (a) What knowledge exists and is generally accepted with regard to the topic?
   (b) Are there important differences or disagreements among scholars?
   (c) Are there significant problems or limitations with any of the research studies?
   (d) What were the research methods employed in the various research studies, which were not, and with what consequences?
   (e) What questions remain unanswered?
   (f) What aspects or approaches seem relatively unexplored?

   This process of reviewing existing knowledge helps to develop a better understanding of the topic. Moreover, it helps to narrow down the topic. For example, if the researcher's area of interest is health problems in a geriatric population, a review on the various aspects of health problems such as physical, social, psychological, and so forth should be performed. Through the review one can find out which problems are more common and need immediate attention. For example, if psychological problems such as feeling of loneliness and depression are found common, then the review can be further focused on these two areas through which the researcher can find out the various interventions used for minimizing these problems, for example, soft music or relaxation techniques. Finally, the researcher can decide on the problem and the intervention that is most relevant and feasible. Another important factor is that while undergoing this review process, the researcher can develop an in-depth understanding about the topic.
3. To identify the gaps in the current state of knowledge or analysis of the topic of interest. When a review of literature is done extensively, it helps the researcher to find out the gaps in the knowledge relevant to the topic of his interest. For example, if the researcher wants to study the reaction of children towards hospitalization, he may find some literature related to this, but the same findings may not be applicable for children from all sectors of the world due to the diversity in cultural practices related to child rearing. The researcher can identify this gap and perform the study.
4. To establish the originality in context of the selected research topic. It is well known that no knowledge exists in vacuum; hence, it is rare that there is no study related to the problem decided by the researcher. Through literature review a researcher can organize these findings, discuss them, and point out their limitations, some of which will be addressed in the research.
5. To compare the methodological approaches to the research problem. A review of literature identifies the various research methods used in similar problems studied by other researchers. It helps the researcher to compare these methods and decide the most appropriate method for the proposed study.
6. To raise questions for further research. A review of literature is done at every step of the research process. Throughout this process, the researcher develops a deeper understanding about the topic and is also able to identify many issues that may have remained unanswered, underexplored, or overlooked. It helps the researcher to recommend the problems for further research.

7. To describe the relationship of each work to the others under consideration. A review of literature helps to describe the work done by others related to the topic. Through this the researcher can compare the work done by other scholars and illustrate other ideas related to the topic, that is, how common or different they are. It also helps to explains why a particular idea or perspective is new.
8. To avoid duplication of work. Through literature review, a researcher can find out whether similar type of study is being done by other researchers, and, if yes, then how to replicate it with a new perspective.
9. To resolve conflicts amongst seemingly contradictory previous studies

For Non-research Purposes

1. As an assignment for an academic course
2. To update current personal knowledge and practice on a topic
3. To evaluate current practices
4. To develop and update guidelines for practice
5. To develop work-related policies

LITERATURE REVIEW IN QUANTITATIVE AND QUALITATIVE RESEARCH

In Quantitative Research

In quantitative research, the researcher begins the review with an extensive literature search on the topic of interest. The researcher includes substantial amount of literature at the beginning of a study to provide the direction for the research questions or hypotheses.

In Qualitative Research

In qualitative research, the purpose and timing of the literature review vary, based on the type of the study to be conducted. In this type of studies, the researcher uses literature with the assumptions of learning from the participants. All types of qualitative design are exploratory in nature, which means that not much has been written about the topic or the population being studied. There are mainly four types of qualitative research, namely phenomenological, ethnography, grounded theory, and historical. Literature review is conducted as per the design of the study.

1. **In Phenomenological Research:** Literature review is done after data collection, in order to avoid the influence of information on the researcher's objectivity while collecting the data. For example, if the researcher is interested in finding out the experience of mothers having a child with chronic illness and is in terminal state, it is possible to get a number of studies through literature review and formulate an opinion about the experience of the mothers, which may or may not be true. So when the researcher does the review after data collection, the findings from the study can be compared and combined with the literature to determine factual information about a phenomenon.
2. **In Ethnographic Studies:** Literature is reviewed early in the research process to provide an early understanding of the background and the variables to be studied and for interpretation of the findings in a particular culture.
3. **In Grounded Theory Approach:** Literature review is performed just to know whether anybody else has done a similar study or not. Literature review also gives a background and motivates the

interest for the particular research area. It is done to compare and contrast the findings before formulating the theory, hypothesis, or any model out of the data collected from the participants.

4. **In Historical Research:** Literature is reviewed to develop research questions and is a major source of data in the study. Historical review requires extensive review of literature that can last for a longer duration. At the end, information collected through the review is analysed and organized to explain the evolvement of a particular phenomenon.

TYPES OF LITERATURE REVIEWS

There are mainly four types of literature reviews: Traditional or narrative review, systematic literature review, meta-analysis, and meta-synthesis.

1. **Traditional or Narrative Review:** This type of review provides an overview of the research findings on a particular topic. It includes a critical summary of the content and is written by experts after examining the published work. The main purpose of this review is to compile a great deal of information in an accessible and concise manner. However, these reviews are prone to bias in many ways; for example, the author may include those studies that support a particular point of view or may focus only on selected indexes or computer database. Often the reviewer does not specify the methodology used for review and may use informal, unsystematic, and subjective methods to collect and interpret information, which is often summarized subjectively and in narrative form. It can lead to bias and may, sometimes, overestimate the value of information.
2. **Systematic Literature Review:** In contrast to the traditional or narrative review, systematic reviews use a more rigorous and well-defined approach for reviewing the literature in a specific subject area. Systematic reviews are used to answer well-focused questions about clinical practice. The word 'systemic' refers to the system adopted by the reviewer, which gives detailed information about the parameters decided by the reviewer in terms of time frame from which the studies are selected, methods used to appraise (e.g., the tools used to evaluate the quality of the studies) and the method of synthesis (e.g. qualitative summaries or statistical calculations). Such studies are also called as 'research on research'. They aim to provide an exhaustive summary of literature relevant to a research question and use explicit methods to identify what can reliably be said on the basis of these studies. Unlike traditional reviews, the purpose of a systematic review is to provide as complete a list as possible of all the published and unpublished studies relating to a particular subject area.

   According to Evans and Pearson, the findings of the systematic review 'frees the decision maker from reliance on the mass of published primary research'. Systematic reviews are helpful for those researchers who do not have the resources and expertise to search and apprise the large number of studies that are relevant for their study.

   For example, a systematic review was conducted by Simkhada et al. on the factors affecting utilization of antenatal care in developing countries. The aim of the review was to identify and analyse the main factors affecting the utilization of antenatal care in developing countries. Data was searched from a range of electronic databases, which was published between 1990 and 2006. English-language publications were searched using relevant keywords, and reference lists were hand-searched. A total of 28 papers were included in the review, and the studies most commonly identified the following factors to be affecting antenatal care uptake—maternal education, husband's education, marital status, availability, cost, household income, women's employment, media exposure, and having a history of obstetric complications. Cultural beliefs and ideas about pregnancy also had an influence on the antenatal care use. Parity had a statistically significant negative effect on adequate attendance. Whilst women of higher parity tend to use antenatal care less, there is interaction with women's age and religion. Only one study examined the effect of the quality of antenatal services on utilization. None identified an association between the utilization of such services and the satisfaction with them. In conclusion, the researcher recommended that more qualitative research is to be performed to explore the effect of women's satisfaction, autonomy, and gender role in the decision-making process. Adequate utilization of antenatal care cannot be achieved merely by establishing health centres; women's overall (social, political and economic) status needs to be considered.

As the current emphasis of nursing research is on evidence-based practice, systematic review is considered to be the best approach for performing literature review.

3. **Meta-analysis:** It is a technique that combines the results of many studies that have been conducted on the same topic. The results of these studies are combined and statistically analysed. According to Anderson, it is a 'rigorous statistical procedure that synthesizes results from multiple primary research studies on a common clinical problem or issue'. While performing the analysis, the exact *p* value is taken into consideration. This helps to draw conclusions and detect patterns and relationships between findings.
4. **Meta-synthesis:** Meta-synthesis is the non-statistical technique used to integrate, evaluate, and interpret the findings of multiple qualitative research studies. Such studies may be combined to identify their common core elements and themes. The findings from phenomenological, grounded theory, or ethnographic studies may be integrated and used. Unlike meta-analysis, where the ultimate intention is to reduce findings, meta-synthesis involves analysing and synthesizing key elements in each study, with the aim of transforming individual findings into new conceptualizations and interpretations. Table 4.1 gives information about the types of literature review.

TABLE 4.1 *Types of Literature Review*

Traditional or Narrative	Systematic	Meta-analysis	Meta-synthesis
Critiques and summarizes a body of literature.	More rigorous and well-defined approach.	A form of systematic review (reductive).	Non-statistical technique.
Draws conclusions about the topic.	Comprehensive; published and unpublished studies relating to a particular subject area.	Takes findings from several studies on the same subject and analyses them using standardized statistical procedures.	Integrates, evaluates, and interprets findings of multiple qualitative research studies.
Identifies gaps or inconsistencies in a body of knowledge.	Details the time frame within which the literature was selected.	Integrates findings from a large body of quantitative findings to enhance understanding (study unit of analysis).	Identifies common core elements and themes.

(*Continued*)

TABLE 4.1 *Types of Literature Review (Continued)*

Traditional or Narrative	Systematic	Meta-analysis	Meta-synthesis
Requires a sufficiently focused research question. Teaching Undergraduate Nursing Research: A Narrative review www.ncbi.nlm.nin.gov/pubmed/11214849.	Details the methods used to evaluate and synthesize findings of the studies in question. Advanced Practice Nurse Outcomes 1990–2008. www.nursingeconomics.net/ce/2013/article3001021.pdf	Draws conclusions and detect patterns and relationships, for example, the effect of exercise on glycaemic control and body mass in type 2 diabetes mellitus by Boule et al. a meta-analysis of controlled clinical trials. JAMA 2001:286(10):1218-27.	May use findings from phenomenological, grounded theory or ethnographic studies; involves analysing and synthesizing key elements with a goal to transform individual findings into new conceptualizations and interpretations, for example, meta-synthesis of 14 qualitative research studies; mothers' experiences of having a pre-term infant in neonatal intensive care unit (www.carlosnayo.net/biblioteca/enfer2008 /mothers.pdf).
Weaknesses • Reviews are influenced by publication bias • In absence of strict protocols, review becomes a subjective judgement of included studies	• Focus of question is narrow. • It lacks comprehensiveness	• Chances of publication bias is more • It can only analyse the role of independent variables in explaining variance in dependent variables if sufficient data is provided in the original studies.	
A large number of studies may make it difficult to draw conclusions.			
The process is subject to bias that supports the researcher's own work.			

LITERATURE REVIEW AND RESEARCH PROCESS

Review of literature is considered an essential and important activity during each step of the research process. It begins with deciding the research problem and continues until the dissemination of research findings. The following is an overview of the use of literature review in relation to steps of quantitative research process.

Problem Statement and Hypothesis

Literature review helps to determine what is known and not known, to uncover gaps, consistencies, or inconsistencies, and/or to reveal unanswered questions in the literature related to the topic, concept, or problem. The review allows for refinement of research problem and hypotheses. Sometimes, it may be observed that a particular topic intended by a researcher is already being studied. The researcher need not be disappointed. There can be further research on the same topic but with other perspectives in terms of setting, data collection methods, population, or partial replication of the same study.

The most important function of literature review is that it helps the researcher to delineate and delimit the problem. For example, if a researcher is interested in studying the health status of children who are residing at orphanages, literature review will help to delineate and delimit the problem by knowing which aspects of health status, such as physical, social, psychological, and spiritual status, are already covered by other researchers.

Study Variables

Identifying and defining the study variables is an important task in the research process. Literature review helps to decide and operationally define the variables. For example, if the researcher is interested in the nursing care of patients admitted in a critical care unit, literature review may reveal various aspects of critical care such as physical, psychosocial, or spiritual and then he can further select one aspect and its related variables of interest. If he selects psychosocial aspects of care, then the review may reveal various studies where variables such as anxiety, coping strategies, perception of illness among patients, or the effect of a particular intervention (therapeutic communication) on anxiety are studied. Literature gives an insight about various variables and the different methods to study those variables.

Theoretical Framework

Literature review helps to reveal various theories related to the topic in nursing and allied fields. It also helps the researcher to justify the findings of the study or for development of a new theory. In the absence of a theory on a study topic, the review can reveal the studies that need to be replicated and the areas of consensus and of dispute.

Design and Method

Exploration of various research designs is an important activity done through literature review. The review reveals the strengths and weaknesses of the designs and methods of previous research studies. It helps the researcher to decide on valid and reliable data collection tools, sample size, and sampling method and to identify the various ethical issues and concerns related to this particular topic. For example, in relation to the data collection tool for assessment of pain, one can use visual analogue scale, 10-point horizontal scale, or verbal expression of pain on a 7-point rating scale. Through review, the researcher can decide on the method that will be best suitable for his study.

Data Analysis Techniques

In relation to data analysis techniques, literature review can give some insight into the various methods used in other studies and help to decide which method will be useful for the present study to make the results of the study meaningful.

Findings, Implications, and Recommendations

Literature review helps to discuss the findings of a study. Through the review, the researcher can relate the findings that may support the previously done studies or new findings, if any. It helps to discuss and implement the findings with respect to its implications in day-to-day practice. Recommendations for further study are based on the study's results and their relationship to the findings of the study.

COMPONENTS OF REVIEW OF LITERATURE

Literature review is a comprehensive summary, which contains the following:

1. An overview of the subject, issue or theory under consideration, along with the objectives of the literature review.
2. Division of works under review into categories (such as those in support of a particular position, those against, and those offering alternative theses entirely).
3. Explanation of how each work is similar to and how it varies from the others.
4. Conclusions as to which parts are best considered in their argument, are most convincing of their opinions, and make the greatest contribution to the understanding and development of their area of research.

SKILLS REQUIRED IN REVIEW OF LITERATURE

To make the literature review effective, and to avoid frustration during the process of review, we need to develop certain skills such as the following:

Critical Thinking Skill: It is the ability to think clearly and rationally. It includes the ability to engage in reflective and independent thinking. A researcher with critical thinking skills will be able to do the following:

1. Understand the logical connections between ideas
2. Identify, construct, and evaluate arguments
3. Detect inconsistencies and common mistakes in reasoning
4. Solve problems systematically
5. Identify the relevance and importance of ideas
6. Reflect on the justification of one's own beliefs and values

Critical Reading Skill: It is an active, intellectually engaging process in which the reader participates in an inner dialogue with the writer. A critical reader actively looks for assumptions, key concepts and ideas, reasons and justification, supporting examples, parallel experiences, and any other structural features of the written text to interpret and assess it accurately and fairly. It enables the reader to read critically and understand the essence of a particular material.

Critical Appraisal Skill: This is the process by which a reader can evaluate a piece of written material and assess whether it possesses validity (i.e., whether it is close to the truth) and applicability (i.e. whether it is clinically useful). If a research is being examined, critical appraisal skills are vital to decide whether the research has been well conducted and whether, ultimately, the results of the research can be implemented into the everyday practice for the benefits of the patients. Critically appraising and reviewing a paper is essentially a process to look for information that is of value.

Information Seeking Skill: It is the ability to scan the literature efficiently using manual or computerized methods to identify a set of potentially useful articles or books.

LITERATURE REVIEW PROCESS

Literature review is a continuous process consisting of various interrelated steps. Before starting the review, the researcher should ask certain questions to self:

1. What is *the specific thesis, problem, or research question* that my literature review helps to define?
2. What type of literature review am I conducting?

3. Am I looking at issues of theory, methodology, or policy? Quantitative research (e.g., the effectiveness of a new procedure) or qualitative research (e.g., studies)?
4. What is the scope of my literature review?
5. What types of sources am I using (e.g., journals, books, government documents, popular media)? What discipline am I working in (e.g., nursing psychology, sociology, or medicine)?
6. How good was my information seeking? Has my search been wide enough to ensure that I have found all the relevant material? Has it been narrow enough to exclude irrelevant material? Is the number of sources I have used appropriate for the length of my paper?
7. Have I critically analysed the literature I used? Did I follow through a set of concepts and questions, comparing items to each other in the ways they deal with them? Instead of just listing and summarizing items, did I assess them, discussing strengths and weaknesses?
8. Have I cited and discussed studies contrary to my perspective?
9. Will the reader find my literature review relevant, appropriate, and useful?

STEPS OF LITERATURE REVIEW

1. Selecting a review topic
2. Searching the literature
3. Gathering, reading and analysing, and synthesizing the literature
4. Writing the review
5. References

Selecting a Review Topic

Selection of the topic for review is a daunting task, especially for students and novice reviewers. A common error that can occur is the selection of a topic that is very broad, for example, pain or obesity in children. Review on these topics may be a useful strategy for determining how much literature is available, but as it generates a large amount of data it makes the review infeasible. Therefore, it is advisable to refine this further so that the final amount of information generated is manageable. For example, if the researcher is interested in conducting a study about the effect of massage on pain during administration of intramuscular injection among paediatric population, he needs to focus the review on various types of massage, technique used, duration, material used, and how the results were measured. Focusing or selection of problem enables the researcher to gather the information that is relevant and manageable. Talking to others, such as clinical specialists or a study population, or reading around a topic can also help to identify the areas of the subject that the reviewer is interested in and may help to indicate how much information exists on the topic, which may help in the selection of the problem and to focus the review.

To summarize, the following needs to be performed for deciding the topic:

1. Decide what exactly you want to find out. A precise question usually works better than a vague one; so, if you are looking at 'The impact of parents' behaviour on children', you might want to think about what exactly you want to find out. A more precise question for this may be, 'Does parental behaviour have any influence on children's eating habits?' or on lifestyle, academic performance and so forth.

2. Decide on the age group (school age, adolescents), socioeconomic background, and gender you would like to study.
3. Identify key words. Keywords are the major concepts or variables that are included in the search. It is an important task as search engines and library databases do not look for your ideas; they just try to match up the words that are used. Words used should really define the research topic such as behaviour, eating habits, or life style. Before starting a key search, it is important to consider synonyms and alternative terms related to the topic. If all possible keywords are not identified, some literature can get omitted from the review, which may adversely affect its quality.

Searching the Literature

After selecting a topic, the next step is to identify, in a structured way, the appropriate and related information. A systematic approach is considered better than a narrative or traditional one. According to F. S. Desmond., literature search can be defined as the process of systematically identifying published materials that meet predetermined criteria. This process is a critical component of research and can be conducted manually or with the aid of computer technology. For searching the literature, certain principles can be followed such as the following:

1. Outline the steps in the search process (Fig. 4.1).
2. Keep a record of the databases included in the research, for example, key words used in each of the database.

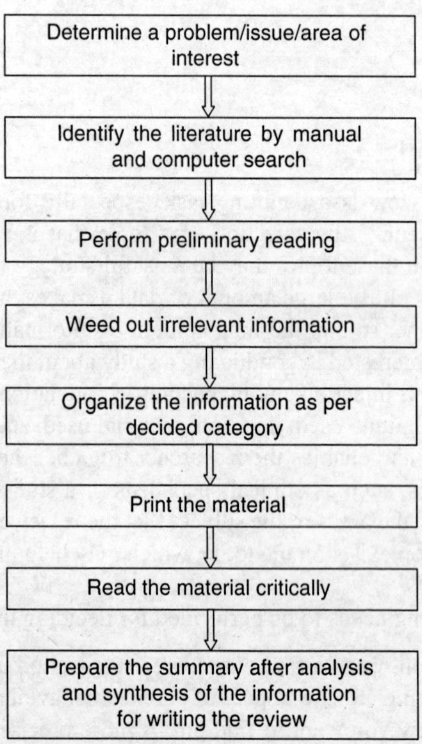

FIGURE 4.1 *Steps for Searching the Literature*

3. Use a table format to identify the databases, number of references retrieved from each database, and the final number of references used for the review.
4. Document the reason for excluding some references.
5. Identify the type of literature source, such as qualitative studies, surveys, or reports.
6. Keep record of all the key journals.

Types of Sources

Usually, primary, secondary and tertiary types of sources are used for the review. Primary sources are considered the best, but secondary and tertiary sources have their own value if used carefully (Table 4.2).

TABLE 4.2 *Types of Sources*

Primary	Secondary	Tertiary
These are original materials that provide first-hand records of events, experiments, creative works, or statistics. They form the basis for subsequent interpretations, analyses, and explanations. Some examples of primary sources are quantitative, qualitative, and empirical research studies. The following is an example of a primary source: Lan, P. T., Faxelid, E., Chuc, N. T., Mogren, I., and Lundborg, C. S. (2008). 'Perceptions and Attitudes in Relation to Reproductive Tract Infections Including Sexually Transmitted Infections in Rural Vietnam: A Qualitative Study', *Health Policy*, 86(2–3): 308–317.	These are descriptions or summary by somebody other than the original researcher, such as a review article that summarizes what is known about a particular phenomenon , materials that provide interpretations, explanations, and descriptions of primary sources, for example, health periodicals such as *American Nurse* or the Health section of the New York Times. The following is an example of a secondary source: Lusk, M. J. and Konecny, P. (2008). 'Cervicitis: A Review', *Current Opinion in Infectious Diseases*, 21(1), 49–55.	These sources synthesize and explain the work of others that might be useful at an early stage but are weak supporters for the researcher's arguments such as books and articles based on secondary sources. Examples include almanacs, directories, fact books, guide books, and manuals. These sources generally give an overview of a topic. Global Health Observatory reports on the current situation and trends for priority health issues.

Initiation of Search

Before initiating the search, it is recommended to prioritize the resources by considering following points:

1. Start with a broad synthesis of literature, such as overviews found in encyclopaedias, journal articles, or abstract series.
2. Turn to journal articles that report research studies. Start with the most recent studies about the topic and then go backward in time. Follow up on references at the end of the articles for more sources to examine.
3. Turn to books related to the topic.

4. Follow this search by looking for recent conference papers on the topic. Make contact with the authors of the papers and ask whether they have an instrument that might be used or modified for use in your study.
5. Look at the abstract of theses/dissertations available at various universities in virtual form.

Once the source is prioritized, selection of an appropriate material is the next important task in literature review. While selecting the material, three major criteria can be used:

1. **Relevance**
   (a) Has the material contributed to the development of required main concepts?
   (b) Does it clarify your position (either by supporting or contrasting with it)?
   (c) Does it provide key interpretations or models you can apply to your design?
   (d) Is the material bound to a particular context or culture?
2. **Authority**
   (a) Is the author qualified to report on the subject?
   (b) Has it been published by a reputable source or can you justify why it is an important source?
   (c) Has the material been critically evaluated or assessed by other authors or colleagues; for example, peer reviewed or professionally edited?
3. **Currency**
   (a) Is the material still influential in the field?
   (b) Is it keeping you up-to-date with new research?

Finding Sources

After finalizing exactly what is needed, the researcher needs to find the sources for the review. It is an important task and requires patience, time, effort, and strategic planning. The following strategies can be used for efficient and effective searches:

1. **Obtain Skills for Online Searching:** There are many sources available on the web to help us to develop these skills. Many of the concepts in using web search engine also apply to searching online library catalogues, and CD-ROMs.
2. **Use Boolean Searching:** It is one of the common methods of searching and is also called as word searching. In this, the words AND, OR, and NOT are used while searching through database. This type of search tells the database to retrieve all of the records in the database that contain a word or a set of words. We can alter the results by using Boolean operators—AND, OR, and NOT. Following are the examples of Boolean operators.

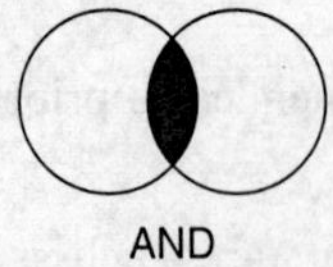

AND

For example, music and depression or steroid resistance and nephrotic syndrome will retrieve records that contain the word music and depression or steroid resistance and nephrotic syndrome.

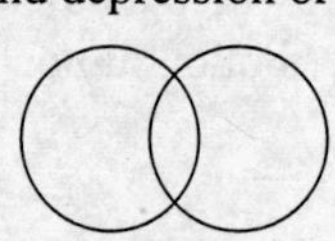

OR

For example, drug resistance or tuberculosis will retrieve records that contain the word drug resistance or tuberculosis. This operator is used to broaden the number of records retrieved.

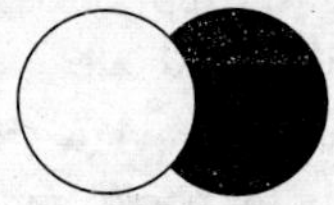

NOT

For example, eating habits not obesity or multi-drug resistance not tuberculosis will retrieve records that contain only the word eating habits but not the word obesity. This operator is used to reduce the number of records retrieved.

(a) **Truncation:** It is used to find different forms of words in a Boolean or keyword search. Some databases use the asterisk and others use the question mark. Check the help function of the database you are using to learn the truncation symbol. For example, *nurs** will retrieve records that contain the words nurse, nurses, nursing in a record. *Isolate** will retrieve records containing words isolate, isolating, isolation. We can use truncated terms with other words using Boolean operators.

For example, *nurs* and education* will retrieve records that include the various forms of nurs* and the word education.

(b) **Nesting:** Nesting is an advanced search strategy that allows us to combine multiple search terms together and utilize Boolean operators and wildcards. It is called as nesting because parentheses are often used to group the main concepts together.

For example, success and (education or employment) will retrieve records that contain the word success and the word education or the word employment. Nesting is often used when search terms have similar meanings, for example, education and (employment or jobs).

(c) **Stop words:** Stop words are commonly used words that will automatically stop a computer keyword search because they occur too frequently in records. Stop words are usually listed in the help screens of whatever database you are using. Some stop words are the, an, at, for, from, then. When constructing a keyword search, it is important to choose the most important words.

For example, If you want to find information about 'What are the effects of stress on physical health among young adults?', the keywords are *effects*, *physical health*, and *young adults*. The words what, is, of, the, are, and on are not descriptive of this topic.

(d) **Thesaurus:** Many databases contain a thesaurus. This is a directory of assigned subject headings (e.g., Medical Subject Headings or MeSH). Searching for a subject heading instead of a word that happens to appear anywhere in a record can reduce the number of irrelevant records retrieved from your search.

Some databases will automatically include synonyms in the search, whether you want them to appear or not, so you have to check the rules. This is called thesaurus mapping. For example, a search for cancer, finds cancer and neoplasm in the PubMed when thesaurus mapping occurs.

3. **Be a Strategic Searcher:** This can be done by using the following methods:
   (a) **Systematic Approach:** To try and find all relevant materials
   (b) **Retrospection:** Find the most recent material and work backwards
   (c) **Citation:** Follow leads from useful articles, books and reading list
   (d) **Targeted:** Restrict the topic and focus on a narrow area of literature

All these strategies are not used in isolation. There is a need to be systematic in looking at everything relevant in the library. Adopt a retrospective approach when looking at journal articles. Use citation searching to get useful leads if the topic crosses various disciplines and targeted when you have a clear picture of what you need to find out.

4. **Evaluate the Source:** All sources used for review should be assessed for its adequacy, relevance, reliability, and authenticity. Especially for books, journal articles and internet sources, the following points should be kept in mind while referring.

    (a) **For Evaluating Books:** Books are initially reviewed by publishers or editors for quality of content and writing style, as well as marketability. Established, reputable publishers take great care in maintaining a certain quality in the titles they publish. When evaluating a book, check these basic points:

    - (i) Author or editor, located on the title page; brief biographical information may be included in the introductory pages or at the end of the book
    - (ii) Publisher, located on the title page
    - (iii) Date of publication, located on the title page
    - (iv) Intended audience, determined by examining the content, preface, and introduction
    - (v) Purpose of the information, determined by examining the content, preface, and introduction

    (b) **For Evaluating an Article:** When evaluating an article, check these basic points:

    - (i) Author(s), usually on the first page of article; position and/or institutional affiliation may be included
    - (ii) Date of publication, most often in the header or footer of an article
    - (iii) Intended audience, determined by examining the content
    - (iv) Purpose of the information, determined by examining the content
    - (v) Author or contact person, usually located at the bottom of the page
    - (vi) Institution, usually a logo or link located in either header or footer
    - (vii) Domain, the last segment of the root or base URL (e.g., .edu, .gov, .com)
    - (viii) Date of creation or revision, usually at the bottom of the page

    (c) **For Internet Source:** In a world overflowing with more and more data, we need to become an intelligent consumer and evaluator of information. As internet is an uncontrolled environment, there is no peer review process of the information it contains and no quality control. Information given on internet is idiosyncratic, unsupervised, and aggregated by anyone with a computer and an internet connection. It can lead to two problems, namely difficulty in finding useful information and the ability of dealing with the overwhelming information on different sites. Another important factor is that the reviewer should not believe whatever he reads on internet. Following questions can help the reviewer to evaluate the internet source.

    - (i) **Purpose:** What is the purpose of the website?
    - (ii) **Accuracy:** How accurate is the information that it contains?
    - (iii) **Authority:** Are the sites' authors or producers authoritative in this subject?
    - (iv) **Coverage:** How much of the subject is covered by the site?
    - (v) **Currency:** How up-to-date is the information that it contains?

(vi) **Objectivity:** Is the information it contains objective or biased?

(vii) **URLs:** How can a URL be a useful tool when evaluating an internet resource?

5. **Locate the Sources:** Computers and electronic databases are the most common source used for literature review. They offer extensive access to information, which can be retrieved more easily and quickly than by a manual search. There are numerous electronic databases, many of which deal with specific fields of information. It is important, therefore, to identify the databases that are relevant to the topic. University and hospital libraries often subscribe to a number of databases and access can be gained using student or staff passwords. Libraries are also an important and valuable source for getting relevant information for the study. The commonly used sources in nursing research are as follows:

(a) **Library:** Library is one of the important sources for review as it has a collection of well-organized printed books and journals, e-journals, and video, and audio materials. The most important factor is that there are people around who can guide and help in searching the appropriate material. There are three major categories of libraries—public, academic, and special libraries.

(i) **Public Library:** It serves the needs of the community in which it is located and usually contains few research reports, for example, Indian Medlars Centre at New Delhi. The purpose of this centre is to index selected peer reviewed medical journals published from India. It also supplements International Indexing Services such as PubMed. It covers 77 journals indexed from 1985 onwards. It was started as an ICMR (Indian Council of Medical Research) funded project.

(ii) **Academic Library:** Usually located within an institution of higher learning, it contains numerous research reports in journals and books. Most academic libraries have an inter-library loan department, which can frequently help you locate and obtain books, booklets, conference proceedings, and articles from other libraries for one or two weeks.

(iii) **Special Library:** It contains a collection of materials on a specific topic or specialty area such as nursing or medicine. Large hospitals, health care centres, and health research centres have special libraries that contain sources relevant to health and research. For example, National Institute of Epidemiology, Chennai, has a library with a collection of latest books, journals, and other documents in various fields of epidemiology, biostatistics, public health, diseases, and clinical trials. It also has inter-library loan facility, a current awareness services, selective dissemination of information, and resource-sharing facility.

(b) **Print_Database_Resources:** It mainly consists of indexes, card catalogues, and abstract reviews. Print indexes are used to find journal sources (periodicals) of Print Database Resources and conceptual articles on a variety of topics, as well as publications of professional organizations and various government agencies.

(i) **Card Catalogues:** A library catalogue is an alphabetical file of authors, subjects, and titles for the material acquired by the library. The card catalogue was a familiar sight to library users for generations, but it has been effectively replaced by the online public access catalogue (OPAC). Some still refer to the online catalogue as a 'card catalogue'. Some libraries with OPAC access still have card catalogues on site, but these are now strictly a secondary resource and are seldom updated. Many of the libraries that have retained their physical card catalogue post a sign advising the year that the card catalogue was last updated. Some libraries have eliminated their card catalogue in favour of the OPAC for the purpose of saving space for other use, such as additional shelving.

They are used to secure books, monographs, conference proceedings, master's theses, and doctoral dissertations.

(ii) **Indexes:** It is a systematic list of book titles or author's names, giving cross-references, and the location of each book or catalogue. It provides assistance in identifying journal articles and other publications relevant to a topic of interest. Indexes are organized into two major sections—subject and author. The research topic's synonymous terms and subheadings identified are used to guide the search through the subject section of index. The subject sections include headings and subheadings, and under these headings several publications are listed. For example, a nursing study on anxiety among parents of children with chronic illness may be listed under the subject heading paediatric nursing with the sub-heading psychosocial aspect of chronic illness. Author section is organized alphabetically by writing first authors' name (not more than three authors), while the second and third authors' names appear as cross reference to the full citation. Indexes are generally produced monthly, bi-monthly, or quarterly and cumulated annually. For example, Index Medicus has a list of 3000 journals, and titles specifically related to nursing are 20, whereas Cumulative Index to Nursing and Allied Health literature covers over 300 periodicals. The choice of index should be done by taking help from librarians and subject experts to save time and get quality information.

(iii) **Abstract Reviews:** It is a brief summary of a research article, thesis, review, conference proceedings, or any in-depth analysis of a particular subject or discipline and is often used to help the reader quickly ascertain the paper's purpose. It contains summaries of databased articles and prepared bibliographies. For example, nursing abstracts, psychological abstracts, and dissertation abstracts international.

(c) **Computer Database Resources:** Computer database is the latest and a valuable source for getting information about the recent trends, issues, and innovative practices emerged through various researches performed by research scholars. It offers up-to-date information for researchers and allows them to keep pace with the ever-changing world of technology. It provides the reviewer a list of references with bibliographic information. Computer databases are especially useful when the researcher is interested in studying multiple variables. Another important advantage is that the reviewer can get the information before it comes in printed form. It includes indexing, abstracts, and full-text articles from more than 800 journals and periodicals, from Computerworld, eWeek, and Wired to PC Magazine, PC World, and Computer Weekly, covering the complete range of fields related to technology. Almost all databases are available through a computer search. Most of the computer databases are available via software programs.

The following are the common databases useful for nursing research:

(i) MEDLINE is a comprehensive database for health literature, which is managed by National Library of Medicine, USA. International Nursing Index and Index Medicus are included in MEDLINE.

(ii) Cochrane Review (http://www.cochrane.org/) is another database that gives extensive search options.

(iii) Cumulative Index to Nursing and Allied Health Literature (http://www.ebscohost.com/cinahl/) is a database of exclusive nursing articles.

(iv) Internet search engine Google has developed Google Scholar (http://scholar.google.com), which helps to confine search options to only academic papers.

(v) Open access journals (http://www.doaj.org) are another source for searching literature. These journals are free to access and can be used without restriction, provided the policies are accepted. Many standard journals provide their archives for free online search access, after a period of time, to developing countries.

(vi) Elsevier publications' internet database for nursing journals is accessible at http://sciencedirect.com/.

(vii) The Nursing Center (http://nursingcenter.com) is the online access site for Lippincott Williams & Wilkins' nursing journals. These journals need subscription and most of them are indexed in MEDLINE and CINAHL (Cumulative Index To Nursing and Allied Health Literature). Many of these journals are published by the organization themselves.

(viii) The Indian Medlars Centre of National Informatics Centre, New Delhi, has designed two databases, IndMED, a bibliographic database of peer reviewed Indian biomedical journals, and medIND, full-text of selected IndMED journals. These are accessible free of cost from the Centre's site (http://indmed.nic.in/).

(ix) CINAHL is published frequently, references a large number of relevant nursing sources, and is the original index for Nursing Literature. It was first published in 1956 and references more than 400 nursing journals, along with publications of American Nurses Association and National League for Nursing.

Regardless of the sources used, an appropriate record of bibliography must be kept. When searching through internet, the online addresses and other pertinent information should be noted so that a search can be duplicated, if necessary. As information can get changed anytime, printing it immediately if possible and keeping a proper record of the source is advised. This will help to avoid duplication of effort and speed up the process of obtaining permission (to use the work of others) when needed. The time required to relocate the source is also reduced. For recording the bibliography and reference material, follow the style recommended by the institution from the beginning itself, for example, Vancouver style or APA style.

(c) **Personal Networking:** Additional resources can be formed by talking to people who are doing work in areas related to the topic of the researcher's interest. This can include people from the same institute or those who meet through professional associations. Talking with people who have completed related work can reveal sources that the researcher may not be aware about, such as unpublished research reports.

(d) **Finding Too Much or Too Less Data:** Very often, it has been observed that the researcher finds either too much or too less information. The reasons for too much information may be that lots of information has been written on the main topic or this topic may have links with other subject areas. In such a case, the researcher can do the following:

(i) Narrow down the topic further by becoming more specific.

(ii) Use more precise terms.

(iii) Concentrate on key authors and books.

(iv) Get the database to help through subject headings and online help.

If too less information is obtained, then the researcher can do the following:

(i) Make the topic more general.

(ii) Think about the comparative or related information that might be helpful.

(iii) Consult the guide, subject expert, or library personnel, as sometimes it may happen that very little is being written on the research topic.

Analysing and Synthesizing the Literature

After identifying and locating the information, it needs to be analysed and synthesized for writing the review. For analysing and synthesizing the review, the researcher must first ensure that it is recorded properly by using various methods such as Endnotes, REFWORKS, 3X5 cards, and Excel worksheet. This makes it easier to analyse, evaluate, and synthesize the information to find patterns, connections, and trends (Table 4.3).

TABLE 4.3 *Methods of Recording the Information*

Endnotes	Endnotes are notes printed at the end of a chapter, rather than at the bottom of the printed page as footnotes.
REFWORKS	REFWORKS is a web-based bibliography and database manager that allows you to create your own personal database by importing references from text files or online databases and other various sources. You can use these references in writing papers and automatically format the paper and the bibliography in seconds.
3X5 cards	Useful for making notes of key information on each article you read. Write the article citation on one side and main points on the other. It can be shuffled as per the need and organized as per themes, methodologies, or trends. It becomes a handy reference when the researcher is writing, rather than having to sift constantly through large stacks of paper or electronic articles.
Excel worksheet	Electronic version of the cards. It takes a little effort to set up and begin using the worksheet, but it really pays off later because you can sort the information quickly and easily.
Procite	It is a programme that manages citations also known as 'reference software'. With Procite one can print bibliographies, change the bibliography style, cite while writing, and import records from electronic databases.

After recording written material, it needs to be analysed and synthesized. The analysis will explore the relationships, major themes, and any critical gaps in the research expressed in the work. It also break-downs a concept or idea into important parts/points, which enables the researcher to draw useful conclusions or make decisions about the topic or problem, whereas in synthesis, information from various sources is combined into a whole.

Synthesis is the basis for developing the literature review for a utilization purpose. Through synthesis of sources, the researcher is able to cluster and interrelate ideas from each research and then paraphrase it. Paraphrasing involves expressing an author's ideas clearly and concisely in his own words.

Most of the published articles contain a summary or abstract at the beginning of the paper. It enables the researcher to decide whether the article is worthy of inclusion or for reading further. At this point, it may be useful to undertake an initial classification and grouping of the articles by type of sources mentioned in Table 4.2.

Once the initial overview has been completed it is necessary to return to the articles to undertake a more systematic and critical review of the content. A researcher should keep in mind that it is not necessary to discuss all studies reviewed during literature search. What is to be reported and how much is to be discussed depend on the relevance of the content in proposed study. The most important aspect is to write the findings of the study in detail. All these findings need to be categorized *to compare*, *to combine*, and *to contrast*. If the available literature is not categorized and presented in a meaningful way, synthesis can be merely a descriptive summary, which will not yield any concrete information and will not help to express the ideas contained in the literature.

Comparing Ideas from the Literature: It means 'to mark or point out the similarities and differences of (two or more things); to bring or place together (actually or mentally) for the purpose of noting the similarities and differences' (Oxford English Dictionary, 2007).

It is an important aspect of synthesis. In this, one can identify the similarities and differences observed in the reviewed literature about a particular aspect of the study. It helps to gain in-depth understanding of the topic and to construct the researcher's argument related to the topic. Similar results reinforce their validity.

The following is an example. 'Whilst Smith et al. (2006) and Wilbert et al. (2006) both reached the same conclusion as Norton (2005), they used different methodology.'

Combining Ideas from the Literature: It means 'to couple or join two or more things together' (Oxford English Dictionary, 2007).

In this, two ideas or concepts are combined. The researcher can combine literature that draws the same conclusions or has used the same methodology. Combining literature can help to create a stronger argument. For example, if you are advocating the use of a particular technique, such as reflexology for reducing stress, it will strengthen your argument if several research papers advocate that technique also, rather than if you based your argument on the results presented in only one research paper.

An example is: 'The literature to date suggests that temperature does have an effect on growth rate (Walker et al., 2006; Knotts et al., 2005; Smith 2005).'

While combining, it is recommended that the researcher should also record the discrepancies observed between the studies. It allows the reviewer to know the topic with all possible comments. While combining the literature, it is advisable to combine it where relevant and not to just cite the most recent or influential paper.

Contrasting Ideas in the Literature: It means 'to set in opposition (two objects of like nature, or one with, rarely to, another) in order to show strikingly their different qualities or characteristics, and compare their superiorities or defects' (Oxford English Dictionary, 2007).

It is important when contrasting literature that consideration is given to why it contrasts and that the reason is explained or postulated. Otherwise, it will simply be comparing the literature, that is, highlighting its similarities and differences. For example, the contrast may be due to a difference in opinion of the authors or in the treatment of subjects in an experiment. It is also possible that no clear explanation for the contrast is possible based on the information contained in the literature. Such contrasts often provide good material on which further research strategies can be developed.

… For example, in one study, massage with oil has shown significant effect on the weight gain and neurobehavioral development among babies with low birth weight. In another study, it has shown only significant weight gain but no effect on neurobehavioral development. This difference may be due to different settings, duration of massage, involvement of mother, skill of researcher in assessing the neurobehavioral development, and so on. Whatever may be the reason, the reviewer should not leave the reader to speculate on contradictory findings but must try to give explanations as only the reviewer has read these studies. The following is another example: '…However, the results presented by Harper et al., (2005) are in stark contrast to this, demonstrating a marked difference between control and test groups. This difference is most likely due to the differing conditions used…'

After categorizing the studies, the researcher should tabulate it as shown in Table 4.4. This table represents on one side the main idea or category and on the other side the literature identified through review as per the name of the researcher or author. This is an example of synthesized review that was done to find out the incidence of needle stick injury and the level of awareness about universal precautions among health care professionals.

TABLE 4.4 *Method of Tabulation*

Main Idea	**Maria Ganczak (2006)**	**Even Drains and Holmes (2004)**	**WHO Report (2002)**	**Kaushik (2004)**
Incidence of needle stick injuries among health care professionals.	Interview with 601 nurses revealed that 50% of nurses had at least one puncture injury during the preceding year. One in five had exposure via mucous membrane and more than half had worked at least once with a recent abrasion or cut on their hands.	Assessed the information from 172 countries. Approximately 461–468 new HIV and 27,472 new Hepatitis C cases were acquired each year among 22.2 million nurses and doctors. Moreover, 18.1–18.4 million had needle stick injuries. 53% were working in developing countries. Out of this, 88% and 86% were sustained with occupational HIV and HCV infections.	Needle stick injury is accountable for 40% of Hepatitis B, 40% of Hepatitis C, and 2% of HIV infections.	A study on 400 nurses working in various hospitals of Delhi revealed that 5.25% of 346 nurses had needle stick injuries in the previous month, 6.3% reported needle stick injuries containing blood, and 24.8% reported an incident involving near miss.
Main Idea	**Valcea (2001)**	**Leliopoulou (1999)**	**Santosh Arora (2005)**	**Maqbool Alam (2002)**
Level of awareness of standard precautions among health care providers.	In this study, 212 nurses from Valcea district were interviewed to identify the knowledge and practice of infection control and blood-borne pathogen transmission. 62% were unaware that following a needle stick, the	In a survey related to nurses' failure to appreciate the risks of infection due to needle stick accidents, most of the nurses thought that the risk of infection from needle stick injury was unlikely or very remote. One in ten nurses thought that special precautions	Attitude of nurses towards HIV patients were assessed. 85% were aware about AIDS but only 15% had shown positive attitude towards HIV positive patients. Reason may be	Knowledge and attitude was assessed in 104 health care workers. Out of this, 70 were nurses and 34 were other health care workers. 21% of nurses and 30% of other health care workers were unaware of the fact that AIDS and Hepatitis C can be transmitted

(*Continued*)

TABLE 4.4 *Method of Tabulation (Continued)*

Main Idea	Valcea (2001)	Leliopoulou (1999)	Santosh Arora (2005)	Maqbool Alam (2002)
	risk for transmission from an infected patient was greater for Hepatitis B virus than HIV infection. 82% had lacerated wounds while opening glass ampoules.	for infection control were necessary only for patients who had full-blown symptoms of HIV or Hepatitis virus.	lack of awareness and fear of risk of infection.	by needle stick injury. 74% nurses had a history of needle stick injury and 67% other health care workers had one to two pricks per year. Only 7% reported the injuries to doctors to get post-exposure treatment. 61 per cent were aware about universal precautions, only 275 were using gloves during phlebotomy. 29% reported that needles should be recapped. In 10–25%, injuries occurred while recapping a used needle.

These findings can be synthesized as follows:

Needle stick injury is one of the important threats for health care workers as it is a major source for acquiring blood-borne diseases such as HIV and Hepatitis B and C. Many studies have reflected its incidence. A study done by Maria Ganczak (2006) on 601 nurses, revealed that 50 per cent of them had at least one puncture injury in the preceding year. Similar findings were noted by Even Drains and Holmes (2004) when they assessed the information from 172 countries; it was observed that out of the 22.2 million nurses and doctors, 18.1–18.4 million had needle stick injuries. Even though 53 per cent were working in developing countries, they sustained 88 per cent and 86 per cent of the occupational HIV and HCV infections, respectively. It was also estimated that every year approximately 461–468 new cases of HIV infection and 27,472–27,941 new cases of Hepatitis C were detected from this population. These findings are further supported by WHO report (2002) where it states that needle stick injury is accountable for 40 per cent of Hepatitis B, 40 per cent of Hepatitis C, and 2 per cent of HIV infections.

The most important reason for these findings could be inadequate knowledge about standard universal precautions. This is evident from the findings of the study performed by Valcea (2001) and Maqbool Alam (2002). Valcea, when interviewing 212 nurses to identify knowledge and practices of infection control and transmission of blood-borne pathogens, found that 62 per cent were unaware that the risk for transmission from an infected patient is greater for Hepatitis B virus than HIV. Similar findings were noted by Maqbool Alam (2002) when he was assessing the knowledge and attitude of 104 health care workers related to universal precautions. He found that 21 per cent of nurses and 30 per cent of other health care workers were unaware of the fact that AIDS and Hepatitis C can be transmitted by needle stick injury. Moreover, 74 per cent of nurses had a history of needle stick injury and only 7 per cent had reported and approached for further management. Poor knowledge not only has imposed a threat for acquiring Hepatitis B and C and HIV, but also has affected the attitude of nurses towards caring of patients with HIV positive status. A study done by Santosh Arora (2005) to assess the attitude of nurses towards HIV positive status revealed that only 5 per cent of the nurses showed positive attitude towards caring for HIV positive patients.

Writing the Review

Once the appraisal of the literature is completed, consideration must be given to how the review will be structured and written. It should be written in a clear and concise manner. Sentences should be small and grammatically correct. Findings of the review should be presented in a meaningful manner. Before initiating the writing of review, the researcher can keep the following tips in mind (Table 4.5).

TABLE 4.5 *Tips on Writing*

Sentences	Express one idea in a sentence. Ensure that all your sentences have a subject, verb, and object.
Paragraphs	Group sentences that express and develop one aspect of your topic. Use a new paragraph for another aspect or another topic.
Consistent Grammar	Use sentences and paragraphs with appropriate use of commas, colons, and semi-colons. Incorrect use of punctuation can affect the meaning.
Transition Words	Use words that link paragraphs and which show contrast and development to your argument, for example, hence, therefore, but, thus, as a result, and in contrast.

Primarily, the written report should include an introduction, body, and conclusion.

Introduction

The introduction should include the purpose of the review and a brief overview of the 'problem'. It is important that the literature sources and the key search terms are outlined. Any limits, boundaries, or inclusion/exclusion criteria should be clearly described. Some comment on what was found in the literature should be offered, that is, whether there was a dearth or wealth of literature on the topic. This gives the reader some insight into the breadth and depth of the literature sourced and also facilitates some judgment as to the validity of the claims being made.

Main Body

The main body of the report presents and discusses the findings from the literature. There are many ways to present the information. It can be presented chronologically, thematically, or methodologically.

Chronological: In a chronological review, the information is organized as per the date of the publication or year. This method is useful for papers focusing on research methodology, historic graphical papers, and other writing where time becomes an important element. For example, a literature review on theories of mental illness might present how the understanding of mental illness has changed through the centuries, by giving a series of examples of key developments and ending with current theories and the direction your research will take. Another example can be the evolution of nursing profession in India where the researcher can organize the data year- or decade-wise.

Thematic: In a thematic review, sources are arranged in terms of the themes or topics they cover. Organizationally, this method is often a stronger one, and it can help us to resist the urge to summarize the sources. Important aspects of similar themes are grouped together to discuss the content under different headings, for example, Pickles et al. did a study on the attitude of nursing towards caring of people with HIV/AIDS thematic review. In this study, the researcher organized the literature review under various themes such as education and knowledge of students related to HIV/AIDS, fear of contracting disease, reluctance towards caring these people, and stigma associated with HIV and AIDS.

Methodological: A methodological approach differs from the other two methods in that the focusing factor usually does not have to related to the content of the material. Instead, it focuses on the 'methods' of the researcher or writer, for example, qualitative verses quantitative methods.

Whatever may be the method the researcher chooses, the content must be presented with logical thinking and clarity and should specify how it relates to the study. According to Polit and Beck, while describing a study's findings, it is best to use a language that indicates the tentativeness of the results rather than making definite statements about the research. Similarly, it is necessary for the reviewer to remain objective about the literature, and personal opinions about the quality of research studies should not be included. It should not be a series of quotes or descriptions. Review should be written in the researcher's own words.

Conclusion

It should summarize major contributions of significant studies and articles to the body of knowledge under review. It should also state any gaps in knowledge which have been identified during review. The researcher should logically present these gaps to justify the topic of proposed study. At the end, it is recommended to give some implications for practice, education, and research.

References

The literature review should conclude with a full bibliographical list of all the books, journal articles, reports, and other media that were referred to in the work. Regardless of whether the review is part of a course of study or for publication, it is an essential part of the process that all sourced material is acknowledged. This means every citation in the text must appear in the reference/bibliography and vice versa. To avoid omissions or errors in referencing, a separate file for it can be added to this list immediately. Some universities offer their students access to referencing systems, such as Endnote. These systems may initially appear difficult to follow, but once the researcher learns the system it saves a lot of time and avoids frustration due to loss of any reference at the end. According to Coughlan et al, (2007), the reference list is a useful source of literature for others who are interested in studying this topic, and therefore, every effort should be made to ensure its accuracy.

The following is an example of literature review written by two research students, in which the second one is a better review:

STUDENT A

Smith (2000) concludes that personal privacy in their living quarters is the most important factor in nursing home residents' perception of their autonomy. He suggests that the physical environment in the more public spaces of the building did not have much impact on their perceptions. Neither the layout of the building nor the activities available seem to make much difference.

Jones and Johnstone (2001) make the claim that the need to control one's environment is a fundamental need of life and suggest that the approach of most institutions, which is to provide total care, may be as bad as no care at all. If people have no choices or think that they have none, they become depressed.

STUDENT B

After studying the residents and staff from two intermediate care facilities in Calgary, Alberta, Smith (2000) came to the conclusion that except for the amount of personal privacy available to residents, the physical environment of these institutions had minimal, if any, effect on their perceptions of control (autonomy). However, French (1998) and Haroon (2000) found that the availability of private areas is not the only aspect of the physical environment that determines residents' autonomy. Haroon (2000) interviewed 115 residents from 32 different nursing homes known to have different levels of autonomy. It was found that physical structures, such as standardized furniture, heating that could not be individually regulated, and no possession of a house key for residents, limited their feelings of independence. Moreover, Hope (2002), who interviewed 225 residents from various nursing homes, substantiates the claim that the characteristics of the institutional environment, such as the extent of resources in the facility as well as its location, are features that residents have indicated as being of great importance to their independence.

CRITIQUING THE LITERATURE REVIEW

A research critique is a careful appraisal of the strength and weakness of a study. A good critique objectively identifies the areas of adequacy and inadequacy, virtues as well as faults. It is always better to involve many people like experts, research scholars, and peer reviewers for critiquing the research articles before publishing it in any journal or conference. It will help to maintain quality in literature. Critiquing of literature helps the reviewers to sharpen their critical thinking skills, which is an essential quality for nursing professionals.

Critiquing of literature that is selected for review is a difficult task as the author of that particular literature would have used the expertise of many sources before finalizing the writing. He is more knowledgeable than the reader related to the information he has presented. So, it is very difficult to pass any judgment about its accuracy and adequacy. Still some guidelines can be used to assess the quality of the content and sources, such as the following:

1. Are relevant studies identified and described?
2. Are relevant theories identified and described?
3. Are primary sources cited in the review?
4. Are the references current?
5. Are relevant landmark studies described?
6. Are the sources paraphrased to promote the flow of the content presented?
7. Is the literature review clearly organized and logically developed?
8. Is the current knowledge about the research problem described?
9. Does the literature review clearly provide a basis for the study conducted?

ETHICAL CONSIDERATION IN LITERATURE REVIEW

The most important ethical aspect of review of literature is plagiarism. It is an act or instance of using or closely imitating the language and thoughts of another author, without authorization, and representation of that author's work as one's own, by not crediting the original author. In academia, plagiarism by students and researchers is considered as academic dishonesty and it can be avoided by appropriate citation.

Another important factor to be considered is that while performing review, the findings of the various studies can become the raw data for analysis and interpretation. All research reports vary in their presentation with respect to details about the methodology used in a particular study, the actual problems faced by the researcher, the highlighting of negative findings, and so forth. So, while carrying out a literature review, if the researcher is going to use the findings, the following ethical questions need to be considered and if necessary should be discussed with the research guide or with the research team:

1. How will you ensure that you treat the work of existing researchers accurately and fairly?
2. Does the research you are reviewing raise ethical questions which need to be addressed?
3. Will you limit yourself to reports and information that is already in public domain or will you contact the researchers for more details?
4. If you ask a study author for more detail, how will you ensure that any exchange respects principles of ethics? For example, will it affect the confidentiality which was promised originally to the participants?
5. How will you incorporate ideas about respecting the participant's consent when deciding whether or not to use an existing study's data? Researchers need to weigh up any risk that participants' data will be used or presented in a way they did not agree to, against any potential benefit from further use of their data. Is it sufficient that they have given permission for using the data for similar activity or purpose but not for the proposed study?
6. Could there be any occasion where the researcher will decide not to include study findings of the research in the review due to the concern about the ethics of that research?

Box 4.1 *Summary of the Information Required in Literature Review*

Title of the study

- Author and year:
- Journal (full reference):
- Purpose of study:
- Type of study:
- Key definitions:
- Credibility:
- Setting:
- Data collection method:
- Appraisal criteria:
- Content:
- Major findings:

(*Continued*)

Box 4.1 *Summary of the Information Required in Literature Review (Continued)*

- Synthesis of studies:
- Coherence:
- Recommendations:
- Summary/Conclusions:
- Recommendations:
- Key thoughts/Comments:
- Strengths/Weaknesses:
- Primary sources:

SUMMARY

A literature review is central to the research process and can help to refine a research question through determining inconsistencies in a body of knowledge. Similarly, it can help to develop greater understanding about the topic and also to think with new perspective. It provides information about various research designs that can be used in the study. Various types of reviews may be used depending on the reason, overall aim, and objectives of the study. Writing a review of the literature is a skill that needs to be learned. By conducting the review, nurses can contribute valuable information towards increasing the body of nursing knowledge and ultimately enhancing patient care through evidence-based practice.

KEY POINTS

- ❑ A literature review in a research report is a summary of current knowledge about a particular problem and includes what is known and unknown about the problem.
- ❑ A good literature review is focused, concise, logical, developed, and integrative and possesses current information.
- ❑ The most important reason for reviewing the literature is to determine the previous knowledge related to the topic, to identify the gaps, and to justify the significance of the proposed study.
- ❑ Primary and secondary sources are commonly used in literature review. Primary sources are referred to the literature written by the original researcher(s). Secondary sources provide a summary or description of a research written by someone other than the original researcher.
- ❑ While performing literature search, it is always better to narrow down the research topic. It avoids waste of time and energy and also frustration. Moreover, it helps to yield relevant information.
- ❑ For searching the literature, different types of sources such as books, printed database, and internet are used.
- ❑ All references must be recorded as per the recommended style of an institution, for example, APA or Vancouver.
- ❑ An effective literature review places each work in the context of its contribution to the topic selected for the review. It also describes the relationship of each work to the others under consideration. It identifies new ways to interpret and shed light on any gaps in previous research.
- ❑ For drawing conclusions from factual information and to make a judgment about its worthiness, it is essential to evaluate every piece of information by using critiquing guidelines.
- ❑ The information documented in a review should be concise and complete (Box 4.1).

QUESTIONS

I. Essay-type Questions

1. Discuss the significance of literature review in nursing research.
2. Differentiate between the types of literature review.
3. Explain literature review as a research process.
4. Explain library as an important source for literature review.
5. What are the common databases useful for nursing research?
6. Discuss how you will determine the creditability of information found on internet.
7. Explain the various methods of writing the information in review of literature.

II. Write Short Notes

1. Primary source of review literature
2. Skills required to search a literature
3. Documentation of a research review
4. Internet as a source of review for nursing research
5. Criteria for critiquing literature review
6. Write an example of a literature review

III. Multiple-choice Questions

Circle the alphabet before the best answer

1. Literature review is a
   (a) brief critical discussion about the merits and weaknesses of a literary work such as play, novel or book
   (b) study-by-study or article-by-article description of studies previously done
   (c) summary of current knowledge about a particular practice or problem and includes what is known and unknown about the problem
2. The purpose of literature review is to
   (a) identify the topic that has not been resolved
   (b) clarify importance of a research problem
   (c) identify the gaps
   (d) all of these
3. Which of the following is not an example of primary source for literature review?
   (a) Scientific journal articles reporting experimental research results
   (b) Dictionaries and encyclopaedias
   (c) Birth certificate
   (d) Census statistic
4. Comprehensive literature review prior to data collection is not recommended in
   (a) experimental research
   (b) historical research
   (c) descriptive research
   (d) grounded research
5. A systematic review
   (a) critiques and summarizes a body of literature
   (b) is a non-statistical technique
   (c) is a rigorous and well-defined approach
   (d) draws conclusions about the topic

6. In Vancouver style
   (a) references are enumerated and listed in the order they appear
   (b) references are written as per author-year system in alphabetical order
   (c) only needed information is given to identify the source
   (d) footnotes are used to provide information about the location of reference
7. Annotated bibliography is a
   (a) descriptive summary often found at the beginning of scholarly journal articles or in periodic indexes.
   (b) list of citations to books, articles, and documents, which are followed by a brief descriptive and evaluative paragraph
   (c) list of references documented at the end of research article
   (d) list of references made for any article
8. The most important ethical concern in writing literature review chapter is
   (a) accuracy
   (b) relevancy
   (c) reliability
   (d) plagiarism
9. Comparing, combining, and contrasting of literature information are the components of
   (a) analysis
   (b) synthesis
   (c) evaluation
   (d) comprehension
10. Drug resistance and tuberculosis is an example of
   (a) truncation
   (b) nesting
   (c) Boolean searching
   (d) stop words

Answer Keys

1. (c) 2. (d) 3. (b) 4. (d) 5. (c) 6. (a) 7. (b) 8. (d)
9. (b) 10. (c)

FURTHER READING

Basavanthappa, B. T. 2007. *Nursing Research*. Jaypee Brothers Medical Publishers (P) Ltd. New Delhi Second edition, pp. 98–99.

Boswell, Carol, Cannon, Sharon. 2007. *Introduction to Nursing Research: Incorporating Evidence Based Practice*. First edition. Canada: Jones and Bartlett Publishers, p. 99.

Burns N, Grove S. K. 2007. *Understanding Nursing Research: Building on Evidence Based Practice* Fourth edition. St Louis: Elsevier Saunders.

Coughlan M, Cronin P, Ryan F. 2007. 'Step-by-step Guide to Critiquing Research. Part 1: Quantitative Research'. *British Journal of Nursing*, 16(11): 658–63.

Cronin, Patricia, Ryan, Frances, Choughlan, Michael. 2008, 'Undertaking a Literature Review: A Step by Step Approach', *British Journal of Nursing*, 17(1): 38–39.

en.wikipedia.org/wiki/library_catlog

Evans Pearson: Ref no. 3

Hart, C. 1998. *Doing Literature Review*. London: Sage.

http://gemini.lib.purdue.edu/core/files/strategies1d.html

http://indmed.nicin

http://philosophy.hku.hk/think/critical/ct.php

http:www.dlsweb.rmit.edu.au/lsu/…/2…/ PG%20lit%20 review.pdf

libguides.library.cqu.edu.au/*litreview*

Libguides.library.usyd.edu.au/content.php?pid

Neuman, W. Lawrence. 2003. *Social Research Methods: Qualitative and Quantitative Approaches*. Fifth edition. Boston: Allyn and Bacon.

Nieswiadomy, Rose Marie. 2009. *Foundation of Nursing Research*. Fifth edition. Dorling Kindersley (India) Pvt. Ltd.

Parahoo, Kader. 2008. *Nursing Research Principles, Process and Issues*. Second edition. Palgrave Macmillan, pp. 135–137.

Pickles, David, King, Lindy. 2009. 'Attitude of Nursing Students Towards Caring for People with HIV/ AIDS: Thematic Literature Review'. *Journal of Advance Nursing*, 65.

Polit, D, Beck, C. 2006. *Nursing Research: Methods Appraisal and Utilization.* Sixth edition. Philadelphia: Lippincott Williams and Wilkins.

ro.uwe.ac.uk

Simkhada, B., Teijlingen, E. R., Porter, M., Simkhada, P. 2008. 'Factors affecting the utilization of antenatal care in developing countries: Systematic review of literature', *Journal of Advanced Nursing* 61(3): 244–260.

Streubert, Helen J., Carpenter, Dona Rinaldi. 1995. *Qualitative Research in Nursing: Advancing the Humanistic Imperative*. First edition. Philadelphia: J. B. Lippincott Company, pp. 21–22.

Thomas, Barbara Schalk. 1990. *Nursing Research: An Experimental Approach*. First edition. Missouri: C.V. Mosby Company, pp. 48–53,110–111, 53–56.

URL: http://libguides.usc.edu/writing

URL: http :// libguides.utoledu.edu/litreview print guide RSS updates

www.commercetuned.co.uk/SEO.../defining-search-strategy.

www.ethicsguidebook/ac.uk/Littreture -reviews and-systematic reviews-99

www.gale.cengage.com/pdf/facts/compdb.pdf

www.helium.com ›... › Colleges & Universities › College Study Tips

www.hospiweb.scotcit.ac.uk/lectures/lit_rev.shtml

www.internettutorials.net/boolean.asp

www.learningcommons.uoguelph.ca

www.library.arizona.edu/tutorials/litrature reviews

www.library.cornell.edu/olinuris/ref/research/skill.28.htm

www.writing.utoronto.ca/advice/specific-types –of …writing./literature review

chapter 5

Theoretical and Conceptual Frameworks

OBJECTIVES

Upon completion of this chapter the learner will be able to:

- Define theory and nursing theory
- Explain the elements, components, role, and functions of a theory
- Understand the meaning of concept, construct, proposition, hypothesis, and model
- Define model, conceptual model, and conceptual map
- Explain the meaning of framework and theoretical, conceptual, and study frameworks
- Differentiate among theoretical, conceptual, and study frameworks
- Describe the basics of framework for research
- Understand the nature of theoretical and conceptual frameworks
- Enlist the purposes of having framework in research
- Explain the framework linking nursing research to nursing practice
- Describe the steps of developing theoretical and conceptual or study frameworks
- Develop theoretical and conceptual or study frameworks
- Critically evaluate theoretical and conceptual or study frameworks

INTRODUCTION

Frameworks are the bases of developing models and theories. A blueprint is required to build a house; similarly, to conduct a research study requires something that is a theoretical or conceptual area in the research literature. Though the theoretical frameworks or the structure is not readily available in the literature, the relevant concepts and their relationships must be identified and selected, which are applicable to the concerned theme. Each research study should have a conceptual base, as it acts as a navigator that helps to remain on the right track to accomplish the purpose of the specific nursing research.

WHAT IS A THEORY?

Definitions

Theory has been defined in a number of ways by different educationists and nursing scholars. In a selected review of literature on theory, there is no one definition of theory that is universally accepted.

The following are the important definitions of theory:

1. 'Theory refers to any systematic ordering of ideas about the phenomena of a field of inquiry.'
2. 'A theory is a set of interrelated construct (concepts), definitions, and propositions that present a systematic view of phenomena of specifying relations among variables, with the purpose of explaining and predicting the phenomena.'
3. 'Theory refers to a set of logically interrelated statement of significance (concepts, propositions, and definitions) that have been derived from philosophic beliefs and scientific data and from which questions or hypotheses can be deducted, tested, and verified.'
4. 'A theory is a set of concepts, definitions, and proposition that project a systematic view of phenomena by designating specific interrelationship among concepts for the purpose of describing, explaining, predicting and/or controlling phenomena.'
5. Meleis describes that a theory enables us to explain a 'maximum number of observable relationships' by setting limits on 'what questions to ask and what methods to use to pursue answers to the questions.'
6. 'A theory is a statement that purports to account for or characterize some phenomena and that pulls out the salient parts of a phenomenon so that one can separate the critical and necessary factors (or relationships) from the accidental or unessential factors (or relationships).'
7. Chinn and Kramer say that a theory is 'a systematic abstraction of reality that serves some purpose'. *Systematic* implies a specific organizational pattern; *abstraction* implies or means that a theory is a representation of reality; and *purpose* includes description, explanation, and prediction of phenomena and control of some reality.
8. 'It is a broad abstract generalization that presents a systematic explanation about the relationship among phenomena.'

Thus, theories are developed from concepts and reveal relationship between the concepts, which are in the form of propositional statements and are connected in a logical system of thought. So, there is a common agreement that a theory shares a common set of elements.

Elements of a Theory

The following are the elements of a theory:

1. Implicit or explicit purpose or goal
2. Concepts or constructs that describe the empirical world
3. Propositions or rational statements that link the concepts and constructs to describe, explain, or predict phenomena of interest

Components of a Theory

The components of a traditional theory as described by Polit and Hungler are listed as follows:

1. A theory comprises a set of concepts that are the abstract characteristics of an object to be studied.
2. It also comprises a set of statements, called propositions, that show the relationship among the concepts under study.
3. It must provide a mechanism that the propositions should be logically interrelated to derive a new statement or hypothesis.

Role and Functions of Theory in Research

Theories play an important role in scientific or empirical investigation and enquiry. They develop a body of knowledge and thus help in the development of a profession. The following are the important functions of a theory:

1. Theories provide an explanation for the observed events and relationships and predict many unobserved diverse phenomena and their relationships.
2. They enable the researcher to isolate a specific problem and to raise new problems for research.
3. They guide the researcher onto the various aspects of a research problem.
4. They organize knowledge or relevant relationships in a systematic, logical, and scientific manner.
5. They give direction to analyse the phenomena.
6. They help the researcher to draw verifiable conclusions.
7. They provide the basis for the construction of a hypothesis, which is useful for an empirical research.
8. They suggest the limits of their application.

DEFINING CONCEPTS, CONSTRUCTS, PROPOSITIONS, HYPOTHESES, DEFINITIONS, AND EMPIRICAL REFERENTS OR INDICATORS

Concepts

Meaning

A concept is an abstract idea of an object and a word picture that strikes in our mind. It is a linguistic label that we assign to an object or event. It is formed by generalizing an object from particular characteristics. The scientific concepts are sharply defined; their relationship with other concepts is classified and empirically validated. These are the basic elements of theory and research that are used to explain and interpret the facts. The concepts may have theoretical or operational definitions. Leininger's theory, which we follow, has 15 major concepts and 85 constructs, Watson's theory 10 carative factors, Henderson's theory 14 basic needs, and Benner's theory 31 competencies and 7 domains of nursing.

Types of Concepts

Concepts are classified according to the levels of abstractions, the levels of categorization, and the levels of measurements as shown in Fig. 5.1.

1. **According to Levels of Abstractions:** It takes into account the degree at which the concept can be observed, the degree at which the meaning of the concept is limited by time and space, and the degree at which the meaning of the concept is limited to a specific reference group. It varies from a high level of abstraction to a high level of concreteness as shown:

Abstract ←——→ Concrete

Constructs ——→ Concepts ——→ Variables

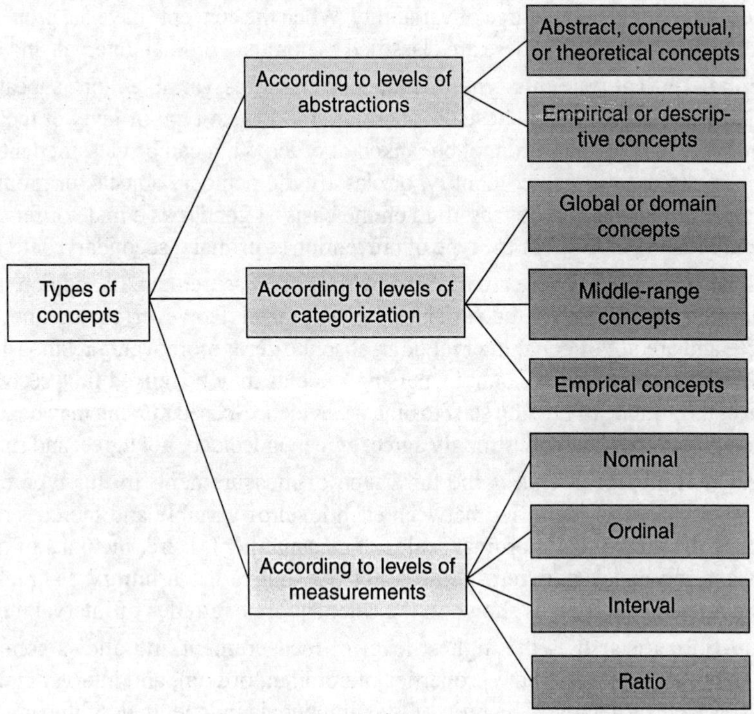

FIGURE 5.1 *Types of Concepts*

(a) **Abstract, Conceptual, or Theoretical Concepts:** The concepts that are not readily observable and the meanings of which are more distant from specific time, space, and referent group are abstract concepts or constructs; when the meanings of the abstract concepts are derived from a theory in which they are embedded, they are known as theoretical concepts, for example, empowering. The abstract concepts are embedded in assumptions and are independent of an individual's perceptions, whereas the assumptions are the statements that are taken for granted or are considered true and make the study logical. Assumptions are the universally accepted truth, embedded in the theories or searched from previous research and nursing practice.

(b) **Empirical or Descriptive Concepts:** These concepts can be observed directly and their meanings are more concrete, for example, self-care.

2. **According to Levels of Categorization:**

(a) **Global or Domain Concepts:** These are broad concepts. They have many interrelated, diverse, and empirical manifestations; for example, the concepts of nursing theory are person, environment, health, and nursing.

(b) **Middle-range Concepts:** These are derived from global concepts and are more refined than the global concepts, for example, self-care, which is derived from the global concept of person.

(c) **Empirical Concepts:** These are the lowest type of conceptual groups. They have specific meaning and can be measured, but they limit the comprehensiveness of the research findings, for example, home visits.

3. **According to Levels of Measurements:** These types of concepts are based on empirical indicators to quantify the existence of a concept—in other words, these are the concepts that can be measured.

The indicators differ in their degree of variability. When the concepts have the property of variability, they are termed as variables. These are classified as nominal, ordinal, interval, and ratio indicators.

(a) **Nominal Indicators:** This type of indicator classifies variables into subcategories that are mutually exclusive and exhaustive. These are the lowest type of level of measurement. They do not vary in degree and cannot be ranked or ordered but can be classified into categories; the numbers are used to name, identify, or classify the persons, objects, or groups; for example, a sample of persons can be classified on the basis of gender as a male or female; religion as a Hindu, Muslim, or Sikh; or the type of prevention as primary, secondary, or tertiary prevention.

(b) **Ordinal Indicators:** These are the second level of measurement. In addition to being mutually exclusive and exhaustive, the variables can be ranked. However, they cannot be quantified in degree and are not of equal interval or an absolute zero; moreover, a relationship 'greater than' or 'lesser than' exists; for example, nursing students may be ranked first, second, and third in a class or the attitude of nursing staff to practise evidence-based nursing may be reflected in a five-point ordinal scale, namely strongly agree, agree, undecided, not agree, and strongly disagree.

(c) **Interval Indicators:** This is the third type of measurement. In this type of indicators, the specific distance is identified between each level of variable and includes all the characteristics of the nominal and ordinal scales of measurement. Here, the units of measurement are constant and equal, and zero point is not true but rather arbitrary. Fahrenheit and Celsius thermometers and time as shown in the calendar are examples of interval measurements.

(d) **Ratio Indicators:** It is the highest level of measurement and allows comparison between variable values. It has all the properties of nominal, ordinal, and interval scales plus an absolute or a true zero value. The ratio of two numbers is independent of the unit of measurement and, therefore, can be equated. For example, the length of two rods is measured in terms of feet and inches and equated in ratio scale.

Constructs

A construct is a cluster of concepts or a newly invented concept that represents an index of behaviour, events, or other phenomena. It is the basic material of which theories are composed of. These are based on the concepts that lend to operationalization and empirical testing, for example, attitude, intelligence, socio-economic status, health-wellness, burnout, and learning ability.

Propositions

These are linkages or relationships that spell out how concepts are interrelated. These lay a foundation for the development of methods that test the validity, strengthen the predicted relationship, or are termed as hypotheses. These are the core of the framework as shown in Fig. 5.2.

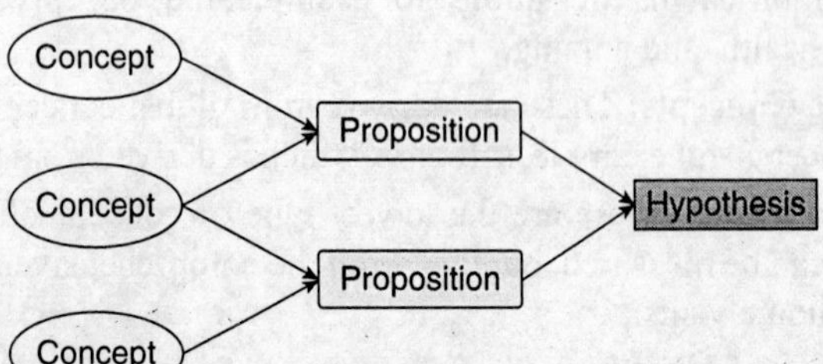

FIGURE 5.2 *Propositions—The Core of Framework*

Hypotheses

The testable proposition is termed as a hypothesis. A hypothesis is a testable or expected relationship between two or more than two variables, which are measurable or potentially measurable. According to Kerlinger, hypothesis is 'a conjectural statement of the relation between two or more variables. Hypotheses are always in declarative sentence form, and they relate, either generally or specifically, variables to variables'. It should be related to the existing body of theory and fact and must be conceptually clear and testable.

Definitions

Concepts must be defined in order to convey the same meaning to the real world. They may have theoretical or operational definitions.

Theoretical Definition

Theoretical definition defines the concept in relation to other concepts as defined in the particular theory. It conveys the general or same meaning of the concept to everyone. It reflects the theory used in the study of that concept; for example, 'recovery' is the degree at which a patient adjusts physiologically, psychologically, and socially to a long-term illness.

Operational Definition

The operational definition links the concept to the real world and identifies empirical referents (indicators) of the concept that can be observed and measured. It specifies the method of observation and measurement adopted by the researcher so that it can convey the same meaning to the audience used in the particular research study; for example, in 'an analytical study on demand and supply of bedlinen in selected wards of Nehru Hospital PGIMER, Chandigarh, 2005', the operational definitions used are as follows:

1. **Demand:** It refers to the quantity of bedlinen required in the wards.
2. **Supply:** It refers to the quantity of bedlinen in the store of the ward sister and linen made available for the use of the patients.
3. **Bedlinen:** It includes bed sheets, draw sheets, blankets, pillows, and pillow covers.
4. **Ward:** It refers to the geographical area where patients are admitted and nursed in Nehru Hospital, PGIMER, Chandigarh.
5. **Ward Sister:** It refers to a professional nurse working as an administrator in charge of the ward.

Empirical Referents or Indicators

These are the categories of actual phenomena that can depict the existence or occurrence of the concept itself; for example, numerical pain-intensity scale is used as an indicator to assess the severity of pain; stress scale or depression scale tested empirically can be used in research studies to assess the stress level or depression level of the individuals. The empirical referent provides a means of measurement of the concept under analysis. These need to be defined and tested for validity and reliability.

WHAT IS NURSING THEORY?

Meaning

Nursing theory is the body of knowledge to define or explain various aspects of nursing. Nursing theories are originated from the nursing concepts and depict the relationship between those concepts.

Development of Nursing Theory

Development of nursing theory began in late 1950s, but it dates back at the time of Florence Nightingale, who used the clinical arena of the hospital as her research laboratory to advance the theory for practice. However, she did not specify propositions or theoretical statements of her vision of nursing and also did not develop the law of nursing. She believed that environment directly affected the health status of the patients. Peplau introduced interpersonal relationships as the core of professional nursing. Later on, various models and theories have been introduced by the nursing scholars. Seaman identified six major categories of theories that nursing has used widely in practice and research. These are as follows:

1. **Learning Theories:** Among the learning theories, theories of conditioning, social learning theories, and Gestalt or cognitive theories are widely used in nursing.
2. **Development Theories:** These are the theories examining the changes occurring through time in physical, mental, psycho-social, and social structure.
3. **Theories of Adaptation, Stress, and Homeostasis:** These are the theories examining how individuals or groups survive and function in a particular environment.
4. **Social Theories:** These theories may focus on social networks, social support, and symbolic interactions.
5. **System Theories:** The diverse theories that may focus on behavioural systems, interaction, communication, and adaptation are also used in nursing research.
6. **Culture Theories:** These are the theories that may overlap with social theories but, in general, focus on cross-cultural practices, culture diversity, value orientation, and so on. They are the theories of discipline of psychology, sociology, anthropology, biology, and education.

There is tremendous growth in the development of the theories and models in nursing in order to improve the nursing practice and have autonomy of the discipline, but it requires a unified theory of nursing.

Paradigm

It is derived from the Greek word *paradeigma*, which means ‘pattern’. Kuhn defines paradigm as a core cluster of concepts (constructs) associated with a recognized scientific achievement that may be identified by a particular scientist or group of scientists. This is also equated with an exemplar, cognitive model, map, or pattern that could be used to guide scientific enquiry. Fawcett and others used the terms *paradigm* and *conceptual model* synonymously.

Nursing paradigms and conceptual models are highly abstract systems of global concepts that may or may not be linked in the form of relational statements and cannot be tested directly through empirical means. Fawcett explains that there are two broad categories used to clarify the world view: mechanism vs. organicism and change vs. persistence. Mechanism is the ‘received view’ and organicism is the ‘perceived view’. Change is perceived view, and persistence or stability is the ‘received view’.

Preparadigms

Paradigms, when in a developing stage and not reached in dominant phase, is termed as preparadigms, for example, the models for solution that are accepted by scientists but not confirmed empirically.

Metaparadigms

These are the paradigms that define the domain of interest and questions to be addressed and identify appropriate theories, methods, and instruments to be utilized. It is the most global perspective of a discipline and serves as a framework, within which more models and theories can be developed. In nursing, these are the most global world view – set of beliefs and values about nursing that are shared by scholars within a discipline.

All the conceptual models or paradigms from nursing, for example, King, Orem, and Roy and so on, share the common domains of focus on metaparadigms: nursing (nursing actions), person (client), environment (society), and health as explained below in Fig. 5.3.

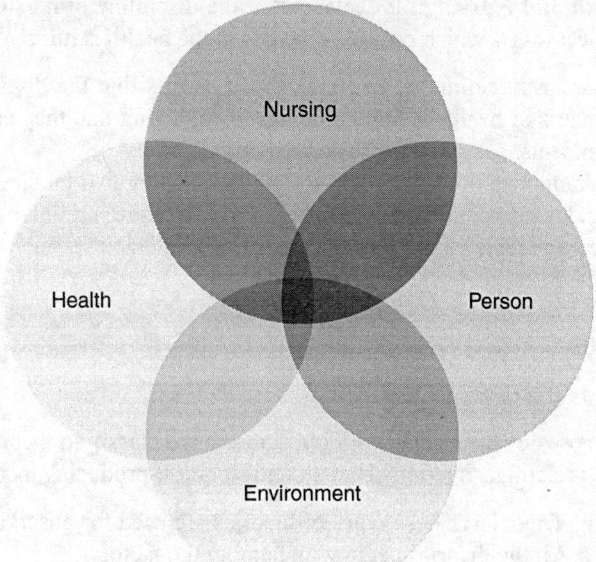

FIGURE 5.3 *Central Concepts or Common Domains of Focus in Nursing Theory*

Central Concepts or Domains

Nursing: Nursing refers to the definition of nursing, the actions taken by the nurses on behalf of, or in conjunction with, the person, and the goals or outcomes of nursing actions. Nursing actions typically are viewed as a systematic process of assessment, labelling, planning, intervention, and evaluation.

Person: Person refers to the recipient of nursing, including individuals, families, communities, and other groups.

Environment: Environment refers to the person's significant others and physical surrounds, as well as to the setting in which the nursing occurs, which ranges from the person's home to the clinical agencies to the society as a whole.

Health: Health is the person's state of well-being, which ranges from high-level wellness to terminal illness.

These domains were first identified in 1978 and formalized along with four relational propositions as the metaparadigms of nursing in 1984 by Fawcett. There are four proposition links: person and health; person and environment; health and nursing; and person, environment, and health.

Relational Propositions or Metaparadigms

Links between Person and Health: It states that the discipline of nursing is concerned with the principles and laws that govern the life process, well-being, and optimal functioning of human beings, sick or well.

Links between Person and Environment: It states that the discipline of nursing is concerned with the patterning of human behaviour in interaction with the environment in normal life events and critical life situations.

Links between Health and Nursing: It declares that the discipline of nursing is concerned with the nursing actions or processes by which positive changes in the health status are affected.

Links between Person, Environment, and Health: It asserts that the discipline of nursing is concerned with the wholeness or health of human beings, recognizing that they are in continuous interaction with their environments.

These four metaparadigm propositions are unique that distinguish nursing from other disciplines, do not reflect the beliefs and values of any country, and, therefore, are international in scope. Meleis identified seven central concepts: nursing client, transitions, interaction, nursing process, environment, nursing therapeutics, and health.

Types of Theories

According to Purposes

According to the purposes of theory, Dickoff and James have classified theories under four headings: factor-isolating, factor-relating, situation-relating, and situation-producing theories.

1. **Factor-isolating Theories:** These types of theories are used for observing, describing and naming the concepts. All the theories begin with naming the factors.
2. **Factor-relating Theories:** The theories showing the relationship among the factors or the concepts once the factors or the concepts are identified are termed as factor-relating theories.
3. **Situation-relating Theories:** These types of theories just depict the proximity in relationship in a given situation and is also termed as situation-depicting theories. When in a situation, causal relationship is formed among concepts; prediction can be made; thereby a prediction theory can be identified.
4. **Situation-producing Theories:** These theories are also known as prescription theories as they prescribe the activities necessary to attain a defined goal.

In 1979, Diers expanded the idea of Dickoff and James and classified theories under four headings: factor-naming, factor-relating, explanatory, and causal hypothesis-testing research.

1. **Factor-naming Research:** This is to describe, name, or characterize a phenomenon, situation, or event to gain insight and is also termed as the factor-searching research.

2. **Factor-relating Research:** The objective of factor-relating research is to develop links among variables and describe the relationships that are discovered after a phenomenon has been explored or described; it is also known as relation-searching research. Many qualitative theories fit into it.
3. **Explanatory or Correlational Research:** In this type of research, no attempt has been made to control or manipulate the environment or situation, rather determine the factors that occur or vary in a given situation.
4. **Causal Hypothesis-testing Research:** It addresses causal relationships among variables in an attempt to predict something.

According to Scope or Breadth (Level)

According to the scope or breadth, the theories are classified into four types: metatheories, grand theories, middle-ranged theories, and practice theories Fig. 5.4.

1. **Metatheories:** It is the analysis of theory or theorizing about theory in a discipline.
2. **Grand or Macro Theories:** These theories address the phenomenon of concern and models. From those models, hypothesis can be derived. These theories are not tested but viewed or assumed as theory-generating models, which then can be tested.
3. **Middle-ranged Theories:** These are the theories which examine the facts and identify a few key variables; propositions are clearly formulated; and tested hypothesis can be derived through inductive or deductive approach. Qualitative studies often derive middle-ranged theories.
4. **Practice Theories:** These theories are very limited in its scope. These may be descriptive, explanatory, and predictive theories.

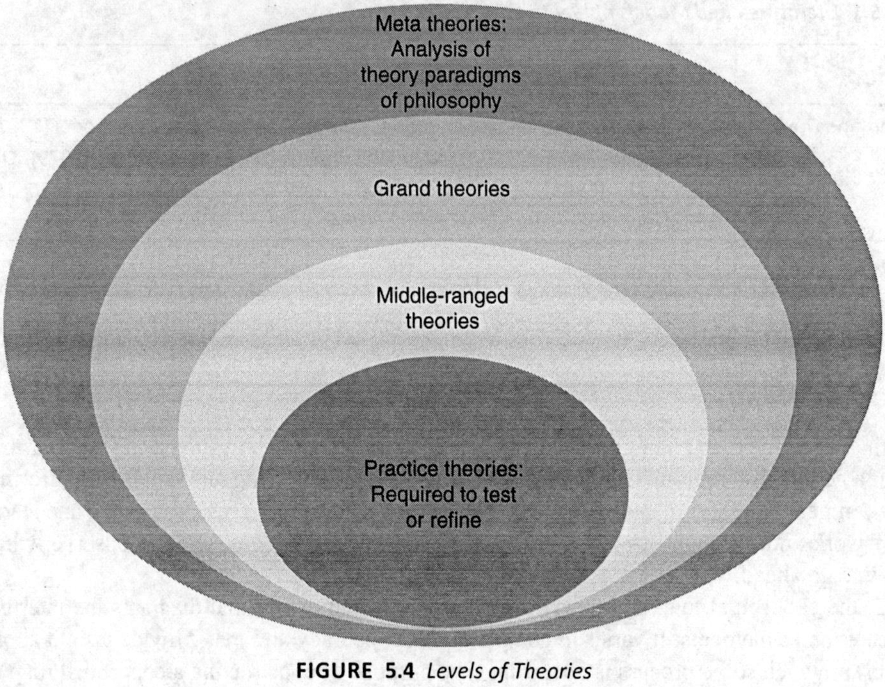

FIGURE 5.4 *Levels of Theories*

MODELS

A model is a symbolic representation of some phenomena and may be concrete or abstract in structural, pictorial, diagrammatical, or mathematical form. It focuses on the structure or the composition of the phenomena under study rather the statement or explanation of the relationships between the phenomena. It provides a more concrete analogy for thinking about the various concepts and how they actually operate.

Conceptual Model

Conceptual model is a symbolic or visual representation of highly abstract cluster of concepts under study based on assumptions and philosophical thoughts in structural, pictorial, or mathematical form. These are also known as schematic models or flow chart that diagrammatically depicts the concepts and its relationships by using boxes, arrows, and other symbols.

There are a number of conceptual models that are developed in nursing, for example, Roy's adaptation model, Orem's self-care model, and other models. Roy's adaptation model focuses on adaptation, identifies the constructs related to adaptation, and depicts the relationships between those constructs; Orem's model focuses on self-care approach and explains how nurses can facilitate the self-care of patients. There are many other examples of conceptual models developed by nurse theorists which have central phenomenon of interest. These conceptual models can be applied in research and other practice areas. A conceptual model may use the same or similar constructs, but their definitions will vary according to the interest of topic or the way taken in that particular philosophical thoughts; for example, the definition of the construct 'health' has been defined differently in different nursing theories. Literature revealed that Fawcett and Down identified 7 conceptual models and Walker and Avant identified 17 conceptual models, which they referred to as grand nursing theories, which are provided in Table 5.1.

TABLE 5.1 *Literature-cited Models of Identified Theories*

Citation	Models in Identified Theories
Fawcett and Down	Johnson's behavioural system model (1980), King's open system model (1981), Levine's conservation model (1973), Neuman's health care system model (1979), Orem's self-care model (1985), Roger's science of unitary human being model (1970, 1980, 1983, 1986), and Roy's adaptation model (1984)
Walker and Avant	Paplau (1952), Orlando (1961), Wiedenbach (1964), Henderson (1966), Levine (1967), Ujheley (1968), Rogers (1970), King (1971), Orem (1971), Travelbee (1971), Neuman (1974, 1979, 1988), Roy (1976), Johnson (1980), Parse (1981), and Watson (1985)

Conceptual Map

Visintainer used the map analogy—the map of a discipline operates in such a way similar to that of the maps of a geographic region. They provide a framework for selecting and organizing information from the environment, whereas in studying a discipline or incorporating in research study, one learns the map or framework and, through mastering the maps, learns what to focus, what to observe, what to think, and how to go ahead.

Thus, the conceptual map is the way of expressing a framework that diagrams the interrelationships of concepts and statements. It varies in complexity and accuracy and may provide insight about different situations in which some process is occurring. The purpose of constructing a conceptual map is to depict the concepts that contribute totally or partially, directly or indirectly, in sequence or cumulatively to cause or may produce an outcome of the study. It may also suggest the hypothesis can be tested in future studies. In short, the conceptual maps are to facilitate building of knowledge related to a particular research study.

FRAMEWORKS

Meaning and Definitions

According to Macmillan dictionary, 'Framework is a structure that supports something and makes it a particular shape'.

It is a set of principles and ideas that can be used to make decisions and judgements when given a meaning to it. It is also viewed as a frame or structure wherein the various parts of an object can be fitted and joined together to give it a particular shape as shown in Fig. 5.5.

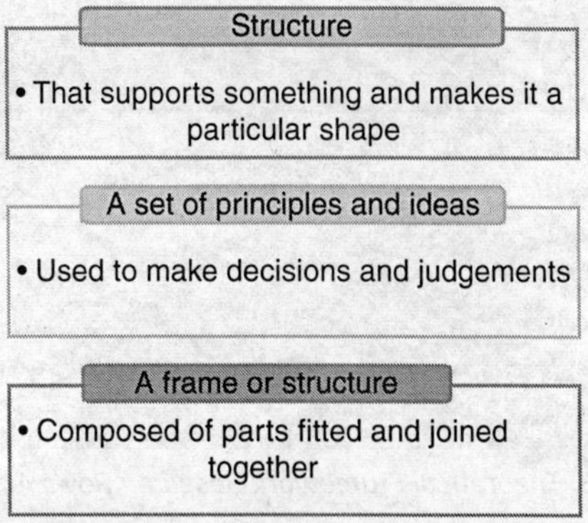

FIGURE 5.5 *Concepts of Framework*

Each research study should have a framework – theoretical, conceptual, or study framework – and should be well integrated within the methodology.

Theoretical Framework

A theoretical framework is a frame to support both qualitative and quantitative research study. As the name indicates, theoretical framework is a collection of interrelated concepts based on one existing theory. It provides a context for examining the problem, frame of reference as a base for observations, definitions of concepts, interpretation, and generalization or defines the overall design of a research study. Framework used to be abstract in nature but provides rationale that guides the researcher in planning a research study. In qualitative studies, a framework is a philosophy or world view and aids in developing a theory; in quantitative studies, it is a testable theory that may emerge from conceptual model or be developed inductively from clinical observations.

It is also viewed as the process of identifying a core set of connectors within a topic of research study and showing how they fit together or related to some way to the subject to get in track. The theoretical framework guides research study, determines which concepts it will measure and what statistical relationship it will look for, and presents a broad, general explanation of relationship between the concepts of interest under research study. The study concepts must be related back to the concepts from an existing theory.

Example: A theoretical framework developed in 'a study on utilization of morning duty hours and influencing environmental stimuli of the operational-level nurses working in selected wards of Nehru

Hospital PGIMER, Chandigarh' to depict and establish the relationship between the study concepts using Roy's adaptation model as shown in Fig. 5.6.

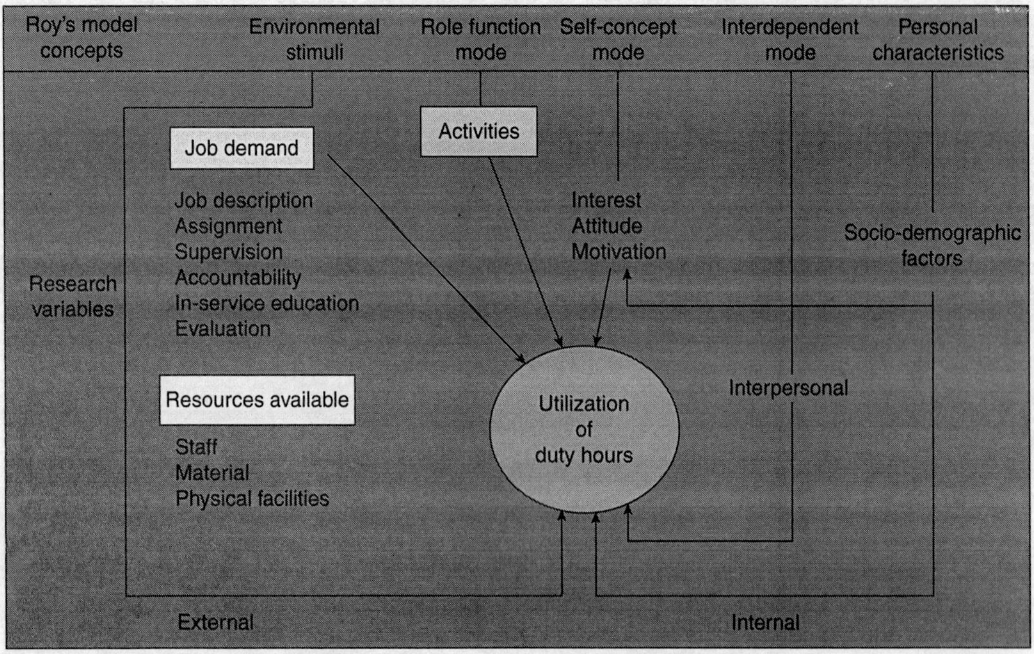

FIGURE 5.6 *Theoretical Framework Based on Roy's Adaptation Model*

This theoretical framework as mentioned above is based on Roy's adaption model. According to Callista Roy, the various concepts are defined as follows:

Adaptation: Adaptation is a process that involves a systematic series of actions directed towards some end.

Environment: Environment is defined as 'all circumstances that surround and affect the behaviour of a person'. Thus, all stimuli, whether internal or external, are part of the person's environment. Change in the environment acts as a catalyst, thus stimulating a person to make adaptive responses.

Person: Person is a bio-psychosocial being as a whole and constantly interacting with the changing environment.

Modes: Modes are explained as the ways of acting labelled as stimuli in the environment. These modes have direct effects on a person's adaptation process, thus called adaptive modes. These are role-performance mode, self-concept mode, interdependent mode, and physiological mode. The role-performance mode is the performance of duties based on a given position in the society. It depends on one's interaction with others in a given situation. Self-concept mode includes one's belief and feelings about oneself at a given time. Interdependent mode involves one's relation with other persons. Physiological mode involves body's basic needs and the ways of dealing with the adaptation in regard to it.

In the study mentioned above, all the modes, except physiological mode, are included in the forms of activities by the operational-level nurses during their duty hours. As depicted, the variables under self-concept mode are interest, attitude, and motivation. Interdependent mode includes the ways of having interpersonal relationship in the health team, and role-performance mode includes all types of activities of nurses at their work place. Personal characteristics comprise socio-demographic variables that influence the self-concept mode of the individual. All these modes are categorized as internal factors of the environment stimuli.

The external factors of environmental stimuli include administrative methods, for example, existence of job descriptions, assignment, supervision, accountability policies, in-service education, performance, and evaluation for job demand within available resources such as staff, material, and physical facilities. Thus, the nurses are constantly exposed to these stimuli during the adaptation process to perform job activities and accordingly utilize their duty hours.

Conceptual Framework

The conceptual framework explains the relationship between concepts and links concepts selected from various theories, from previous research results, and from researcher's own experiences.

Example: The conceptual framework developed for a study on 'a randomized controlled trial to assess the effect of low Fowler's position on back pain and vascular complications following transfemoral diagnostic cardiac catheterization in Advanced Cardiac Centre, PGIMER, Chandigarh' based on Ludwig Von Bertalanffy's general systems theory and Ida Jean Orlando's nursing process theory as shown in Fig. 5.7.

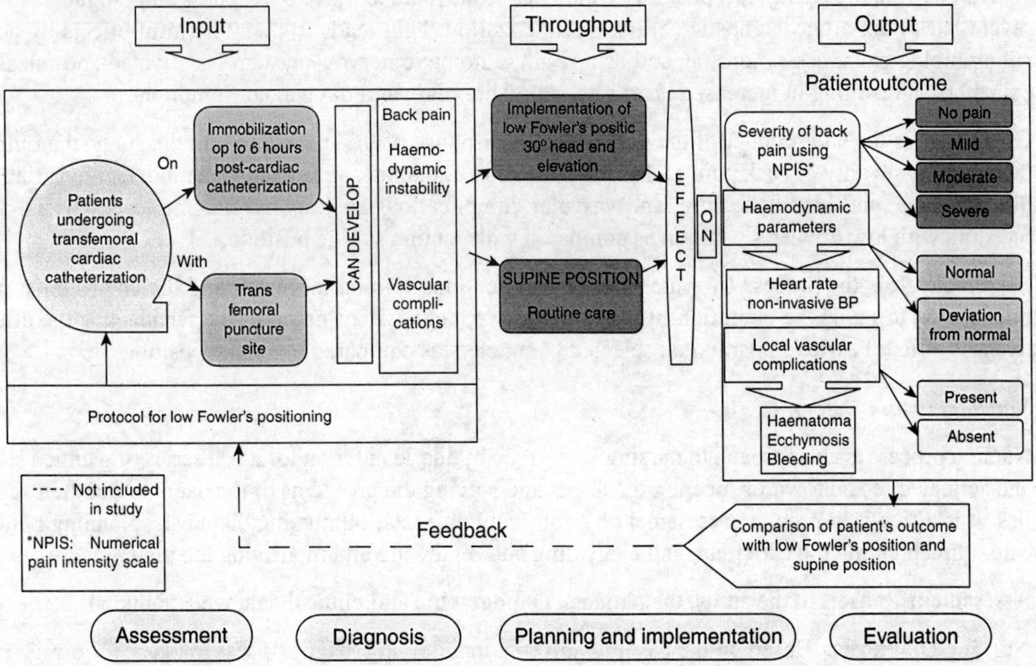

FIGURE 5.7 *Conceptual Framework Based on Ludwig Von Bertalanffy's General Systems Theory and Ida Jean Orlando's Nursing Process Theory*

General System Theory

General system theory pioneered by Ludwig Von Bertalanffy in 1969 serves as a model for viewing man as interacting with the environment. A system is a group of elements that interact with one another to achieve a goal. It can be either open or closed. In open system, there is continual and varying degree of interaction with the environment from which the system receives input and gives back output in the form of matter, energy, and information. The closed system does not interact with the environment. In the research study, a patient is continually interacting with the environment and thus constitutes an open system. The model also specifies that the universe consists of hierarchy of systems and each system may be received as having one or more suprasystems and subsystems. In view of this concept, suprasystem is the region around the patient, that is, mattress, position in the bed, and duration of bed rest; and subsystems are different organs within the body of the patient.

The main concepts of this model are input, throughput, output, and feedback.

Input: Matter, energy, and information that enters a system are called input. According to this concept, the input is the low Fowler's position (elevating the head end of bed to 30°) given to one group of patients who have undergone transfemoral diagnostic cardiac catheterization, meeting the inclusion criteria, and the accessories for providing low Fowler's position are bed, long ruler, and D (angles protector). The other group remained in routine (supine) position without any intervention.

Throughput: The system's part or subsystems that use the input in a process are referred as throughput. Throughput is the implementation of low Lowler's position and its effect on the severity of pain, haemodynamic variables, and local vascular complications (haematoma, ecchymosis, and bleeding).

Elevating the head end of the bed to 30° is associated with reduction in stress on back muscles as compared to supine (lying flat) position, which may contribute to muscle weakness and fatigue, leading severe back pain after diagnostic cardiac catheterization. Pain leads to many harmful effects by activating biological stress syndrome, and as a result, automatic nervous system is activated and releases epinephrine, resulting in increased heart rate, blood pressure, and oxygen consumption.

Output: It is the end product of the system or the response of the throughput. In the study, the output included the severity of back pain such as no pain, mild, moderate, and severe; haemodynamic variables like heart rate and blood pressure; and vascular complications such as haematoma, ecchymosis, and bleeding with low Fowler's position as compared with routine supine position.

Feedback: It is the process by which the system continually monitors itself and the environment for information to guide the operation. It may be positive, negative, or neutral. The feedback is the effectiveness of low Fowler's position on selected parameters as compared to supine position.

Nursing Process Theory

Nursing process is an approach to nursing care given by Ida Jean Orlando. It is a series of planned steps and actions directed towards meeting the needs and solving the problems of the patients and their families. It is a five-step process: assessment by gathering data, stating nursing diagnosis, planning patient care, implementing the care plan, and evaluating and reviewing and modifying the plan.

Assessment Phase: In the study, the patients' demographic and clinical data were gathered.

Nursing Diagnosis: Based on the baseline information, nursing diagnosis was made as follows:

1. Pain related to immobilization
2. Alterations of haemodynamic variables such as heart rate and blood pressure related to pain
3. Imminent local vascular complications (haematoma, ecchymosis, and bleeding) due to puncture of femoral access site during catheterization procedure.

Planning: During the planning phase, it was planned to have and develop a protocol on elevation of the head end of the bed to an angle of 30°; standardized numerical pain intensity scale; vascular complication assessment tool, and a record pro-forma to record the selected variables.

Implementation: As per the plan, the implementations were carried out to assess the effectiveness of low Fowler's position or head end elevation.

Evaluation: It is the final step of the nursing process. In the study, in order to evaluate the effectiveness of the selected protocol, the patients were assessed on selected parameters: back pain, haemodynamic variables, and vascular complications.

Study Framework

Study framework explains the relationship between variables or concepts and links variables or concepts selected from the research problem. The variables need to be operationally defined, that is, what meaning the particular variable or concept has in the research study undertaken; for example, in an analytical study on 'demand and supply of bedlinen in selected wards of Nehru Hospital, PGIMER, Chandigarh, 2005', the framework for the study as shown in Fig. 5.8 involves the integration of concepts regarding the method of estimating demand of bedlinen, analysis of supply, and their comparison in terms of balance and imbalance between demand and supply. Imbalance may be in the form of shortage or surplus supply of bedlinen.

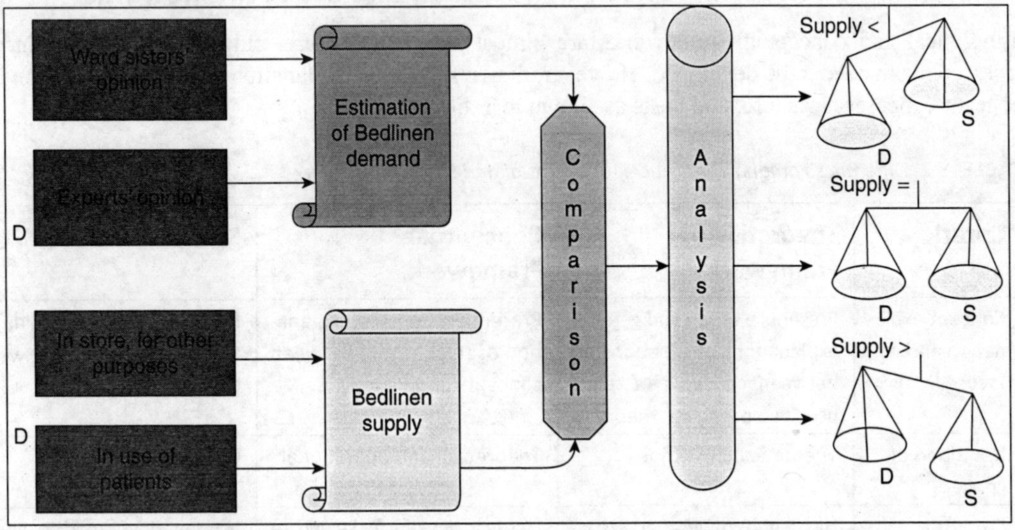

FIGURE 5.8 *Study Framework for an Analysis of Demand and Supply of Bedlinen*

These concepts have been related to the research problem, identified from the field of nursing science, economics, general management, and hospital management, and operationally defined as in how much was explored in the study by the researcher.

Estimation of Demand of Bedlinen

To estimate the demand of bedlinen, the following approaches were considered:

Ward Sisters' Opinions: This is based on ward sisters' opinions for the demand of bedlinen or the requisition sent to get the required number of bedlinen per bed.

Experts' Opinions: This includes the opinions of 10 experts from the field of nursing service, hospital administration, and nursing education regarding requirement of bedlinen for selected units.

Bedlinen Supply: To get the exact record of bedlinen supply, information were gathered regarding bedlinen in stock, in use and unused, or available in store.

Comparison and Analysis

This is third concept depicted in the study framework and is based on comparison between demand and supply of bedlinen. The following possibilities can be predicted:

1. **Supply < Demand:** This indicates that the available quantity of bedlinen is less than the bedlinen required. Hence, there is a state of imbalance. This also means that there is a shortage of bedlinen.
2. **Supply = Demand:** This means that supply is equal to demand, that is, the available quantity of bedlinen is equal to the bedlinen required in the ward. Hence, this is a state of balance.
3. **Supply > Demand:** This indicates that supply is more than demand, that is, the available quantity of bedlinen is equal to the bedlinen required in the ward. Hence, this is also a state of imbalance. This also means that there is a surplus or an excess of bedlinen.

Differences among Theoretical, Conceptual, and Study Frameworks

Theoretical and conceptual frameworks are almost similar in nature, purposes, and importance in research. Both need to be developed. However, they differ in the explanation of relationship among the concepts, focuses, structure, and basis as shown in Table 5.2.

TABLE 5.2 *Differences among Theoretical, Conceptual and Study Frameworks*

Criterion	Theoretical Framework	Conceptual Framework	Study Framework
Concept explanation and its focuses	Presents a broad and general explanation of relationship between concepts of focus used in a particular theory	Presents a specific explanation of relationship between concepts under study	Presents a specific explanation of relationship between concepts under study
Definition of concepts	Theoretical definitions	Theoretical and operational	Operational
Structure	Has highly developed structure	Has less developed structure	Has less developed structure
Basis	Based on one existing theory	Based on two or more theories, from previous research results and researcher's own experiences	Based on identified study constructs, concepts or variables, design, measurement, and outcome of the study

BASICS TO FRAMEWORK FOR RESEARCH

Framework for research can be developed through the deductive or the inductive approach as shown in Fig. 5.9.

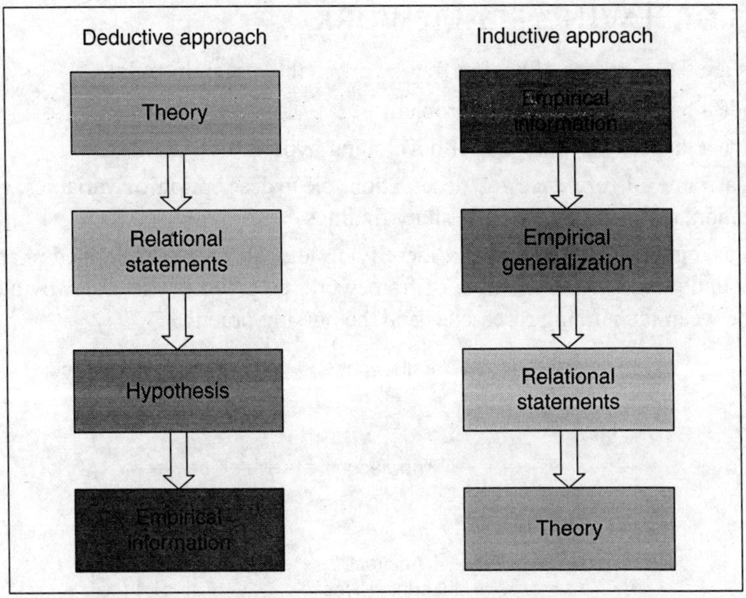

FIGURE 5.9 *Basics to Framework: Deductive and Inductive Approaches*

Deductive Approach

Deductive is a logical process from the complexities or the whole observed situation to arrive at a particular or certain single idea. Before stating finally the propositions or the relational statements deducted, test them or compare them with available propositions and ideas. The researcher starts with the theory, theoretical framework, or model from which testable propositions and hypotheses are deducted and then tested through the collection of empirical data. It is the process of drawing conclusions as to specific events from generalizations.

Inductive Approach

It is also a form of logical reasoning, where a generalization is drawn from several observations and specific instances, or the process of reasoning from particular to a whole group of ideas, phenomena, or situation. In research studies, it is necessary to isolate certain elements within the complexities and reconstruct them on a simpler conceptual model or framework before they are examined.

NATURE OF THEORETICAL AND CONCEPTUAL FRAMEWORKS

The characteristics of the theoretical and conceptual frameworks are as follows:

1. Theories and conceptual frameworks are not discovered, rather created or developed.
2. They cannot be proved and never considered final and thereby can be modified or discarded.
3. The frameworks have multiple roles in developing new knowledge to lighten the path and keep in track.
4. There is a direct relationship between a theory and a research.
5. The frameworks can depict relationship by using conceptual map.

PURPOSES OF HAVING FRAMEWORK

The followings are the purposes of having framework in the research study:

1. To provide a base for examining a problem
2. To provide a theoretical rationale for developing hypothesis
3. To have a frame of reference for observation, clear description of variables, research designs, interpretation, and generalization of study findings
4. It serves as a guide to systematically identifying logical, precisely defined relationship between variables under study. The example of framework, as given in Fig. 5.10, by clearly depicts the linking between the nursing researches and the nursing practice.

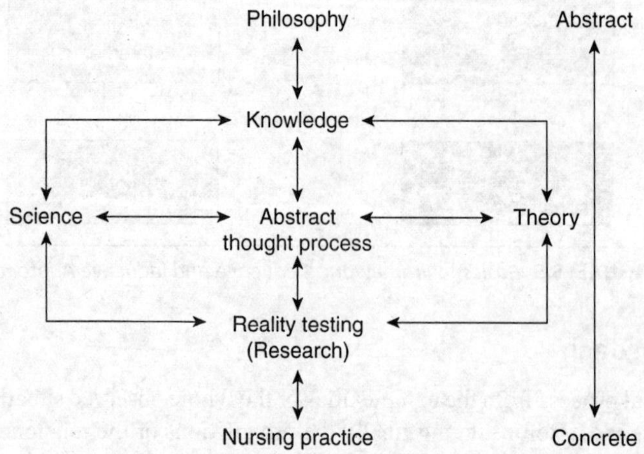

FIGURE 5.10 *Framework Linking Nursing Research to Nursing Practice (Adapted from Burns and Grove, 1993)*

DEVELOPING THEORETICAL AND CONCEPTUAL OR STUDY FRAMEWORKS

There are mainly four steps that are being followed: selecting and developing concepts, developing relational statements, developing hierarchical statement sets, and constructing a conceptual map expressing framework as shown in Fig. 5.11.

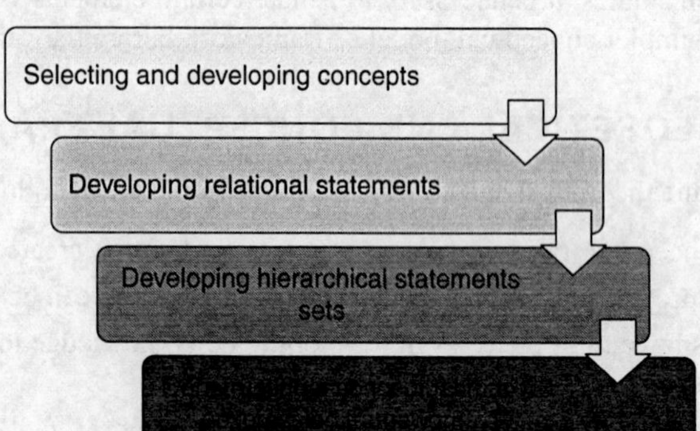

FIGURE 5.11 *Steps for Developing Framework*

Developing and Defining Concepts

1. Define the concepts appropriately and clearly from existing theoretical work if available, either operationally or theoretically, depending on the type of study undertaken. It will be helpful to tell the researchers what exactly they want to measure and how they are going to measure the variables of interest.
2. Search published concept analysis for definitions, previous studies using concepts, or other literature defined after the scholarly work.

Developing Relational Statements

1. Link all the concepts through relational statements.
2. Note that the relational statements must describe its characteristics in terms of direction, shape, strength symmetry, sequencing, probability of occurrence, necessity and sufficiency of relationship as shown in Fig. 5.12.
3. Note that the type of statements expressed determines the objective, the question or the hypothesis formulated, the design, the statistical analysis, and the type of findings of the study.

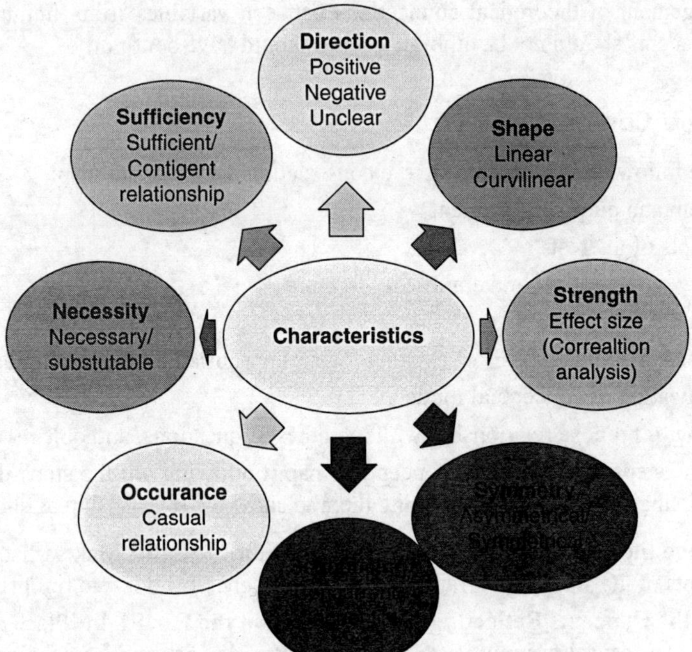

FIGURE 5.12 *Characteristics of Relational Statements*

Developing Hierarchical Statement Sets

Arrange Hierarchical Statements

Arrange the statements in hierarchy from a high level to a low level of abstraction as shown in Fig. 5.13:

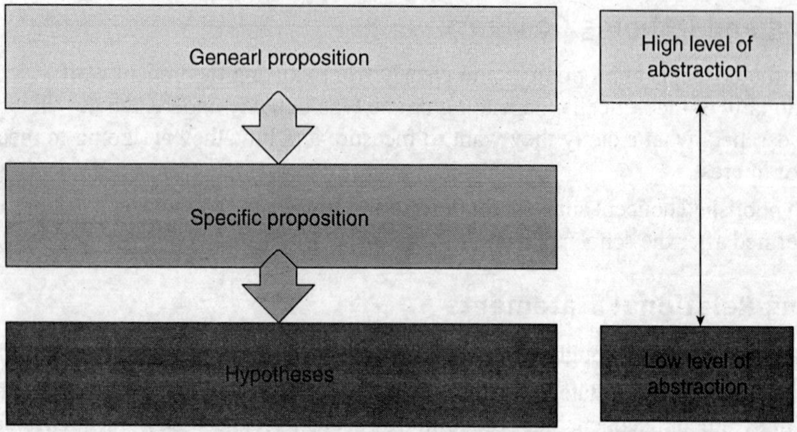

FIGURE 5.13 *Developing Hierarchical Statements*

Formulate Theoretical Rationale

Verify the arrangement of theoretical connections between variables from literature. Make sure that definitions of concepts should not be ambiguous and should have continuity.

Constructing a Conceptual Map

1. Gather the following information before constructing a conceptual map:
   (a) Problem and purpose statement
   (b) Concepts of interest
   (c) Review of theoretical and empirical literature
   (d) Relational statements
   (e) Identification and analysis of existing theory appropriate to the concerned research problem
   (f) Identification of conceptual models
   (g) Linking of propose relationship with hypotheses, questions, and objectives
2. Perform the steps to construct a conceptual map. Following are the steps that should be taken while depicting the concepts and linking them to show the relationship as shown in Fig. 5.14:

   (a) **Arrange the Concepts in a Sequence from Left to Right:** Make a list of all the identified concepts of the study and arrange them in a sequence from left to right (Figs 5.6–5.8).

   (b) **Place the Concepts Reflecting the Outcomes on the Far Right:** Place the concepts that are included as causal or input variables on the left side of the conceptual map (diagram or flow chart) and the concepts reflecting the effects or outcomes on the far right as shown in Figs 5.7 and 5.8.

   (c) **Place the Concepts of More Abstract in a Frame or Box:** As depicted in Fig. 5.6, the more abstract concepts, for example, job demand and job responsibilities, are in boxes, and variables are not enclosed in a box or frame.

   (d) **Interrelated Concepts can be Linked by Enclosing Them in a Frame or Circle:** Link all the interrelated concepts by enclosing them in a circle or frame.

(e) **Link the Concepts by Using Arrows:** Use arrows or other symbols to show the link or relationship between the concepts. The researchers usually show link, but 'not included in the study', by drawing dotted line as shown in Fig. 5.7.

(f) **Examine the Map for Completeness:** Before finalizing the conceptual map, check that it is complete from all aspects as per the framework.

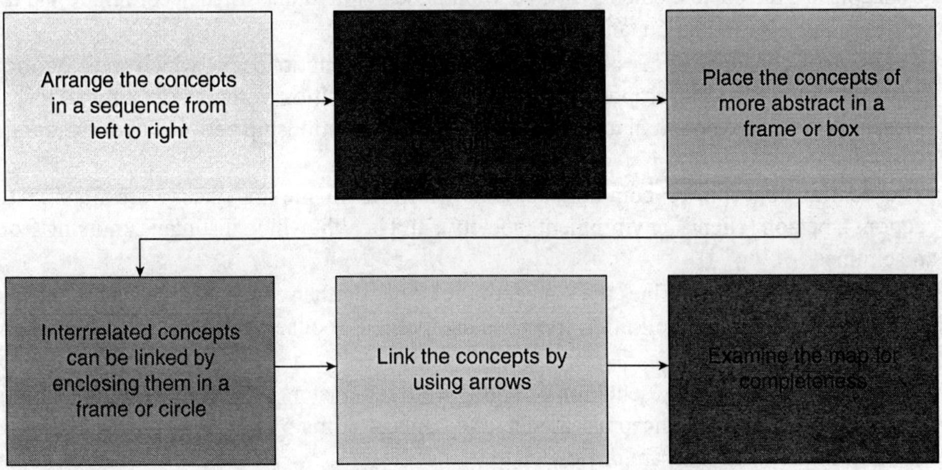

FIGURE 5.14 *Steps for Constructing Conceptual Map*

CHECKLIST TO EVALUATE THEORETICAL OR CONCEPTUAL FRAMEWORK

The criteria to evaluate a theoretical or a conceptual framework are as follows:

1. Is the theoretical framework clearly identified and selected as per the research study?
2. Is the framework appropriate for the study?
3. Are the concepts clearly identified and selected?
4. Are the concepts operationally or theoretically defined clearly?
5. Are the concepts showing proposed relationship clearly?
6. Are the proposition statements written clearly?
7. Is there a theoretical rationale related to the interrelationships among the concepts?
8. Can the propositions help to guide the research questions or hypotheses?
9. Is the framework based on nursing theory or theory from other discipline?

KEY POINTS

- Framework serves as a guide to systematically identifying logical, precisely defined relationship between concepts or variables both in qualitative and quantitative studies. These are the bases of developing models and theories.
- A theory is a set of interrelated construct (concepts), definitions, and propositions that present a systematic view of phenomena of specifying relations among variables with the purpose of explaining and predicting the phenomena.

- Theories are developed from the concepts and reveal relationship between the concepts which are in the form of propositional statements and are connected in a logical system of thought to explain and predict the phenomena under study.
- Nursing theory is the body of knowledge to define or explain various aspects or concepts of nursing.
- Concepts are the basic elements of theory and research and classified according to the levels of abstractions, categorization, and measurements.
- A cluster of concepts forms construct and linkages or relationships, which spell out how concepts are interrelated in proposition. The testable proposition is termed as a hypothesis, which measures or has the potential to measure the expected relationship between two or more than two variables.
- The central concepts or common domains of focus in nursing theory are nursing (nursing actions), person (client), environment (society), and health, which distinguish nursing from other disciplines.
- Theoretical definition defines the concept in relation to other concept as defined in the particular theory, and operational definition specifies the method of observation and measurement adopted by the researcher.
- A symbolic or visual representation of highly abstract clusters of concepts and depicting its relationships is known as conceptual model, and conceptual map is the way of expressing a framework in the form of diagram or flow chart.
- Theoretical framework is a collection of interrelated concepts based on one existing theory and highly abstract in nature; conceptual framework is a collection of concepts selected from various theories, from previous research results and from researchers' own experiences; and study framework explains the relationship between variables or concepts and links variables or concepts selected from the research problem.
- There are four steps for developing framework: selecting and developing concepts, developing relational statements, developing hierarchical statement sets, and constructing a conceptual map. It is developed through inductive or deductive approach.

QUESTIONS

I. Essay-type Questions

1. Define a theory and a nursing theory? Describe four central concepts of nursing theory.
2. Enlist the elements and components of a theory.
3. Discuss the different levels of measurement and give appropriate examples.
4. What do you mean by framework? Differentiate between theoretical and conceptual frameworks.
5. Describe, with examples, the concept of study framework. Make a distinction between study framework and theoretical framework.
6. Justify how inductive and deductive reasoning are basic to develop a framework.
7. Discuss the nature and purposes of having framework in research.
8. Describe the general steps in developing theoretical and conceptual frameworks.
9. Explain the different aspects taken into consideration while constructing a conceptual map.
10. Enlist the criteria to evaluate a theoretical or a conceptual framework.

II. Short Notes

1. Write a short note on the following:
   (a) Concepts
   (b) Construct
   (c) Proposition
   (d) Hypothesis
   (e) Conceptual model
   (f) Conceptual map
   (g) Paradigm
   (h) Metaparadigm

III. Multiple-choice Questions

Circle the alphabet before the best answer

1. The basic elements of a theory or research that are used to explain and interpret the facts are
   (a) empirical indicators
   (b) variables or concepts
   (c) relational statements
   (d) hypotheses
2. Which of the following indicator specifies the ratio of two numbers is independent of the unit of measurement?
   (a) Nominal (c) Ordinal
   (b) Interval (d) Ratio
3. The term *hypothesis* is defined as
   (a) a cluster of concepts that represent an index of phenomena
   (b) the relationship that explains how concepts are interrelated
   (c) a testable relationship between two or more variables that can be measured or has the potential to measure
   (d) an abstract or concrete idea of a phenomenon
4. The basic approach important to develop framework for research is
   (a) inductive
   (c) deductive
   (b) both inductive and deductive
   (d) none
5. The core of framework is
   (a) concept (c) proposition
   (b) construct (d) hypothesis
6. The framework that explains relationship between concepts and links concepts from various theories, research findings, and experiences of researchers is termed as
   (a) conceptual framework
   (b) study framework
   (c) both conceptual and study framework
   (d) theoretical framework
7. The conceptual and theoretical framework differ in one of the following:
   (a) Nature
   (c) Importance
   (b) Purpose
   (d) Focuses and structure

Answer Keys

1. (b) 2. (d) 3. (c) 4. (b) 5. (c) 6. (a) 7. (d)

IV. Rearrange the steps of developing a framework in sequence:

(a) Selecting the concepts
(b) Developing hierarchical statements
(c) Defining the concepts under study
(d) Developing relational statements
(e) Constructing a conceptual map

Answer Keys

(a) Selecting the concepts
(b) Defining the concepts under study
(c) Developing relational statements
(d) Developing hierarchical statements
(e) Constructing a conceptual map

FURTHER READING

Barnum, B. J. S. 1990. *Nursing Theory, Analysis, Application, Evaluation* (3rd ed.). Glenview, Illinois: Scott, Foreman/Little, Brown, 1–18.

Berger, P. L. and Kellner, H. 1981. *Sociology Reinterpreted: An Essay on Method and Vocation*. Garden City NY: Anchor Press/Doubleday Books.

Bertalanffy, L. von, 1969. *General System Theory*. New York: George Braziller Inc.

Briggs, E. 2002. 'The Nursing Management of Pain in Older People'. *Nursing Older People*, 14(7), 23–29.

Burns, N., and Grove, S. K. 1993. *The Practice of Nursing Research, Conduct, Critique and Utilization* (2nd ed.). Philadelphia, PA: W. B. Saunders.

Chinn, P. L., and Jacobs, M. K. 1983. *Theory and Nursing: A Systematic Approach*. St. Louis: CV Mosby.

Chinn, P. L., and Kramer, M. K. 1991. *Theory and Nursing* (4th ed.). St. Louis: CV Mosby, 5.

Dickoff, J., and James, P. 1968. 'A Theory of Theories: A Position Paper'. *Nursing Research*, 17, 197–203.

Diers, D. 1979. *Research in Nursing Practice*. Philadelphia: J.B. Lippincott.

Fawcett, J. 1989. *Analysis and Evaluation of Conceptual Models of Nursing* (2nd ed.). Philadelphia: FD Davis.

Fowcett, H.,Downs, F. 1986. *The Relationship of Theory and Research*. Norwalk, Connecticut: Appleton-Century-Crofts.

Gage, N. L. (ed.), 1963. Paradigms for research on teaching. In *Handbook of Research on Teaching*. Chicago: Rand McNally and Company, 100.

Hardy, M. E. 1974. 'Theories: Components, Development, Evaluation'. *Perspectives on Nursing Theory* (Nicoll, L., ed.), pp. 342–51. Boston: Little, Brown and Co., 1986. (Reprinted from Theoretical Foundations for Nursing, NY: MSS Information Systems. Originally titled *The Nature of Theories*).

Kaur, K. 2005. 'An Analytical Study on Demand and Supply of Bedlinen in Selected Wards of Nehru Hospital, PGIMER, Chandigarh, 2005'. Chandigarh: An Unpublished Theses of M.Sc. Nursing. Panjab University, Chandigarh.

Kerlinger, F. 1973. Foundations of Behavioural Research (3rd ed.). New York: Holt, Rinehart and Winston.

Koziol-McLain, J. K., and Maeve, M. K. 1993. Nursing Theory in Perspective. *Nursing Outlook*, 41(2), 79.

Mathew, T. K. 2012. 'A Randomized controlled trial to assess the effect of low Fowler's position on back pain and vascular complications following transfemoral diagnostic cardiac catheterization in Advanced Cardiac Centre, PGIMER, Chandigarh. An Unpublished Thesis of M.Sc. Nursing. Panjab University, Chandigarh.

Meleis, A. I. 1985. *Theoretical Nursing: Development and Progress*. Philadelphia: J.B. Lippincott.

Meleis, A. I. 1991. *Theoretical Nursing, Development and Progress* (2nd ed.). Philadelphia: JB Lippincott, pp. 25–70.

Morton, P. G., and Fontaine, D. K. 1996. *Critical Care Nursing: A Holistic Approach* (8th ed.). Philadelphia: Lippincott Williams and Wilkins, pp. 393–61.

Orem, D. 1985. *Nursing: Concepts of Practice* (3rd ed.). New York: McGraw-Hill.

Peplau, H. 1952. *Interpersonal Relations in Nursing*. New York: Putnam; 1952.

Polit, D. F. and Beck, C. T. 2006. *Nursing Research–Principles and Methods* (7th ed.). New Delhi: Wolters Kluwer Health (India) Pvt. Ltd (1st Indian reprint).

Polit, D. F., and Hungler, B. P. 1995. *Nursing Research: Principles and Methods* (5th ed.). Philadelphia: JB Lippincott Company.

Roy, C. 1984. *Introduction to Nursing: An Adaptation Model* (2nd ed.) Englewood Cliffs, NJ: Prentice- Hall.

Seaman, C. H. C. 1987. *Research Methods: Principles, Practice, and Theory Nursing*. (3rd ed.). Los Alton, California: Prentice-Hall.

Sharma, N. B. 2001. A study on utilization of morning duty hours and influencing environmental stimuli of the operational level nurses working in selected wards of Nehru hospital PGIMER, Chandigarh. An Unpublished Thesis of M.Sc. Nursing. Panjab University, Chandigarh.

Silva, M. C. 1981. 'Selection of a Theoretical Framework'. Krampitz, S.D. and Pavlouch, N. (eds.), *Readings for Nursing Research* (pp. 49–53). St. Louis: Mosby.

Urden, C. J., Keeling, A. W., Turner, M. 2006. 'Predictors of Vascular Complications Post-diagnostic Cardiac Catheterization and Percutaneous Coronary Interventions. *Dimension of Critical Care Nursing*, 25(3), 138–42.

Visintainer, M. 1986. 'The Nature of Knowledge and Theory in Nursing'. *Image*, 18(2), 10, 13.

Walker, L.O., Avant, K. C. 1988. *Stretegies for Theory Construction in Nursing* (2nd ed.). Norwalk, Connecticut: Appleton-Lange.

www.macmillandictionary.com/dictionary.com.

chapter

6 Ethics in Research

OBJECTIVES

Upon completion of this chapter the learner will be able to:

- Define ethics and code of ethics
- Get acquainted with historical background of ethics in nursing research
- Enumerate the ethical principles
- Understand the importance of ethical consideration in research
- Analyse and evaluate the risk/benefit ratio as a researcher
- Get sensitized and improve attention towards ethical issues in planning and conduct of research
- Constitute and understand the role of ethics committee
- Enlist the rights and responsibilities of researchers and institutions
- Consider ethical dilemma of nurse scientists and contemplate solving them

INTRODUCTION

The consideration of ethics in research is of growing importance. It is, therefore, critical that the researcher understands the basics of ethics in research and how this might affect the research project. This is especially important if the research involves interaction with members of the general community who involve themselves as participants (that is, respondents) in a research project.

Research that involves human subjects or participants raises unique and complex ethical, legal, social, and political issues. The clinical research in health sciences involves clinical trials of drugs or treatments and medical or nursing interventions; hence, it is important for health-care professionals to be aware of the ethical issues concerned with such interventions in a research.

Research ethics are a set of principles or guidelines that will assist the researcher in making difficult research decisions and in deciding which goals are most important in reconciling conflicting values. Ethics are a set of moral and social standards that includes both *prohibitions against* and *prescriptions for* specific kinds of behaviour in a research.

When humans are used as study participants, care must be taken that their rights are protected. Legal and ethical issues in research revolve around this concept.

HISTORICAL BACKGROUND

During the Second World War, in the 1940s, a number of experiments were conducted on the prisoners of war in the name of medical research, totally disregarding ethical conduct. Nazis used the prisoners of war and racial enemies as experimental subjects. They tested human endurance and reaction on untested drugs (unethical because the medicines were harmful and people could not refuse to participate). Similar war-time experiments happened in Australia and Japan.

In 1960, in a school for mentally retarded children, the inmates were deliberately infected with a mild form of hepatitis virus. Tuskegee syphilis study, in Alabama, was done during 1932–1972 by US Public Health Service. In this study, more than 400 African American men with latent syphilis were followed for the natural course of the disease rather than being provided with treatment. This was done though penicillin was available for the treatment of syphilis. During this period, 40 wives of these men got infected with syphilis and 19 children were born with congenital syphilis.

In the light of many such instances and in response to human rights violation, a *code of ethics*, called the NUREMBERG code, has been developed for research, which came into being after Nazi atrocities were made public in the *Nuremberg Trials*. In 1947, trials were conducted in Nuremberg, Germany, where physicians were convicted of crimes against humanity.

Another code of ethics is the 'Declaration of Helsinki'. Based on these, the international set of standards for medical ethics was adopted in 1964 by the World Medical Association, which was most recently revised in 2008. Most disciplines like psychology, sociology, and medicine have their own code of ethics.

In India, drug trials are controlled by the Drug Controller General of India (DCGI). Clinical trials are controlled by the Clinical Trial Registry of India (CTRI) of ICMR. Indian Good Clinical Practices (IGCP) are the code of ethics based on World Health Organization's international guidelines. Besides following the code of ethics, medical research has to have its roots in competency, integrity, and honesty of the researcher and in welfare of the humanity. At no stage should a patient's safety be risked, nor should his ignorance be exploited knowingly.

Though all researchers (student, professional, or academic) have no intention to harm the research subjects, there are possibilities that interaction with participants may inadvertently harm them in some unintended way. This could include the following besides physical harm:

1. Psychological harm
2. Financial harm
3. Social harm

It is, therefore, essential that the researcher carefully evaluates the potential for harm through the intended research study, ensures that he is well aware of the ethical standards, and takes every step such that no harm is caused to the study participants.

Clinical research attempts to address a relatively straightforward and extremely important challenge. Those who are the first to undergo potential new medical or nursing interventions invariably face some possibly serious risks, no matter how much prior testing has occurred in the laboratory and in animals. The benefits of the research may, however, be uncertain and may not be experienced by the person participating in the research. In addition, the risk involved for research participants may be difficult to identify or assess in advance or prior to research study.

IMPORTANCE OF ETHICAL CONSIDERATIONS IN RESEARCH

There is a growing need of ethical considerations in research as participants are becoming increasingly aware of their rights. National and international human rights commissions have been established in a number of countries for the promotion and protection of their citizens' human rights. In such a climate, the key responsibility for ethical awareness and for the status of the profession rests with each individual researcher and also the funding agency. It is important to ensure compliance with good ethical practice across all sectors of research.

The reasons for ethical considerations in research are as follows:

1. **Validate the Aims of Research:** Ethical norms validate the aims of research such as acquiring new knowledge, truth, and avoidance of error.
2. **Support Ream or Collaborative Work:** Research often involves a great deal of cooperation and coordination among various people or researchers in different disciplines and institutes. Ethical standards promote the values that are essential for collaborative work such as trust, accountability, mutual understanding, and fairness.
3. **Enhance Accountability:** Various ethical norms help a researcher to ensure that he or she is accountable to public for the research trials. For example, policies on research misconduct on human subject protection and use of new techniques or interventions are necessary in order to make sure that researchers who are funded by public money can be held accountable to the public.
4. **Promote or Preserve Moral and Social Values:** Consideration of the ethical issues in conducting research studies promotes a variety of moral and social values.

RISK TO STUDY SUBJECTS IN QUANTITATIVE RESEARCH OR CLINICAL TRIALS

1. The use of a placebo (a dummy treatment) in clinical trials has become one of the most controversial issues in biomedical sciences. Much discussion has been generated as to whether the use of placebos should be permitted at all in the face of the existence of accepted treatment or intervention. Patients do not know whether they are receiving the experimental drug or treatment, a previously approved drug or treatment, or even a placebo. However, the use of placebos is permissible under certain conditions.
2. There may be harmful and unpleasant side effects or outcomes of the research studies. They may last for only a short time, or they may affect the study subject for the long duration of his life.
3. The treatment modalities or nursing interventions being studied may have no positive effect on the health of the study subjects.
4. The time and attention required for participants for clinical trials and interventions may be long. It may require many hours of testing, miles of travel, hospital stays, or complicated dosing.
5. New interventions or treatment modalities may not always mean better for the health of an individual.

ETHICS IN QUALITATIVE RESEARCH

Qualitative research aims at an in-depth understanding of an issue, including an exploration of the reasons and context for participants' beliefs and actions, so it is often designed to be probing in nature. Although, interviews, the commonest qualitative method in health services research, are particularly well suited to the collection of data on sensitive social health issues, however, these may produce anxiety or distress in participants.

RISKS TO THE PARTICIPANTS IN QUALITATIVE RESEARCH

Anxiety and Distress

In-depth exploration of sensitive issue is a characteristic of the qualitative research approach, which may produce anxiety or distress in the participants. The questions which lead to anxiety and distress depend on the personal biography and experiences of an individual.

Identification of the Participant by Self or Others

Qualitative research studies collect large amounts of information about participants related to health and illness, lifestyles, and views or beliefs about health care, as well as information about members of their families and social groups. If identification occurs, it potentially may lead to serious harm such as prejudice and reprisal to the participant or their wider social group. Interview transcripts contain multiple clues to the person's identity such as their name, employment details, place of residence, and events which have occurred in their communities. It is, therefore, impossible to anonymize interview data at the stage of analysis, and the identity of the participants often will be known to the person carrying out the transcription. Even after the protocols of anonymization are applied, quotations, speech mannerisms, and context may provide enough information for the participants to be identified by themselves or others, and it is not always easy to predict which data will lead to identification.

Misrepresentation

The analysis of qualitative data inevitably is influenced by the theoretical framework, personal characteristics, and preconceptions of the researcher. The interpretative nature of qualitative research means that the published results are only a version of 'the truth', and the validity of the findings must be judged in relation to the care with which the data were analysed. Although all research is, to some extent, socially constructed, it is in qualitative studies that the participants are more likely to feel that their views have been misrepresented or taken out of context. These issues are particularly relevant to health services research.

Inconvenience and Opportunity Costs

In addition to the serious potential risks outlined above, the inconvenience and opportunity costs involved in participating in qualitative research are often underestimated. Most qualitative studies in the health services involve in-depth interviews with the participants. Such interviews normally last for hours and necessitate the participant travelling to a research centre or allowing the interviewer into their home. In some studies, the participants will be asked to take part in a second interview.

CODE OF ETHICS IN NURSING SCIENCES

Nursing is a profession as old as human civilization. The beginning of professional nursing can be traced to nineteenth century England to the school that was founded by Florence Nightingale. Professional development and shaping the ethical precept or values were communicated since that time.

By the end of the nineteenth century, modern nursing had been established, and ethics in nursing was seriously being discussed. The international council of nurses (ICN) was established in 1899, and it took lead in forming the code of ethics developed by Indian Nursing Council. A primary value of ethical consideration in nursing has been the determination of focus on nurse's work. Ethical codes are systemic guidelines for shaping ethical behaviour that answer the normative questions of what beliefs and values should be morally accepted. However, it must be noted that no code can provide absolute or complete rules that are free of conflict and ambiguity. Professional codes, however, do serve a useful purpose in providing direction to health-care professionals. Ultimately, one must remember that codes do not eliminate moral dilemmas and are of no use unless the professionals are motivated to act morally.

American Nurses Association issued ethical guidelines in the conduct, dissemination, and implementation of nursing research. The American Nurses Association (ANA) also published, in 2001, a revised code of ethics for nurses with imperative statements.

Canadian Nurses Association and Australian Nurses Associations have developed their own code of ethics for nursing research.

Belmont Report (1978) provides model for many disciplinary guidelines for biomedical and biochemical research most recently revised in 2005.

Belmont Report gives three basic ethical principles: beneficence, respect for human dignity, and justice.

To safeguard the justice to the participants of the research, an elaborated informed consent should be obtained.

The following chart will assist nurses to translate the standards into action. Nurses and nursing students can, therefore, do the following:

1. Study the standards under each element of the *code*.
2. Reflect on what each standard means to you. Think about how you can apply ethics in your nursing domain: practice, education, research, or management.
3. Discuss the *code* with co-workers and others.
4. Use a specific example from experience to identify ethical dilemmas and standards of conduct as outlined in the *code*. Identify how you would resolve the dilemmas.
5. Work in groups to clarify ethical decision-making and reach a consensus on standards of ethical conduct.
6. Collaborate with your national nurses' association, co-workers, and others in the continuous application of ethical standards in nursing practice, education, management, and research.

ETHICAL PRINCIPLES

Ethical principles actually control professionalism in nursing practice much more than ethical theories. Principles encompass basic premises from which rules are developed. Principles are the moral norms that nursing, as a profession, both demands and strives to implement to everyday clinical practice.

Lachman created a clever acronym to help nurses remember to have moral courage in situations and to remind nurses of the code of ethics for nurses. The acronym is CODE, which means the following:

C: Courage to be moral requirers
O: Obligations to honour (What is the right thing to do?)
D: Danger to manage (What do I need to handle my fear?)
E: Expression and action (What action do I need to maintain my integrity?)

Definition

Ethics are acts of moral principles that the researcher must follow while conducting nursing research to ensure rights and welfare of the individuals, groups. or community under study.

Principles

Ethical principles provide a foundation for nursing practice. They are defined as basis for nurse's decisions on consideration of consequences and of universal moral principles when making clinical judgements. The most fundamental of these principles is respect for persons.

The *primary* and basic ethical principles are the following:

1. Respect for persons
2. Respect for autonomy
3. Non-maleficence
4. Beneficence
5. Justice

The *secondary* ethical principles that can be incorporated with the primary principles when interpreting ethical issues and making clinical decisions are the following:

1. Veracity
2. Confidentiality
3. Fidelity

Respect for Persons: According to ANA, the most fundamental principle of professional behaviour is respect for persons. This principle applies not only to the clinical settings but to all life situations. This principle emphasizes that all people should treat others as worthy individuals. In nursing practice, this principle should be simplified. Thus, respect for persons generally means respecting a client's autonomy.

Respect for Autonomy: Respecting a client's rights, values, and choices is synonymous to respecting a person's autonomy. Informed consent is a method that promotes and respects a person's autonomy. For a client to make an autonomous decision and action, he or she must be offered enough information and options to make up his or her mind free of coercion or external and internal influences. In clinical settings, this is promoted by obtaining informed consent from the client. Therefore, it requires that health personnel obtain a patient's informed consent, not only for the treatment but also for the participation in a research.

Non-maleficence: Non-maleficence means duty to do no harm. This is promoted by doing the following nursing interventions:

1. Avoiding deliberate harm or the risk of harm that occurs during the performance of nursing actions.
2. Considering the degree of risk permissible.
3. Determining whether the use of technological advances provides benefits that outweigh risks.

Beneficence: Beneficence is doing actions for the promotion of good. Beneficence principles state that the actions one takes should promote good. It requires the balancing of harms and benefits. Benefits promote the clients' welfare and health, whereas harms or risks could cause deterioration in health and welfare. This is done by the following:

1. Providing health benefits to the clients
2. Balancing the benefits and risks of harm
3. Considering how a client can be best helped

Justice: Justice is the promotion of equity or fairness in every situation a nurse encounters in the care of the client. One of the crucial and distinctive features of this principle is avoiding exploitation and abuse of participants. The researcher understands that the application of the principle of justice in research studies is demonstrated by recognizing vulnerability of the participants and their contributions to the study.

The following nursing implications promote justice:

1. Ensuring fair allocation of resources among the patients
2. Determining the order in which clients should be treated

The following are the secondary principles of ethical conduct:

Veracity: It concerns telling the truth and incorporates the concept that individuals should always be told the truth. It requires professional caregivers to provide with accurate, reality-based information about their health status and care or treatment prospection. Truth telling is an ethical concern for nurses because truth is the basis for mutual trust between the patient and the nurse, and trust is the basis for patient's hope of benefits from nursing services.

Confidentiality: Maintaining confidentiality means that a nurse by legal and ethical standards keeps the information private, which the patients or the families have discussed, unless the information falls under a limit of confidentiality. Confidentiality is at the core of nurses, establishing trusting relationship with other nurses, patients, families, and others. The principle of confidentiality provides that caregivers should respect a patient's need for privacy and use personal information about him or her only to improve care.

Fidelity: Fidelity is keeping one's promises or commitments. The principle of fidelity holds that a person should be faithful towards his or her duties and obligations. Fidelity is important in a nurse because a patient's hope for relief and recovery rests on evidence of caregivers' conscientiousness.

CODE OF ETHICS FOR NURSES IN INDIA (CODE OF ETHICS AND PROFESSIONAL CONDUCT, INDIAN NURSING COUNCIL)

Introduction

The code of professional conduct for nurses is critical for building professionalism and accountability. Ethical consideration is vital in any area dealing with human beings because it represents values, rights, and relationship. A nurse must have professional competence, responsibility, and accountability with moral obligations. Nurses are obliged to provide services even if they are in conflict with their personal beliefs and values.

Purposes

The purpose of the code of professional conduct is to inform both the nurses and society of minimum standards for professional conduct. It provides the regulatory bodies a basis for decision-making regarding standards of professional conduct. The code of ethics helps to protect the rights of individuals, families, and community as well as the rights of nurses.

Uses of the Code

1. Acknowledges rightful place of individuals in the health care delivery system
2. Contributes towards empowerment of individuals to become responsible for their health and well-being

3. Contributes to quality care
4. Identifies obligations in practice, research, and relationship
5. Informs the individuals, families, communities, and other professionals about the expectations of a nurse

Code of Ethics for Nurses in India

1. Respect the uniqueness of individuals in provision of care. A nurse must perform the following:
   (a) Provide care for individuals without consideration of caste, creed, religion, culture, ethnicity, gender, socioeconomic or political status, personal attributes, or any other ground.
   (b) Individualize the care considering the beliefs, values, and cultural sensitivities.
   (c) Appreciate place for individuals in family and community and facilitate the participation of significant others in care.
   (d) Develop and promote a trustful relationship with individuals.
   (e) Recognize the uniqueness of response of an individual to interventions and adapt accordingly.
2. Respect the rights of individuals as partners in care and help in making informed choices. A nurse has the following responsibilities:
   (a) Appreciate individuals' right to make decisions about their care and therefore give adequate and accurate information for enabling them to make informed choices.
   (b) Respect the decision made by individuals regarding their care.
   (c) Protect the public from misinformation and misinterpretation.
   (d) Advocate special provisions to protect vulnerable individuals and groups.
3. Respect individuals' right to privacy, maintain confidentiality, and share information judiciously. A nurse must perform the following:
   (a) Respect the individuals' right to privacy of their personal information.
   (b) Maintain confidentiality of privileged information except in life threatening situations and use discretion in sharing information.
   (c) Take informed consent and maintain anonymity when information is required for quality assurance, academic, or legal reasons.
   (d) Limit the access to all personal records, written and computerized, only to authorized persons.
4. Maintain competence in order to render quality nursing care. A nurse must strive for the following:
   (a) Ensure nursing care is provided only by a registered nurse.
   (a) Maintain quality nursing care and uphold the standard of care.
   (b) Value continuing education initiatives and utilize all opportunities for self-development.
   (c) Value research as a means of development of nursing profession and participate in nursing research adhering to ethical principles.
5. Practise nursing in the framework of clinical, professional, and legal boundaries. A nurse is obliged to do the following:
   (a) Adhere to the code of ethics and code of professional conduct for nurses in India developed by the Indian Nursing Council.
   (b) Practice according to laws.

6. Work harmonically with members of the health team.
   (a) A nurse must appreciate the team's efforts in rendering care.
   (b) A nurse must cooperate, coordinate, and collaborate with the members of the health team to meet the needs of the patients.
7. Commit to reciprocate positive trust invested in nursing profession by society. A nurse must demonstrate personal etiquettes and attributes in all dealings.

Code of Professional Conduct for Nurses in India

1. **Professional Responsibility and Accountability:** A nurse has the following responsibilities:
   (a) Appreciate the sense of self-worth and nurture it.
   (b) Maintain standards of personal conduct reflecting credit upon the profession.
   (c) Carry out responsibilities within the framework of professional boundaries.
   (d) Be accountable for maintaining practice standards set by the Indian Nursing Council.
   (e) Be accountable for own decisions and actions.
   (f) Be compassionate.
   (g) Be responsible for continuous improvement of current practices.
   (h) Provide adequate information to individuals that allow them informed choices.
   (i) Practise behaviour that promotes health.
2. **Nursing Practice:** A nurse must ensure the following in nursing practice:
   (a) Provide care in accordance with set standards of practice.
   (b) Treat all individuals and their families with dignity in providing physical, psychological, emotional, social, and spiritual aspects of care.
   (c) Respect individuals and their families in the context of traditional and cultural practices, promoting healthy practices and discouraging harmful practices.
   (d) Present realistic picture truthfully in all situations, facilitating autonomous decision-making by individuals and families.
   (e) Promote participation of individuals and significant others in care.
   (f) Ensure safe practices.
   (g) Consult, coordinate, collaborate, and follow-up appropriately when individual care needs exceed the competence of the nurse.
3. **Communication and Inter Personal Relationships:** A nurse has the following duties:
   (a) Establish and maintain effective IPR with individuals, families, and communities.
   (b) Uphold dignity of team members and maintain effective Inter Personal Relationship (IPR) with them.
   (c) Appreciate and nurture professional role of team members.
   (d) Cooperate with other health professionals to meet the needs of the individuals, families, and communities.
4. **Valuing Human Beings:** A nurse needs to perform the following:
   (a) Take appropriate action to protect individuals from harmful unethical practices.
   (b) Consider relevant facts while taking decisions in the best interest of individuals.

(c) Encourage and support individuals in their right to speak for themselves on issues affecting their health and welfare.

(d) Respect and support the choice made by individuals.

5. **Management:** A nurse has the following responsibilities:
   (a) Ensure appropriate allocation and utilization of available resources.
   (b) Participate in supervision and education of students and other formal care providers.
   (c) Use judgement in relation to individual competence while accepting and delegating responsibility.
   (d) Facilitate conducive work culture in order to achieve institutional objectives.
   (e) Communicate effectively following appropriate channels of communication.
   (f) Participate in performance appraisal.
   (g) Participate in education of nursing services.
   (h) Participate in policy decisions, following the principles of equity and accessibility of services.
   (i) Work with individuals to identify their needs and sensitize policy makers and funding agencies for resource allocation.
6. **Professional Advancement:** A nurse must ensure the following:
   (a) Provide protection of human rights while pursuing the advancement of knowledge.
   (b) Contribute to development of nursing practice.
   (c) Participate in determining and implementing quality care.
   (d) Take responsibility for updating own knowledge and competencies.
   (e) Contribute to the core of professional knowledge and competencies.

Vulnerable Individuals

The following are the vulnerable individuals:

1. Children
2. Mentally or emotionally disabled people
3. Physically disabled people
4. The terminally ill
5. Institutionalized people
6. Pregnant women

Ethical Issues

Ethical issues are listed as follows:

1. Coercion of subject to participate
2. Withholding benefits from control subjects
3. Invasion of privacy
4. Proxy consents in research

5. Balancing potential benefits against actual cost
6. Maintaining anonymity and confidentiality

WAYS TO IMPROVE ATTENTION TOWARDS ETHICAL ISSUES IN PLANNING AND CONDUCT OF RESEARCH

Pay Attention to Study Design: For a research to be ethical, the study design must be scientifically sound. It should have sufficient power to test the hypothesis. A poorly designed and underpowered study would fail to provide an accurate and reliable answer to the research question, even though the question has been well framed. It is unethical to conduct a study with major flaws in its design.

Choose the Subjects without Bias: The principles of benevolence and justice require that we must choose our subjects without any bias. We must safeguard the rights of the poor, illiterate, disadvantaged, and vulnerable patients—the population that houses general wards of a public hospital. Fearful of the fact that the rich and the powerful can be 'problem subjects', researchers selectively exclude them in their study. For a study to be ethical, the inclusion and the exclusion criteria need to be described properly. When the subjects in a study are well chosen, its results can be applied to the population that will receive the interventions.

Enhance Benefits; Minimize Risks: Researchers are often confronted with difficult decisions that go well beyond the choice of drugs, devises, and interventions. They do not tell the subjects that during the study, some tests or procedures may harm them and that they might have to take more tests, pay more, and stay longer in the hospital because the study design demands so. Researcher should not callously disregard their welfare for the sake of research goals. According to the principles of nonmaleficence and beneficence, a researcher should minimize the risks by using procedures which are consistent with sound research design. He or she must ensure that the benefits from the research outweigh the risks.

Maintain Confidentiality: Inform the subjects about the extent to which personal information would be disclosed. Do not divulge identity and records of test subjects as far as possible. The investigator must make clear how privacy and confidentiality concerns will be approached. Researchers must be sensitive to not only how information is protected from unauthorized observation but also if and how participants are to be notified of any unforeseen findings from the research that they may or may not want to know. Avoid indirect exposure of identity. Providing information which will allow identity to be guessed should be discouraged. Ensure that the subject does not have to undergo any discrimination or stigmatization due to disclosure.

Have the Protocol Reviewed: Before a study begins, it must be approved by a research ethics committee (institutional review board). This ensures that the people who enroll in trials are informed what the study is about and how their welfare and rights will be protected.

Respect the Subject's Rights: The first principle of medical ethics (autonomy) requires us to respect people and their rights. Informed consent ensures that individuals can decide to participate only when the research is consistent with their values, interests, and preferences. Though written consent forms are used to document the consent, the process of informed consent is more important than a subject's signature on the form.

Special Considerations in case of Vulnerable Groups: Research involving vulnerable persons, which may include children, persons with developmental or cognitive disabilities, persons who are institutionalized, the homeless, or those without legal status, also raises unique issues in any research context. In case of pregnant women, ensure that there is no risk to the foetus or the mother.

Clinical Trials on Children as Subjects: Research involving children and youth raises unique ethical issues. These result primarily from related ideas of competence, autonomy, and vulnerability. Children have traditionally been considered as more vulnerable than adults because of their lack of competence to take part in decision-making around complex issues such as health care and inclusion in research. This vulnerability means that others (parents, legal guardians, health-care professionals, and educators) must be trusted to act in their best interests and make decisions for them.

ANALYSIS OR EVALUATION OF RISK/BENEFIT RATIO BY THE RESEARCHER

In designing a research study, carefully assess the risks and the benefits that would be incurred. The degree of risk should not exceed the potential benefits or knowledge to be gained. All researches involve some risks, but in many cases, risk is minimal. Minimal risk means risk anticipated to be no greater than those ordinarily encountered in daily life or during routine physical or psychological tests.

Major Potential Benefits to Participants

The following are the major benefits to the participants:

1. Access to an intervention that might otherwise be unavailable to them
2. Increased knowledge about themselves or their conditions, either through opportunity for introspection and self-reflection or through interaction with researchers
3. Escape from normal routine and excitement of being a part of a study
4. Satisfaction that information they provide may help others with similar problems or conditions
5. Direct monetary or material gains through stipends or other incentives

Major Potential Risks to Participants

Major potential risks to the participants are listed below:

1. Physical harm, including unanticipated side effects due to research interventions
2. Physical discomfort, fatigue, or boredom
3. Psychological or emotional distress resulting from self-disclosure, introspection, fear of the unknown, discomfort with strangers, anger, or embarrassment at the type of questions asked
4. Social risks such as the risk of stigma, adverse effects on personal relations, and loss of status
5. Loss of privacy
6. Loss of time
7. Monetary cost, for example, for transportation, child care, and time lost from work

Risk and Benefits (Algorithm)

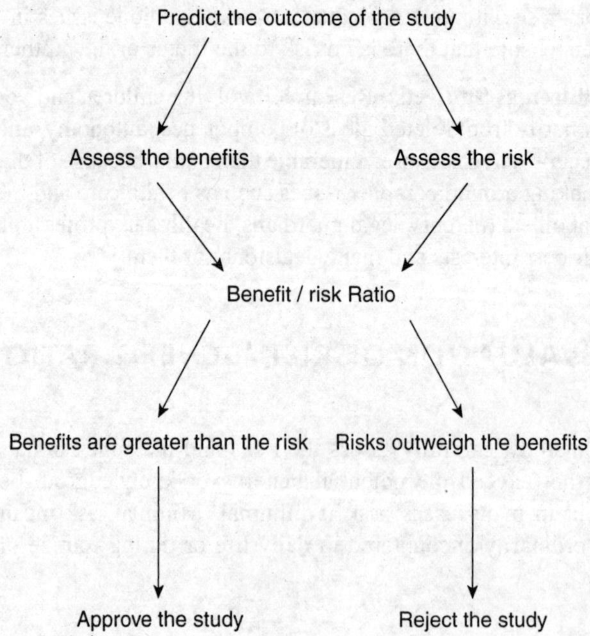

Informed Consent

Informed consent is one of the most important ways of legally protecting the research participants from any harm that is likely to occur during their participation in a research.

Informed consent means the participants have full information about the nature of research and its potential risks and benefits and are in a position to make rational decision about participating in a study.

Content of Informed Consent

Before signing the consent form, the following points must be discussed with the participants:

1. **Participant Status:** Prospective participants need to understand clearly the distinction between a research and a treatment.
2. **Study Goals:** The overall goals of the research should be stated in simple language.
3. **Type of Data:** Prospective participants should be told about the data that will be collected.
4. **Procedures:** Prospective participants should be given a description of the data collection procedures and procedures to be used in any innovative treatment.
5. **Nature of Commitment:** Information should be provided regarding the participant's estimated time commitments at each point of contact and number of contacts within specified time frames.
6. **Sponsorship:** Information on who is sponsoring or if the research is part of an academic requirement should be shared.
7. **Participant Selection:** Explain how prospective participants were selected for recruitment and how many will be participating in the research study.

8. **Potential Risks:** The participants should be informed about any foreseeable risks (physical, psychological, social, or economic).
9. **Potential Benefits:** Potential benefits should be described, as well as benefits to others.
10. **Alternatives:** If appropriate, researchers should provide information about alternative procedures or treatments that may be advantageous to participants.
11. **Compensation:** If stipends are to be paid, these should be discussed with the participants.
12. **Confidentiality Pledge:** Participants should be assured that their privacy will at all times be protected.
13. **Voluntary Consent:** Researcher should indicate that participation is strictly voluntary and failure to volunteer will not result in any penalty or loss of benefits.
14. **Right to Withdraw and Withhold Information:** Prospective participants should be told that even after consenting, they have the right to withdraw from the study and refuse to provide any specific information.
15. **Contact Information:** The researcher should give information on whom to contact in the event of further questions, comments, or complaints.

Documentation of Informed Consent

1. Researcher usually documents the informed consent after taking the participant's signature on the consent form.
2. Consent form should contain all required information essential for the participant.
3. Prospective participants should be given ample time to review the written document before signing it.
4. Document should also be signed by the researcher, and a copy should be retained by both the parties.

ETHICS COMMITTEE OR INSTITUTION REVIEW BOARDS

Ethics committees involve groups of individuals from diverse backgrounds who support health-care institutions with three major functions: providing ethics consultation, developing and/or revising select policies pertaining to clinical ethics.

Ethics committee or the institution review boards (IRB) have numerous protection responsibilities that include initial and continuing review of the study protocol and related documents, review of the documentation of informed consent, and review of reports of unanticipated problems (UAPs) and of adverse events (AEs).

The reporting of UAPs and AEs is an important mechanism of ensuring subject safety. The AE report needs to present an accurate and expanding picture of harms occurring during the study. When first formed, IRBs were expected to be able to monitor the progress of a clinical trial at their site, but such expectations have become unreasonable for multicentre studies and complex single-centre studies.

Role of Ethics Committee

The ethics committee is expected to play the following roles:

1. To promote the rights of the patients
2. To promote shared decision-making between the patients (or their surrogates if study participant is incapacitated) and their clinicians
3. To promote fair policies and procedures that maximize the likelihood of achieving good, patient-centred outcomes

Ethics committee comprises an eminent medical or nursing scientist, dean academics, head of the department of pharmacology, retired high court judge, a biomedical ethicist, non-medical person, social scientist, two clinicians, and a member secretary. There should be at least one female member.

This committee will examine all research projects involving human subjects directly or indirectly. It will also examine the complaints related to malpractice and issues related to 'conflict of interest' in scientific publications. This committee may also give opinion regarding ethical issues in matters referred to it from the government, state government, Indian Nursing Council (INC), State Nursing Council, and other statutory bodies. Due to enormous increase in the workload for the ethics committee, there are various sub-committees with a different set of members. As under Baba Farid University of Health Sciences, there is a sub- committee in University College of Nursing, Faridkot, with a set of members that examines the thesis and dissertation proposals for masters and PhD programs.

RIGHTS AND RESPONSIBILITIES OF RESEARCHERS AND INSTITUTIONS

Relationship between Researchers and institutions

1. Institutions have the responsibility to respect the autonomy of researchers and the ethical guidelines for a research.
2. Institutions should create and maintain an environment with adequate support system to enable researchers to follow ethical guidelines.
3. Institutions have the responsibility to take appropriate and adequate steps for protection against pressures to the observance of ethical guidelines for a research.

Protection and Promotion of Integrity in Research

1. Researcher should select a research project that he or she is interested in and one that will be useful for the society.
2. Researcher should not undertake classified research or research whose findings are to be kept confidential. Researcher has the right as well as the responsibility to make all necessary efforts to bring the research and its findings to the public domain in an appropriate manner.
3. Researcher has a responsibility towards the interest of those involved in or affected by this work. All concerned should make reasonable efforts to anticipate or to guard against possible misuse and undesirable or harmful consequences of a research.
4. Researcher should ensure that there is honesty and transparency at every stage of the research as these are indispensable for a good and ethical research.
5. Researcher should ensure that there is no fabrication, falsification, plagiarism, or unethical practices at any stage of the research and that the findings of the research are reported accurately and truthfully.
6. Researcher must ensure respect, protection, and promotion of the rights of the participants.

Relationship among Researchers

1. A principal researcher is responsible for the ethical conduct of research by all juniors, assistants, students, and trainees. At the same time, juniors, assistants, students, and trainees have an equal responsibility for ethical conduct.

2. No researcher should engage personally or professionally in discriminatory, harmful, or exploitative practices or any perceived form of harassment.
3. In addition to researchers, other individuals such as administrative staff of the organization conducting research or setting that may be associated, all of them should be briefed on ethical issues and guidelines, including the need to protect the rights of the participants and confidentiality of identifiable data.

Data Sharing

1. Sharing of data should be done in the form which is consistent with the interests and rights of the participants.
2. By sharing data with the other researchers involved in particular research, all necessary measures to maintain the confidentiality should be taken and followed.

ETHICAL DILEMMAS FOR NURSES

1. Vulnerable groups include children, mentally sick, severely ill, physically disable, terminally ill, pregnant women, and institutionalized individuals. How to safeguard them is nurse's concern.
2. Nurses mainly undertake nursing procedure which would benefit the recipient. Interventional studies pose a dilemma that to exclude individuals in control group is to deprive them of the benefits of the intervention; therefore, nurses, to deal with this type of dilemma, mostly take up 'one group pre- and post-test design' instead of a true experimental study.
3. Health education to experimental group and the control group is deprived of the benefits.
4. Nurses face psychological probing in qualitative studies such as how they cope up. Children of parents with terminal illness may cause mental trauma to the parents.
5. Testing a new drug on one-group testing may have enhancement of life spam. This group is exposed to potential side effects, whereas the other group is denied of potential beneficial effects.
6. Faith in the nurses leads the participants to share the secrets of their lives such as Alzheimer's disease or old age issues.

GUIDELINES FOR CRITICIZING ETHICAL ASPECT OF A RESEARCH

1. Was the study approved by the ethics committee?
2. Did the researcher take appropriate steps to minimize harm and maximize benefits?
3. Did the benefits overweigh the risks or actual comfort?
4. Was any pressure used to recruit the participants into the study?
5. Was the Informed consent taken?
6. Were adequate steps taken to safeguard the participant's privacy?
7. Were vulnerable groups involved? If yes, were special precautions taken?
8. Was any other ethical reason relevant to the study taken into the consideration?
9. Were the subjects told how could they get the results of the study?
10. Were the subjects provided the opportunity to ask questions and ensured the contact means of the researcher if other questions to ask or any complication arise?

KEY POINTS

- Research ethics are a set of principles or guidelines that will assist the researcher in making difficult research decisions and in deciding which goals are most important in reconciling conflicting values.
- In the light of many atrocities which were done on vulnerable human beings in the name of medical research and in response to human rights violation, 'code of ethics', called the NUREMBERG Code, was first developed for research in 1947.
- Research participants can be exposed to a number of risks while going through the research such as physical harm, psychological harm, financial harm, and also social harm. Research can also benefit the participant in some way.
- It is, therefore, essential that the researcher carefully evaluates the potential for harm through the intended research study and ensures that he or she is well aware of the ethical standards and takes every step not to cause any harm to the study participants.
- Informed consent is one of the most important ways of legally protecting the research participants from any harm that is likely to occur in a research on them. It means the participants have full information about the nature of the research and its potential risks and benefits and are in a position to make rational decision about participating in a study.
- Ethics committee or the Institution Review Boards (IRB) has numerous protection responsibilities that include initial and continuing review of the study protocol and related documents, review of the documentation of informed consent, and review of the reports of unanticipated problems (UAPs) and of adverse events (AEs).
- Nurse scientists confront many dilemmas in conducting research, which they need to thoughtfully solve.

QUESTIONS

I. Essay-type Questions

1. (a) Define ethics and code of ethics.

   (b) Discuss briefly the importance of ethical consideration in research.
2. Describe the risk/benefit ratio of research.
3. Describe the ethical principles to be considered in planning and conducting the research.
4. Chalk out the format of an informed consent form for interventional study?
5. Describe in brief the rights and responsibilities of researchers and institutions?

II. Short Notes

1. Types of ethical principles
2. Historical development of ethics in nursing research
3. Content of informed consent
4. Constitution of ethical board or committee
5. Potential benefits to study subjects

III. Multiple-choice Questions

Circle the alphabet before the best answer

1. ICN was established in
   (a) 1699 (b) 1799
   (c) 1899 (d) 1999
2. Example of recent disregard for ethical consideration is
   (a) Gazi experiments
   (b) Nazi experiments
   (c) Kazi experiments
   (d) None of above
3. An international code of ethics for nurses was first adopted by ICN in
   (a) 1943 (b) 1953
   (c) 1963 (d) 1973
4. Which one of the following is the primary ethical principle?
   (a) Veracity (b) Fidelity
   (c) Justice (d) Confidentiality
5. Which one of the following is the secondary ethical principle?
   (a) Beneficence (b) Justice
   (c) Fidelity (d) All of the above

Answer Keys

1. (c) 2. (b) 3. (b) 4. (c) 5. (a)

FURTHER READING

Field P. A., Morse J. M. 1985. *Nursing Research: The Application of Qualitative Approaches*: Taylor & Francis.

Holloway I, Wheeler S. 'Ethical Issues in Qualitative Nursing Research'. *Nursing Ethics*. 1995; 2(3): 223.

http://icmr.nic.in/ethics_SOP.pdf

http://nursingcrib.com/nursing-notes-reviewer/fundamentals-of-nursing/ethical principles/

http://www.columbia.edu/~mvp19/RMC/M5/QualEthics.pdf

http://www.icn.ch/images/stories/documents/about/icncode_english.pdf

http://www.jblearning.com/samples/0763748986/48986_ch03_pass3.pdf

http://www.who.int/ethics/topic/en

Kerr Ross C. Janet, Wood J. Marilynn. 2006. *Basic Steps in Planning Nursing Research*, Jones and Barlett Publishers.

Munhall L. Patricia. 2001. *Nursing Research: A Qualitative Perspective*, Jones and Barlett Publishers.

Polit D. F., Beck C. T. 2003. *Nursing Research: Principles and Methods*. Lippincott Williams and Wilkins.

Potter P. A., Perry A. G. 2005. *Fundamental of Nursing*. St.Louis: Mosby.

Raj Bhaskara. 2010. *Nursing Research and Biostatics*. Emmess Medical Publishers.

Tolsma Hastings T. Marie, Brockopp Young Dorothy. 2003. *Fundamentals of Nursing Research*. Jones and Barlett Publishers.

Williamson G. R., Prof. S. 'Action Research: Politics, Ethics and Participation'. *Journal of Advanced Nursing* 2002; 40(5):587.

chapter 7

Quantitative and Qualitative Research Approaches and Designs

OBJECTIVES

Upon completion of this chapter the learner will be able to:

- Define qualitative and quantitative approaches
- Describe the terms used in these approaches
- List the main types of qualitative and quantitative research designs
- Discuss methods of qualitative and quantitative research approaches in nursing
- Explain the advantages and disadvantages of these approaches

INTRODUCTION

After going through the descriptions of various types of researches, one fact that comes to light is that there are two basic approaches to research, namely quantitative approach and qualitative approach. This chapter deals briefly with these two approaches to research. An attempt has been made to relate them with examples from nursing research.

Research design is the researcher's overall plan for obtaining answers to the research questions. It spells out the basic strategies that the researcher adopts to gather information that is accurate and interpretable. Research design comprises methodological decisions that the researcher makes to accomplish the objectives of the research project.

QUANTITATIVE RESEARCH APPROACH

What is Quantitative Research?

Quantitative research is a formal, objective, and systematic process. It is used to describe variables, test relationships between variables, and examine cause and effect interactions among variables. The quantitative research process involves conceptualizing, planning, implementing, and communicating the findings of a quantitative research project. It involves generation of data in quantitative form, which can be subjected to vigorous quantitative analysis in a formal and rigid fashion. Quantitative research is conducted to describe new situations, events, or concepts, for example, determining the effectiveness of home remedies on the health of post-natal mothers and newborns.

Review of the Terms Relevant to Quantitative Research

In order to understand quantitative research, it is necessary to comprehend the following important terms:

1. **Basic Research or Pure Research:** According to Miller (1991), this is scientific investigation that involves pursuit of 'knowledge for knowledge's sake'. Basic scientific investigation is undertaken to seek new knowledge about health phenomenon with the hope of establishing general principles.

The purpose of basic research is to generate and refine theory; thus, the findings, often, are not directly useful in practice. Basic nursing research on physiological variables might include laboratory investigations in animals or humans to develop principles regarding physiological functioning, pathological processes, or the effects of treatments on physiological and pathological functioning. These studies might focus on the increasing understanding of oxygenation, perfusion, fluid and electrolyte balance, acid–base status, eating and sleeping patterns of comfort status, and patho-physiology of the immune system. Basic research is often implemented in laboratories with animals to examine the effects of the proposed intervention and usually precedes or is the basis for applied research.

2. **Applied Research or Practical Research:** This is scientific investigation undertaken to generate knowledge that will directly influence or improve clinical practice. The purpose of applied research is to solve problems, make decisions, and predict or control outcomes in real-life practice situations. The findings from applied studies can also be invaluable to policy makers as a basis for making changes to policies that address health and social problems. For example, the treatment of bedsore with insulin dressing is a result of applied research. Many of the studies conducted in nursing are applied because the nurse researchers have chosen to focus on clinical problems and testing of nursing interventions to improve patient outcomes. Applied research is also used to test theory and validate its usefulness in clinical practice. Often, the new knowledge discovered through basic research is examined for usefulness in practice by applied research, thus making these approaches complementary.

Rigour in Quantitative Research

Striving for excellence in research is rigour. It requires discipline, adherence to detail, and strict accuracy. It is essential for a tightly controlled study design for development of quantitative studies to have logical, deductive, or inductive reasoning. Meticulous details are logically linked, and specific steps are used to develop the research process. These steps, such as design, measurement, sample, data collection, and statistical analysis, must be examined for weaknesses and errors. Precision, which encompasses accuracy, detail, and order, is another important aspect of rigour. It is evident in the concise statement of research purpose and detailed development of the study design. The measurement or quantification of the study variables is most important in precision. For example, a researcher might use a glucose strip to measure and record the presence of sugar in the urine rather than doing a urine test with Benedict's solution and recording it on a data collection sheet. Other important elements are the precise measuring tools and a representative sample.

Type and Designs of Quantitative Research

Quantitative research is classified into various types as follows:

1. Non-experimental or descriptive
   - (a) Comparative
   - (b) Correlational
   - (c) Survey
   - (d) Developmental studies
     - (i) Longitudinal
     - (ii) Cross-sectional
   - (e) Epidemiological studies
     - (i) Case control
     - (ii) Cohort

Some other non-experimental researches are evaluation research, impact analysis, implementation analysis, outcome analysis, cost–benefit analysis, need assessment, meta-analysis, and meta-synthesis.

2. Experimental or interventional
   (a) Experimental
   (b) Quasi-experimental

The type of research conducted is influenced by the current knowledge of a research problem. Descriptive studies are often conducted when little knowledge on the problem is available. With the increase in knowledge level, correlational, quasi-experimental, and experimental studies are conducted.

Non-experimental or Descriptive Research

The following are the salient features of a non-experimental or descriptive research:

1. It is the exploration and description of phenomenon in real-life situations. It provides an accurate account of the characteristics of particular individuals, situations, or groups. It attempts to describe what exists, determine the frequency with which something occurs, discover new meaning, and categorize the information obtained. Development of theory or description, which provides a basis for future quantitative research, is the outcome of descriptive research, which also includes the description of concepts and identification of relationships.
2. Descriptive research relies on observation as a means of collecting data. Depending on the type of information sought, participants can be interviewed, questionnaires distributed, and visual records, including sounds and smells, made. It is also important that the observations made are written down or recorded in an organized form and presented in a clear and systematic way for subsequent analysis of data, resulting in valid and accurate conclusions.
3. To save unnecessary work and to give accurate information on the subject of research, the sample of people or events surveyed must be carefully selected and delineated so that specific objectives can be formulated. It does not involve manipulation of variables, and variables are studied as they exist in the real world.
4. Since descriptive research depends on human observations and responses, there is a danger of distortion of data, which can be caused by inadvertently including biased questions in the questionnaires and interviews or through selective observation of events. The researcher needs to be aware of these facts. In order to reduce the element of bias, operational definitions of variables, large sample size, random sampling techniques, valid and reliable research tools, and formal data collection methods should be adopted.

Examples of Descriptive Research Studies: The following are examples of descriptive research studies:

1. A descriptive study on the incidence of constipation among patients admitted in the orthopaedic wards of Safdarjung Hospital, New Delhi
2. A descriptive study on the prevalence of back ache among nurses working in the critical care units of Devi Shetty Hospital, Kolkata, West Bengal

Comparative Research: Comparative designs are the same as descriptive but the researcher tries to compare data between certain populations such as rural and urban, males and females, or between age groups. Comparative research is carried out in experimental studies as well.

Correlational Research: *Correlation* is a word used to describe the measure of association or the relationship between two phenomena. Correlational research involves systematic investigation of relationships between or among variables. The information sought in correlational research is expressed in numbers, and depending on the nature of data, various statistical techniques are used to find the meaning of the numerical data. The researcher measures the selected variables in a sample and then uses correlational statistics to determine the relationships among variables, whereby the researcher is able to determine the degree or strength and type (positive or negative) of relationship between variables. The strength of relationship varies ranging from –1 (perfect negative correlational) to +1 (perfect positive correlational), with '0' indicating no relationship. A positive relationship indicates that the variables vary together, that is, both variables either increase or decrease together. For example, research has shown that an increase in the amount of alcohol consumed increases the risk for liver damage. A negative relationship indicates that the variables vary in opposite directions, that is, as one variable increases the other will decrease. For example, research has shown that an increase in the quantity and duration of alcohol intake is correlational with decrease in life span.

In general, correlational studies have independent and dependent variables, but the effect of the independent variable on the dependent variable is observed without manipulating the independent variable.

The primary intent of correlational studies is to explain the nature of relationship in the real world and not to determine the cause and effect. However, correlational studies are the means for generating hypothesis to guide quasi-experimental and experimental studies that do focus on examining cause and effect relationships. One of the advantages of correlational research is that it allows for the measurement of a number of characteristics (technically called variables) and their relationships. Unlike other research approaches, correlational research produces a measure of the amount of relationship between the variables being studied, and when used in prediction studies, it gives an estimate of the probable accuracy of the predictions made.

Surveys, developmental studies such as longitudinal and cross-sectional, and epidemiological studies such as case control and cohort fall under the descriptive and comparative non-experimental designs.

Advantages and disadvantages of non-experimental research:

Advantages: Non-experimental research designs are better depictive of the real-life situation as the variables under study are not subjected to any kind of experiment. Furthermore, there are certain cases in which conducting an experimental study is not practically feasible (may be on account of ethical reasons or others); in such cases, non-experimental researches are more suitable.

Disadvantages: The main disadvantage of non-experimental research design is that it involves non-random selection of study subjects. Hence, the results obtained are not completely error free and this ultimately affects the authenticity and generalizability of the findings.

Experimental or Interventional Research Design

Experimental designs have the following three essential properties:

1. **Randomization:** The experimenter assigns the subjects to control or experimental group on a random basis.
2. **Control:** The experimenter introduces control over the experimental situation and makes a control group, which does not receive the intervention.
3. **Manipulation:** The experimenter does something (manipulate or treat) to at least some of the subjects (experimental group) in the study. There is some type of intervention done to the experimental group.

Experimental designs are objective, systematic, and highly controlled investigations carried out for the purpose of predicting and controlling phenomena in nursing practice. In the experimental study, the causality between the independent and the dependent variables is examined under highly controlled conditions. Because of vigorous control of variables, experimental research is considered the most powerful quantitative method of research.

Advantages of Experimental Design: The following are the advantages of experimental design:

1. It is most scientific in nature.
2. It gives the most reliable *cause and effect* relationship.
3. It is the most authentic method.
4. Randomized controlled trial (RCT) is placed at the highest level on the evidence-based practice pyramid.

Disadvantages of Experimental Design: Despite the advantages of experimental research, this type of design has several limitations.

1. There are a number of constraints that make a true experimental approach impractical or impossible in most nursing situations.
2. Experiments are sometimes criticized for their artificiality.
3. Random controls are not always possible in human interaction.
4. Hawthorne effect or the knowledge of being included in a study may be sufficient to cause people to change their behaviour. The same is the case with placebo effect.

Quasi-experimental Design

Quasi-experimental research design looks quite similar to an experimental design. It also involves manipulation of an independent variable. However, quasi-experimental designs lack at least one of the two other properties, that is, either randomization or control.

Quasi-experimental research design is undertaken to examine the causal relationships or to determine the effect of one variable on another. It has an element of manipulation of independent variable to observe the effect on the dependent variable. As mentioned already, this approach lacks at least one of the two other essential characteristics of a true experiment, that is, random assignment of the subject or a control group. Quasi-experimental studies involve implementing a treatment and examining the effects of the treatment using selected methods of measurement. These studies usually lack a certain amount of control over the manipulation of the treatment, management of the setting, or selection of the subjects. When studying human behaviour, especially in clinical settings, researchers are often unable to randomly select the subjects or to manipulate or control certain variables related to the subjects or the setting. Thus, nurse researchers conduct more quasi-experimental studies than experimental studies. Since not all the conditions of true experimental study designs can be fulfilled in a quasi-experimental study, the nature of the shortcoming is recognized and steps are taken to minimize them or predict a level of reliability of the result.

The study varies according to the population studied, the variables examined, the environment of the study, and the degree or control achieved in the experiment. A researcher using an experimental design is an active agent rather than a passive observer. The study is undertaken in a laboratory or research facility and must take into account the extent to which it is possible to control the variables. The application of control is difficult when studies are conducted in natural settings on human subjects. Hence, experiment design is not feasible to use in nursing research. Quasi-experimental, pre-experimental, or non-experimental designs are undertaken more frequently.

Types of Quasi-experimental Research: The following are the various types of quasi-experimental research:

1. Pre-test–post-test design
2. After only design or post-test only design

3. Solomon four-group design
4. Pre-experimental study, non-equivalent control group post-test only design
5. Time series design

Why do Nurse Scientists Mostly Opt For Non-experimental Approach?

The following are the reasons for nurse scientists opting for the non-experimental approach of research:

1. A vast number of human characteristics are inherently not subject to experimental manipulation (health beliefs, personality, cultural effect, etc.). Therefore, the effect of these on response to treatment cannot be studied experimentally or objectively.
2. Human behaviour is of primary interest to nurses, but for ethical reasons, many a times it is not possible to use experimentation on humans.
3. Administrative and financial constraints and inconvenience of staff also make experimental research impossible.
4. Some research questions are not suitable for experimental design, for example, finding out prevalence.

Control in Quantitative Research

Control in quantitative research is achieved by the researcher imposing rules to decrease the possibility of error, thereby increasing the probability of the study's findings being an accurate reflection of reality. The rules used to achieve control in research are referred to as design. Various degrees of control ranging from *mildly controlled* or *not controlled* that is, descriptive, to *highly controlled*, that is, experimental, are included depending on the type of the study. Descriptive and correlational studies often are designed with little or no researcher control, because the subjects are examined as they exist in their natural setting such as office, home, or school. The focus of quasi-experimental studies is on determining the effectiveness of a treatment (independent variable) in producing a desired outcome (dependent variable) in a partially controlled setting. So, these studies are conducted with more control in the selection of study subjects, implementation of the treatment planned, and the measurement of dependent variables.

Through control, the researcher can reduce the influence of extraneous variables, which exist in all studies and can interfere with obtaining a clear understanding or insight of the relationships among study variables. For example, if a study is focused on the effect of relaxation therapy on perception of labour pain, the researcher would have to control the extraneous variables such as the administration of drugs for relief of pain, frequent disturbance in care, noise, and facilities in the labour room to prevent their influence on the women's perception of labour pain. Selecting women with labour pain who are admitted in a separate cabin and administering no drug for pain relief would control some of these extraneous variables.

In quantitative research, both random and non-random samples are used. Descriptive studies are often conducted on non-probability samples in which the subjects are selected on the basis of convenience. Since a randomly selected sample is very difficult to obtain in nursing research, quantitative studies are often conducted with convenience sample.

In quasi-experimental and experimental studies, the subjects who are a part of convenience sample are often randomly assigned to the treatment group or to the control group (no treatment). This is done to increase the control and rigour of a study. The research setting, that is, the location in which a study is conducted, is either natural, partially controlled, or highly controlled.

Steps in Quantitative Research

The quantitative research process involves conceptualizing a research project, planning and implementing that project, and communicating the findings. There is a logical flow of the research process as one step builds progressively on another.
Figure 7.1 is an example of a quasi-experimental research design.

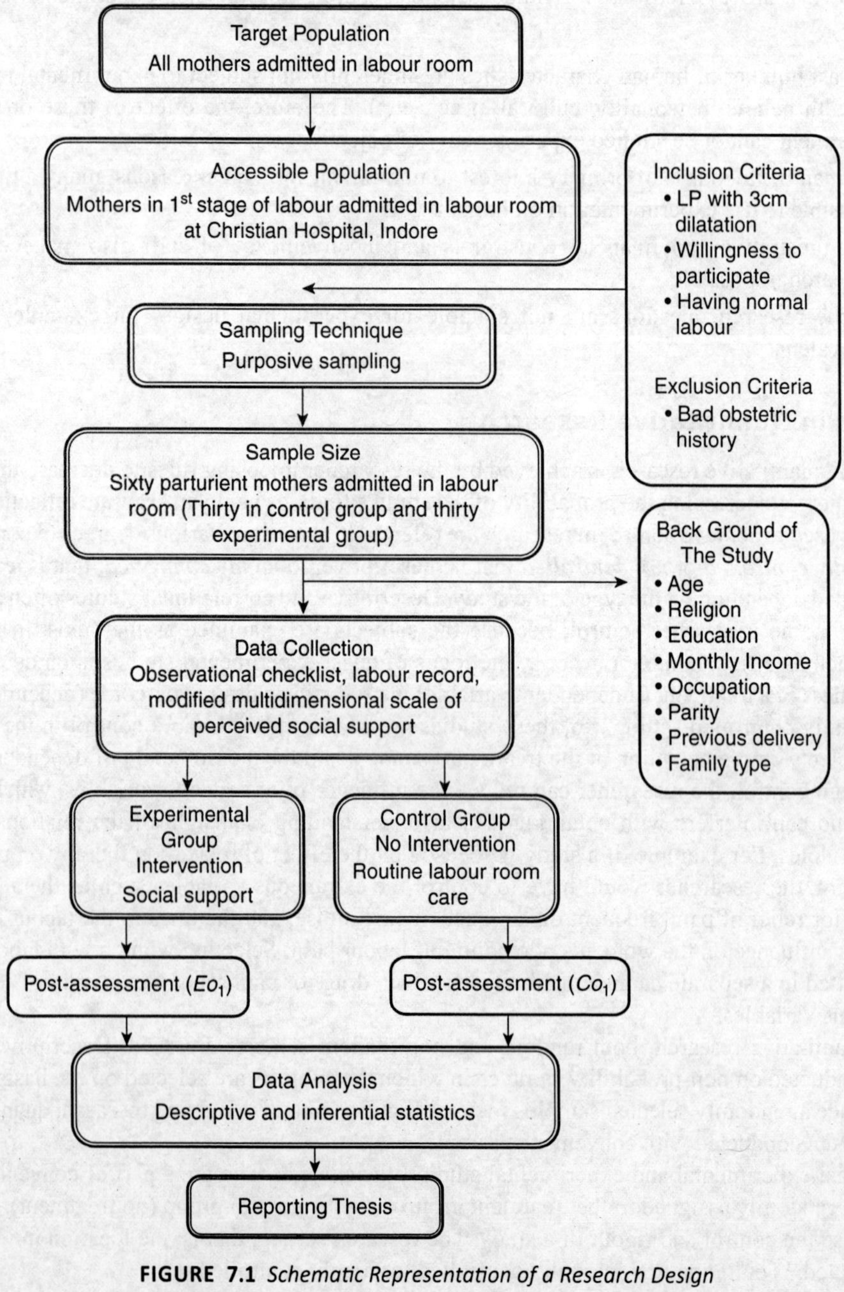

FIGURE 7.1 *Schematic Representation of a Research Design*

QUALITATIVE RESEARCH APPROACH

Qualitative research approach is concerned with the subjective assessment of attitudes, opinions, and behaviours. It is a systematic, subjective, and methodological approach used to describe life experiences and give them meaning. This approach to research generates results either in non-quantitative form or in the forms that are not subjected to rigorous quantitative analysis. The qualitative research approach is not a new idea in social or behavioural sciences. Nursing profession's interest in qualitative research problems began in the late 1970s.

The terminology and methods of reasoning used in qualitative research differ from those used in more traditional quantitative research methods and reflect alternative philosophical orientations. The specific philosophical orientation of each approach directs the research methods. Although qualitative approach is unique, there are many commonalities between this approach and the quantitative approach.

Philosophical View of Qualitative Research Approach

Qualitative research approaches are based on a world view that is holistic and may incorporate the following beliefs:

1. There are multiple constructed realities.
2. The knower and the known are inseparable.
3. Enquiry is value bound.
4. All generalizations are bounded by time and context.

Qualitative research provides a process in which nurses can examine a phenomenon outside traditional views.

Characteristics of Qualitative Research Design

The following are some of the characteristics of qualitative research design:

1. The approach tends to be holistic in nature, striving for an understanding of the whole.
2. The researcher's intense involvement is needed, which demands commitment for longer periods in the field of study.
3. Qualitative research design emerges as study advances.
4. The designs are flexible and can be adjusted to the information being gathered during data collection. Sometimes, when it is not feasible to collect the data as planned, the same can be rescheduled according to the convenience of the study subjects, facilities available, and so on.
5. For collecting useful, detailed information on qualitative research, the designs typically merge the various strategies of data collection.
6. The designs require ongoing data analysis for the formation of subsequent strategies and to determine when further field work should be done. As mentioned earlier, this requires the researcher's involvement in the collection of data, and thus, one might have to spend more time than planned.
7. At times, qualitative research designs also require the researchers to become research instruments for data collection.

Phases of Qualitative Research Approach

The exact form of a qualitative research design cannot be known and be specified in advance. The researcher generally goes through three main phases when embarking upon a qualitative research design.

First Phase: This phase involves the orientation and overview of the problem at hand, and the researchers only presume the type of knowledge that is expected to be obtained by undertaking this particular study. They are also not familiar with the phenomenon that will drive the enquiry forward. To understand better, the researchers initially attempt to get an overview of the salient features of interest. They have to go through various literature reviews, which will enable further understanding of the research study.

Qualitative data collection is usually done by three main methods:

1. Participants are asked verbally to describe their experiences of the phenomenon by *interactive interviewing.*
2. Participants are asked to *write descriptions* of their experiences of the phenomenon.
3. *Descriptive observation* of verbal and non-verbal behaviour of the study participants is done.

One may be surprised by the sheer volume of data and the detailed level of analysis that result even when the research undertaken involves a small number of participants.

Second Phase: This phase involves focused attention given on the salient aspects of the phenomenon under study, followed by an in-depth exploration of the prominent, conspicuous aspects of the phenomenon. During this phase, a variety of people related to the field are invited to participate in the study. They are asked more questions to gather more information about the phenomenon. The questions are asked based on the understanding developed during the first phase of the design.

Third Phase: This is the final phase of qualitative design. Much effort is undertaken to ensure and to establish that the findings gathered are trustworthy. Furthermore, the researchers confirm their understanding and findings by analysing and discussing with study participants to reaffirm the authenticity, or correctness, of their findings, following which the study is finally closed.

Importance of Qualitative Research

Qualitative research is important for the following reasons:

1. The methodology undertaken in qualitative research contributes a great deal in nursing studies. Nursing researchers have appreciated the contribution of qualitative research approach, because it is a discipline that helps and encourages the building of a knowledge base in the process of clarifying how nursing sciences should be developed.
2. The methods followed in qualitative research enable the researchers to study social and cultural phenomena, thus contributing to social sciences.
3. Being an inductive approach for discovering and expanding knowledge, it includes the researcher's involvement in the identification of meaning or relevance of a particular phenomenon to the individual.
4. Qualitative strategies are useful for exploring facts and developing concepts about an area that has received very little research attention.

Types of Qualitative Research

Six approaches to qualitative research used in nursing are briefly discussed here. They are historical, phenomenological, ethnographic, grounded theory, case study, and action research.

Historical Research in Nursing

One of the assumptions of historical philosophy is that it is possible to learn from the past. The philosophy of history is a search for wisdom in which the historians examine what has been, what is, and what ought to be. An attempt is made by a historical philosopher to identify a developmental scheme for history to explain all events and structures as elements of the same social process.

Historical research has been defined 'as the systematic and objective location, evaluation, and synthesis of evidence in order to establish facts and draw conclusions about past events'.

One of the criteria of a profession is that knowledge of the history of the profession is transmitted to those entering the profession. Until recently, historical nursing research was not considered a valued activity. Few nurse researchers had the skills or desire to undertake a historical research. Therefore, knowledge of nursing history is sketchy. However, there is a growing interest in the field of historical nursing research.

Lusk suggests the following about nursing research: The topics should be significant with a potential to illuminate or place a new perspective on current questions, thus contributing to scholarly understanding. They should also be feasible in terms of data and resource availability. Finally, the topics should be intriguing and capable of sustaining the interest of the researcher.

Historical approach is past-oriented and is used if the researcher believes that the answer to the question lies in the past. Relevant data of the past occurrence are systematically gathered and critically evaluated. Historical research approach provides a better understanding of what has happened in the past and thus gives an insight into present happenings.

Historical research examines the events of the past and explores the meaning and relationship of events. As its resource, primary historical data in the form of historic artefacts, records, writings, minutes of the meeting, photographs, and documentary films are used for data collection. Firstly, primary historical data must be scrutinized to ascertain whether the artefact or document to be studied is genuine. Secondly, the written evidence in the form of historic documents needs to be examined for authenticity of the content. This is important because many medieval texts are known to be very inaccurate and vague in their description of events. Secondary sources of data, such as encyclopaedias, textbooks, and almanacs, are second-hand accounts of past events provided by someone other than a reliable observer or witness.

The following are some of the values of historical research:

1. It provides solutions to problems that have occurred in the past and the findings obtained may shed light on the contemporary problems.
2. It throws light on present and future trends.
3. It allows the scope for revaluation of data, supporting hypotheses, theories, and generalizations that are presently held about the past.
4. It stresses the relative importance and the effects of the interactions that are found within all cultures.

Historical research is not purely based on scientific method, because the data used are seldom based on direct observation or experimentation. However, it should share many of the disciplines of scientific methods, such as objectivity, minimizing the scope of bias, distortion, use of chemical and radioactive analysis, and statistics. It must be noted that mere collection of historic facts or the setting up of chronological events does not constitute research.

The research students, whatever may be their field of study, must undertake a review of literature, because it helps the researcher to be aware of what has been done and written in the past. So, the principles of historic research can be seen to be of direct work relevance to this part of their research.

Developing an Inventory of Sources: Many of the materials for historical research are available in private archives and libraries or are privately owned. The researcher must take written permission to gain access to the library archives. The private materials are often difficult to locate, and even when they are discovered, access to them may be a problem.

Letters, memos, handwritten materials, and mementoes of significant nursing leaders are being discarded, because no one recognizes their value as an important source of data for historical research in nursing; the same applies to institutions and agencies with which nursing has been involved. Sometimes, when such materials are found, it is in such a poor condition that much of the material is unclear or completely lost, broken, rusty, and dilapidated; many ancient papers may crumble into dust while being handled as a source of primary data. Conduct of historical research can be both depressing and stimulating. It is depressing because of the lack of care provided to the priceless material and is stimulating because a rich mine of data is available.

Determining the Validity and Reliability of Data of Historical Research: The validity and reliability concerns in historical research are related to the sources from which the data are collected. A primary source of material—material written by a person who experienced an event and the letters and other mementoes saved by the person being studied—is most likely to shed true light on the information the researcher seeks. The secondary source is written by someone who previously read and summarized the primary source material. Textbooks and history books are secondary source materials. Primary sources are considered more valid and reliable than secondary sources.

To consider the validity and reliability, authenticity and accuracy, of primary sources of data in historical research, two strategies have been developed, viz. external and internal criticism. External criticism is used to determine the validity of the source material. The researcher needs to know where, when, why, and by whom a document was written. This may involve verifying the handwriting or determining the age of the paper on which it was written. Internal criticism is the examination of the reliability of the document. The researcher must determine the possible biases of the author. Two independent sources that provide the same information are needed to verify the accuracy of a statement. In addition, the researcher must ensure that he or she understands the statements made by the writer because words and their meanings change across time and across culture. It is also possible to read into a document a meaning not originally intended by the author.

Collecting the Data for Historical Research: Data collection for pertinent material may require months, years, or even a decade of dedicated searching. This is because there is no clear, obvious end to data collection. The researcher with the help of the guide has to make a decision to discontinue the collection of data. The researcher has to be persistent and optimistic and use patience in the long and sometimes discouraging search. One also has to be very skilful in the meticulous recording of data with every detail being complete. Logical classification of the data is necessary to help in analysis, drawing inferences, and so on.

Areas of historical study may be undertaken on periods of development (nursing during Mughal period) or particular geographical location (cities, continents, countries, areas, etc.); military nursing history studies the various weapons used during wars and riots and the military strategies used, including the effect of these events on the health services of the society.

Writing the Research Report: Traditional formalized style that is mostly used in writing a research report is not followed in historical research. The report may appear to be deceptively simple. The reader may not recognize the extensive work that was required to write the paper, as the studies are designed to attract the interest of the reader.

Disadvantages of Historical Research: Although historical study is a challenging task for a researcher, its value to nursing has been recognized of late. There is an attempt by nurse researchers to undertake historical research, though they are aware of some of its disadvantages such as the following:

1. The investigator must rely on finding data that already exist and cannot develop new data.
2. The researcher cannot alter the form in which the data appear but must attempt to understand them in their existing form.

3. The investigator must analyse and interpret the meaning of data without the advantage of being able to ask clarifying questions.
4. The data available may be incomplete, having gaps in critical areas; the investigator must be able to translate terms, concepts, and ideas in the light of their historical period and context.
5. The researcher must overcome obstacles of time, resources, freedom of movement, and language to search for and evaluate data resources.
6. One cannot predict an accurate timetable for the completion of a historical study. The researcher must not only locate and evaluate the data but also develop insights that tie together these masses of data.

Examples of Historical Research Studies: The following are examples of historical research studies:

1. A historical study on the development of Tamil Nadu Nursing Council
2. A study (historical) on the development of military nursing
3. A study on the historical development of midwifery in India

Phenomenological Research

Phenomenon is an occurrence or a circumstance that impresses the observer as unusual or extraordinary or a thing that appears to and is constructed by the mind. Phenomena occur only when a person experiences them. An experience is considered unique to the individual.

Phenomenology as a philosophy has been the basis for a number of approaches to research. According to phenomenologists, a person is intrigued with the environment; the world shapes the self and the self shapes the world.

Phenomenological research approach to qualitative research is to trace out precisely the lived experiences of people and generate theories or models of phenomenon being studied. It is inductive, descriptive, and qualitative methodology developed from phenomenological philosophy for the purpose of describing experience as they are lived by the study participants.

Phenomenological research has mainly two approaches, namely descriptive and interpretive.

The purpose of descriptive phenomenological research is to describe experiences as they are lived and capture the lived experience of the study participants. It also involves the researchers' experience in collecting data for a study and in analysing the data.

The interpretive phenomenological study is to deal with or answer the query: 'What is the meaning of one's lived experience?' Because a person is self-interpretive, the only reliable source to answer this question is the person himself/herself. The central concern of nursing is *understanding human behaviour or experience*. It requires that the person interpret the action or experience for the researcher; the researcher then interprets the explanation provided by the person.

The primary sources of data collection in phenomenological research are the real-life situations of the individuals being studied. The most common means of data collection are in-depth interviews, that is, semi-structured audio-taped interviews with the participants. These are recorded in interview notes or audio tapes. Furthermore, the emerging themes are frequently validated with the participants because their meanings of that lived experience are central to the phenomenological study. People who have recently had the experience are selected. For example, a woman who has recently been diagnosed as a case of breast cancer can be interviewed for a study of psychological impacts of this medical condition. To assist the participants in describing lived experiences while at the same time setting aside researchers' own personal feelings, the *bracketing* technique is used. This technique involves building rapport, encouraging, listening while preparing what to ask next, keeping discussion on tract, and handling emotions.

Characteristics of the Phenomenological Approach: The following are the characteristics of the phenomenological approach:

1. It tends to withstand the acceptance of those situations that are not observable and are based on speculative thinking.
2. It tends to oppose naturalism, that is, objectivism and positivism.
3. It tends to justify knowledge with reference to the existing awareness of a substance (as narrated by itself). It is disclosed comprehensively, distinctively, and in a suitable way for something of its kind.
4. The primary source of data collection is the real-life situations of the subjects being studied. In-depth interviews and audio-taped interviews with participants are the common methods used. Emerging themes are frequently validated with participants, because their personal lived experiences are central to the phenomenological study.
5. The process of data analysis involves the difficult and tedious task of comparing and contrasting the final data in order to determine what patterns, themes, or trends emerge. While in the final analysis stage, the researcher attempts to seek further knowledge about that lived experience of the subject in a concise manner. To make the knowledge relevant to other researchers, it must be understandable and clear, detailing the relationship that exists.

Examples of Phenomenological Research Studies: The following are examples of phenomenological research studies:

1. A phenomenological study on lived experience of earthquake victims in selected areas of Bhuj, Gujarat.
2. A phenomenological study on psychological experience of victims trapped in the Uphaar cinema tragedy in New Delhi.

Ethnographic Research

The following are the salient features of ethnographic research:

1. This approach or method was developed by anthropologists as a mechanism for studying culture. It is a method of conducting enquiry of a life process by studying individuals, artefacts, or documents in their natural settings and includes both anthropology and historical forms of research. Ethnographic enquiry facilitates understanding about cultural behaviour and practices affecting the health of people. In health care research, ethnography provides access to health beliefs and health care practices in particular cultural or sub-cultural groups. Macro-ethnography is the study of broadly defined culture, whereas micro-ethnography is the study of more narrow aspects of a culture.
2. Ethnographic research in nursing is used to increase ethnic cultural awareness and also to enhance the quality of health care for persons of all cultures.
3. Madeleine Leininger has used the phrase ethno-nursing research, which 'focuses mainly on observing and documenting interactions with people of their daily life conditions and patterns influencing human care, health, and nursing care practices'.
4. Ethnographic research is a time-consuming labour-intensive work, which may take months or years of field work, because the researcher learns about the cultural groups in which they are interested through extensive field work.
5. To study the culture, a certain level of intimacy is required, which can only develop over time and by working together directly with the cultural group members who are active participants in

the study. Rather than using a formal tool for data collection, the researchers use themselves as instruments, spending time with group members to collect data through informal interactions and observations. Information on three major aspects of cultural life is sought in ethnographic studies: cultural behaviour (what members of culture do), cultural artefacts (what members of the culture make and use), and cultural speech (what members of the cultural group say). Sources of data collection in ethnography studies include in-depth interviews, record analysis, and observation of physical evidences (photographs, diaries, letters, etc.)

Examples of Ethnographic Research Studies: The following are examples of ethnographic research studies:

1. An ethnographic study on the features and critical attributes, processes, and beliefs of self-help groups of women living with chronic substance abuse husbands in selected villages of Nadia District, West Bengal.
2. An ethnographic study on socio-cultural beliefs of people about child marriage in selected rural communities of Rajasthan.

Grounded Theory Research

The following are the important aspects of grounded theory research:

1. The term *grounded* means the theory that developed from the research has its roots in the data from which it was derived. Grounded theory research is an inductive technique that emerged from the discipline of sociology. This theory has become an important research method for the study of nursing theories of phenomena relevant to nurses. It is different from other methods because of its particular approach to theory development. Grounded theory suggests that there should be a continuous interplay between data collection and data analysis. The main focus is on developing social experience that involves social and psychological stages and phases that characterize a particular event or episode.
2. The characteristics of grounded theory begin with a research situation within the situation. The task of the researcher is to understand what is happening there (core variable and how the players manage their role). Reality is created by attaching meanings to situations. Meaning is expressed in symbols such as words, religious objects, and clothing. These symbolic meanings are the basis for actions and interactions. Group life is based on consensus and share meanings. Interactions may lead to redefinition or new meanings, which can result in redefinition of self.
3. The steps of the grounded theory research occur simultaneously. Constant comparison is an important methodological technique undertaken in grounded theory. Here, inductive process is used. For example, suppose a community health nurse is using grounded theory methodology to study family dysfunction in inter-religious marriage; the nurse limits the study to those families that are experiencing such marriages. For the purpose, data collection is done both in the homes of the participants (through observations, interviews, and role plays) and in their work environment (through observations and interviews). The nurse begins to categorize and code the data gathered, which helps her in thinking and conception of the families. To verify the theory, the nurse plans to study other dysfunctional families who are scapegoating.
4. The sources of data collection in grounded theory are formal and informal interviews, documents, participants' observation diaries, audio tape-recordings, case studies, and art works. The sources

of data collection vary with the focus of enquiry, the purpose of investigation, and the guidelines suggested by the research approach being used.

5. A sample of 25–50 people are usually included in grounded theory research. The research projects are conducted by in-depth interviews, data collection notes, typed interviewer transcripts, and video-taped or audio-taped conversation, which contain various processes of data to be stored and analysed, initiated by loading and categorizing the data.

Examples of Grounded Theory Research Studies: The following are examples of grounded theory research studies:

1. A study on the response and adaptation of patients diagnosed with AIDS in Safdarjung Hospital, New Delhi.
2. A grounded theory research on the adaptation levels of people with quadriplegia at LNJP Hospital, New Delhi.

Case Study

The following are the important features of case study method of research:

1. The research on a phenomenon by studying in-depth a single case is a case study approach. The case can be an individual person, an event, a group, an institution, or a place. It is concerned with an in-depth analysis and a systematic description of one point or a group of points to promote understanding of nursing interventions.
2. Case study methodology in nursing sciences has been in use for a long time for in-depth study of a single point or a group of points to generate knowledge to solve nursing problems of patients suffering with specific disease. For example, how does a patient of myocardial infarction manage the *dietary regime* prescribed for him? Data for case study are collected by observation or by the personal interview method. In general, analysis in case study design does not involve sophisticated, qualitative, and statistical techniques, since the stress is more on the analysis of the collected data. Basically, case studies are considered as qualitative research studies; however, they could be either quantitative or qualitative research study based on the purpose and phenomenon under study.

Examples of Case Study Design: The following are examples of case study method of research:

1. A case study on the availability of emergency services in RML Hospital, New Delhi.
2. A case study on the organization and functioning of SSKM Hospital, Kolkata, West Bengal.

Action Research

A basic definition of this type of research is 'a small scale intervention in the functioning of the real world and a close examination of the effects of such an intervention'. The main characteristic of this type of research is that it is essentially an *on-the-spot* procedure, principally designed to deal with a specific problem evident in a particular situation. No attempt is made to separate a particular feature of the problem from its context. In order to study it in isolation, action research depends mainly on observation and behavioural data; constant monitoring and evaluation are carried out, and the conclusions of the findings are applied immediately and monitored further. It is a practical form of research, which aims at a specific problem situation with little or no control over independent variables. It cannot fulfil the scientific requirement for generalizability.

The method of data collection involved in action research is interview, observation, socio-drama, plays, skits, drawings and painting, story-telling, and so on. The importance of action research in nursing is based on the fact that it has the ability to exert power, especially when the research involves collaboration between study participants and the researcher. The research process can help to improve nursing practice and will result in the ability to work harmoniously with others and improve cooperation among caregivers, thereby resulting in the improvement of professional spirit. Action research in nursing will help in recognizing strength and areas of improvement, nursing knowledge, actions, and consciousness, thus benefitting the client of the organization. Future organizational changes can be made possible by taking action through planning and fact finding.

Action research in nursing, especially in the Indian set-up, has particular importance because of the following reasons:

1. It helps to solve a problem by enriching the field of application of a discipline.
2. It facilitates collaboration with several other disciplines for solving the problem.
3. It helps to study individual cases without the objective to generalize.
4. It tries to say how things can be changed.
5. It reports in a common language.

An action study is conducted in the practical situation, which helps to solve the problem of patient care. Action studies can help in the training of nursing students, bridging the gap of classroom demonstrations of nursing procedures and their practical applications to the real clinical situations, which mostly have insufficient infrastructure, supplies, facilities, and so on to provide good care.

Examples of Action Research Studies: The following are examples of action research studies:

1. An action research on the practicability of providing care by nurses trained in private organizations and appointed or working in several hospitals.
2. An action research on the use of proposed well-being support program to solve somatic morbidity among chronic mentally ill women suffering from post-natal depression.

FACTORS AFFECTING SELECTION OF RESEARCH DESIGN

The following are the factors that affect the selection of a research design:

1. **Nature of Research Problem:** Does the study require exploration or implementation of a new technique? If a new technique is needed to be initiated, an experimental research design will be more appropriate. In some cases, an explorative study may be required before the experimental research to explore the need or capacity of the nurses to adopt the new technique.
2. **Purpose of the Study:** Why is the research required? Does the researcher wish to develop an in-depth understanding of the phenomenon under consideration or does he just want to know the extent of an existing problem? If the investigator develops an insight into the problem, a qualitative approach will be more applicable.
3. **Researcher's Knowledge and Experience:** A novice researcher should undergo further training or develop thorough knowledge and skills in interviewing and recording qualitative data before attempting to do a qualitative study.
4. **Researcher's Interest and Motivation:** This is important to conduct the study successfully until the end. Motivated researchers will carry out the investigation on the topic of their interest

wholeheartedly enjoying every step of the research process and will feel proud and confident about the outcome.

5. **Research Ethics and Principles:** The selection of research design will depend on whether it will be ethical to conduct an experimental study on the samples selected, such as children. The new drug or technique may be likely to cause certain amount of harm but is also likely to provide some benefits. The researcher has to find the ratio of benefit to harm and also obtain an informed consent.
6. **Subjects or Participants:** Availability of the subjects is an important factor in selecting the research design. A researcher might plan to perform a study on some topic of interest but might find that, during a particular time period, the subjects are not available. For example, suppose a researcher wants case studies of bronchitis among infants in the months of May and June, even a single case may not be found.
7. **Resources, Time, and Possible Control of Extraneous Variables:** To conduct a study following a specific research approach and selecting an appropriate design, the researcher needs to see whether resources (money, men, and material) are available and time is suitable to carry out the study. Moreover, if it is an experimental study, the researcher should determine whether it will be possible to control the extraneous variables.
8. **Users of the Research Study:** Before taking up a study, the researcher should consider to whom is the study going to be useful. Any research taken up by the researcher should be socially relevant and useful to someone in the society. In the case of nursing research, the study should contribute towards improving the body of nursing knowledge and benefit the people the nurses serve.

CRITIQUING RESEARCH DESIGN

Once the research design is selected and the research process completed, the following questions need to be answered:

1. Was the design selected appropriate to the research question?
2. Did it involve experimental intervention?
3. If so, was it true or quasi-experimental?
4. What were the types of comparisons undertaken?
5. Was the number of samples or data appropriate?
6. What were the procedures used to control external factors (experimental)?
7. To what extent is the study valid internally or externally?
8. To what extent could the study be used as evidence-based practice?
9. What were the major limitations of the study?
10. If the design was non-experimental, would an experimental design have been more appropriate?

KEY POINTS

- The quantitative research process involves conceptualizing, planning, implementing, and communicating the findings of a quantitative research project.
- Basic scientific investigation is undertaken to seek new knowledge about health phenomenon with the hope of establishing general principles.

- The purpose of applied research is to solve problems, make decisions, and predict or control outcomes in real-life practice situations. The findings from applied studies can also be invaluable to policy makers as a basis for making changes to policies that address health and social problems.
- Striving for excellence in research is rigour. It requires discipline, adherence to detail, and strict accuracy.
- The type of research conducted is influenced by the current knowledge of a research problem. Descriptive studies are often conducted when little knowledge on the problem is available. With the increase in knowledge level, correlational, quasi-experimental, and experimental studies are conducted.
- Descriptive research relies on observation as a means of collecting data. Depending on the type of information sought, participants can be interviewed, questionnaires distributed, and visual records, including sounds and smells, made. It is also important that the observations made are written down or recorded in an organized form and presented in a clear and systematic way for subsequent analysis of data, resulting in valid and accurate conclusions.
- Correlational research involves systematic investigation of relationships between or among variables. The information sought in correlational research is expressed in numbers, and depending on the nature of data, various statistical techniques are used to find the meaning of the numerical data.
- Quasi-experimental studies involve implementing a treatment and examining the effects of the treatment using selected methods of measurement. Quasi-experimental studies usually lack certain amount of control over the manipulation of the treatment, management of the setting, or selection of the subjects.
- In the experimental study, the causality between the independent and the dependent variables is examined under highly controlled conditions.
- The terminology and methods of reasoning used in qualitative research differ from those used in the more traditional quantitative research methods and reflect alternative philosophical orientations. The specific philosophical orientation of each approach directs the research method. Qualitative research provides a process in which nurses can examine a phenomenon outside traditional views.
- Six approaches to qualitative research are used in nursing. They are historical, phenomenological, ethnographic, grounded theory, case study, and action research.
- Action research and case study are the most common forms of qualitative research conducted by nurses.

QUESTIONS

I. Essay-type Questions

1. Discuss historical research.
2. Define briefly the qualitative research approach. Explain any one of the two common approaches to qualitative research used in nursing.

II. Short Notes

1. Case study as a research method
2. Quantitative research approach
3. Descriptive research

III. Multiple-choice Questions

Circle the alphabet before the best answer

1. The value of historical research is that it
   (a) throws light on the contemporary problems
   (b) throws light on the present and future trends
   (c) allows scope for re-evaluation
   (d) stresses the relative importance of research
2. The validity, reliability, authenticity, and accuracy, of primary sources of data in historical research can be achieved by
   (a) external criticism
   (b) discussing with fellow researchers
   (c) internal and external criticism
   (d) collecting secondary data
3. Descriptive research study is concerned with
   (a) exploration and description of phenomena
   (b) observation
   (c) systematic way of subsequent analysis of data
   (d) valid accurate conclusions
4. One of the characteristics of qualitative research designs is that it
   (a) needs explanation of terminology and methods
   (b) is concerned with field work
   (c) is flexible and can be adjusted to the information being gathered during data collection
   (d) demands team approach
5. Experimental studies differ from the other research approaches because of the
   (a) controlled manipulation of at least one treatment variable
   (b) exposure of all the subjects to the treatment
   (c) conduct of the study in a laboratory
   (d) easy availability of human subjects

Answer Keys

1. (b) 2. (c) 3. (a) 4. (c) 5. (a)

FURTHER READING

Bloor, Michael, Word, Fiona. 2006. *Keywords in Qualitative Methods. A Vocabulary of Research Concepts*. New Delhi: Saga Publications.

Burns, Nancy, Grove, Susan K. *Understanding Nursing Research: Building an Evidence-based Practice*. Fourth edition. New Delhi: Elsevier Publications.

Kothari, C. R. 2007. *Research Methodology: Methods and Techniques*. New Delhi: New Age International (P) Limited Publishers.

Kovacs, Alberta R. 1987. *The Research Process: Essentials of Skill Development*. Philadelphia: F. A. Davis Company.

Polit, Devise E., Beck, Cheryl T. 2008. *Nursing Research: Generating and Assessing Evidence for Nursing Practice*. Eighth edition. Lippincott Williams and Wilkins.

Sharma, Suresh K. 2011. *Nursing Research and Statistics*. New Delhi: Elsevier Publishers.

Treece, Eleanor Walters, Treece Jr, James William, 1986. *Elements of Research in Nursing*. Saint Louis, Toronto: C.V. Mosby Company.

Walliman, Nicholas. 2005. *Your Research Project*. New Delhi: Vistaar Publications.

Wilson, Holly Skodol. 1989. *Research in Nursing*. Second edition. Redwood City, California: Addison-Wesley Publishing Company.

chapter

8 Population, Sampling and Data Collection Methods in Qualitative Research

OBJECTIVES

Upon completion of this chapter the learner will be able to:

- Provide a brief overview of qualitative research and its concept and characteristics
- Explain about population, sample, and sampling in qualitative studies
- Emphasize on the types of sampling used in qualitative research and how they differ from those used in quantitative research
- Clarify the concept of sampling size required for qualitative studies
- Explain the criteria for when to stop sampling.

INTRODUCTION

Qualitative research designs are becoming increasingly popular among researchers in different spheres. However, researchers face challenges mostly while using the qualitative research designs on account of the unfamiliarity with the core concepts of qualitative research. The present chapter aims to provide a basic understanding of the concept of population and sampling in qualitative research.

DEFINITION OF QUALITATIVE RESEARCH

According to Munhall and Boyd (1999), 'Qualitative research is a systematic interactive, subjective approach used to describe life experiences and give them meaning.'

WHY TO USE A QUALITATIVE METHODOLOGY?

There are various reasons based on which one may decide to use a qualitative research methodology. Strauss and Corbin (1990) claim that qualitative methods can be used for the following purposes:

1. To better understand any phenomenon about which little is yet known
2. To gain new perspectives on things about which much is already known
3. To gain more in-depth information that may be difficult to convey quantitatively

Hence, qualitative methods are usually adopted in situations where an extensive and in-depth study or information is required to discover a new phenomenon or to unveil some unknown dimensions of a phenomenon. This 'rich' information so obtained cannot usually be obtained by the use of quantitative methods. As qualitative studies are more descriptive in nature, they tend to provide a more elaborate and extensive understanding of the problem under study.

Distinct Characteristics of Qualitative Research

1. Qualitative researches have a holistic approach to questions—a recognition that *human realities are complex*. Different people can have different perspectives, thinking, or views on a particular issue.
2. Qualitative researches are *emergent* and *flexible* in nature.
3. Qualitative researches make use of *naturally occurring data* so that the situation can be observed and analysed as it is.
4. The researcher acts as the *human instrument* of data collection.
5. Qualitative researchers predominantly use *inductive data analysis*.
6. Unlike quantitative research summaries that are predominantly statistical (numerical), qualitative research reports are usually *descriptive*, involving statements and verbatim from the participants.

POPULATION, SAMPLES, AND SAMPLING

According to Polit and Hungler (2004), population, sample, and sampling are defined as follows:

'A *population* is the entire aggregation of cases that meets a specified set of criteria.'

'A *sample* is a subset of the population.'

'*Sampling* is the process of selecting a portion of the population to represent the entire population.'

Sampling Strategies for Qualitative Researchers

Sampling strategy for qualitative researches is different from that used in quantitative studies. The main aim is to select as samples those who can be the best source of information. Mostly qualitative researches use small, flexible, and purposefully selected samples rather than those selected randomly. The samples thus selected are those who can best describe the phenomenon under study. At the same time, since beginning there has been a lot of debate on the issues of researchers' biasness in selection of samples and thereby problems in generalization of the findings. However, this remains an inherent feature of qualitative designs and is therefore not considered as a weakness. Moreover, there are ways to enhance the credibility and transferability of the findings.

There is no hard and fast rule regarding the sample size in qualitative researches. An appropriate sample size is one that adequately answers the research question. This may range from single figures to larger numbers depending upon the aim of the study. Usually the sample size is determined by the information obtained from the participants. Once the purpose of the study is achieved and newer themes, categories, and sub-categories stop emerging, which is known as the point of data saturation, the information is considered to be complete and no more samples are looked for.

The Logic of Qualitative Sampling

Quantitative research is concerned with the measurement of attributes and relationships in a population, and therefore, a representative sample is needed to ensure that the measurements accurately reflect and can be generalized to the population. In contrast, the aim of most qualitative studies is to discover the meaning and to uncover multiple realities, and therefore, *generalizability* is *not* the guiding criterion in *qualitative researches*.

The qualitative researcher asks such questions as the following:

1. Who would be an information-rich data source for my study?
2. Whom should I talk to first or what should I observe to maximize my understanding of the phenomenon?

It is clear with these types of questions that the critical first step in qualitative sampling is the selection of a setting with high potential for *information richness*.

As the study progresses, new sampling questions such as the following emerge:

1. Whom can I talk to or observe to confirm my understandings?
2. Whom can I talk to or observe to challenge or modify my understandings?
3. Whom can I talk to or observe to enrich my understandings?

Hence, in qualitative research, sampling design is an emergent one.

Types of Qualitative Sampling

In quantitative enquiry, the dominant sampling strategy is probability sampling, which depends on the selection of a random and representative sample from the larger population. The purpose of probability sampling is subsequent generalization of the research findings to the population. In contrast, *purposeful sampling* is the dominant strategy in qualitative research. Purposeful sampling seeks *information-rich cases*, which can be studied *in depth*.

Qualitative researchers may begin with a *convenience sample* (sometimes referred to in qualitative studies as a *volunteer sample*). Although qualitative sampling may begin with volunteer informants, most qualitative studies eventually evolve to a purposive sampling strategy. In qualitative research, purposive sampling is often referred to as *theoretical sampling* (especially in grounded theory studies) or *purposeful sampling*.

The main goal of purposive sampling is to focus on particular characteristics of a population that are of interest and will best enable the researcher to answer the research questions. The sample being studied is not representative of the population, but for researchers pursuing *qualitative* or *mixed method research designs*, this is not considered to be a weakness.

Types of Purposeful Sampling

There are about 16 different types of purposeful sampling. They are briefly described as follows:

1. **Extreme and Deviant Case Sampling:** This involves learning from highly unusual manifestations of the phenomenon of interest, such as outstanding successes, notable failures, top of the class, dropouts, exotic events, and crises.
2. **Intensity Sampling:** This involves information-rich cases that manifest the phenomenon intensely, but not extremely, such as good students, poor students, and above or below average.
3. **Maximum Variation Sampling or Heterogeneous Sampling:** This involves purposefully picking a wide range of variation on dimensions of interest. This documents unique or diverse variations that have emerged in adapting to different conditions. It also identifies important common

patterns that cut across variations. Like in the example of interviewing students of Saint Joseph University (SJU) the researcher may want to get samples of students from different nationalities, professional backgrounds, cultures, work experience, and the like.

4. **Homogeneous Sampling:** This one reduces variation, simplifies analysis, and facilitates group interviewing. For example, instead of having the maximum number of nationalities as in the case of maximum variation, it may focus on one nationality, say Americans only.
5. **Typical Case Sampling:** It involves taking a sample of what one would call typical for a particular phenomenon.
6. **Stratified Purposeful Sampling:** This illustrates the characteristics of particular subgroups of interest and facilitates comparisons between the different groups.
7. **Critical Case Sampling:** This permits logical generalization and maximum application of information to other cases, for example, if it is true for this one case, it is likely to be true of all other cases. One must have heard statements such as if it happened to so and so, then it can happen to anybody. Or if so and so passed that exam, then anybody can pass.
8. **Snowball or Chain Sampling:** This particular one identifies cases of interest from people who know people who know what cases are information-rich, good examples for study, and good interview subjects. This is commonly used in studies that may be looking at issues such as the homeless households. What the researcher does is to get hold of one and he/she will tell where the others are or can be found. When those others are found, they will tell where one can get more others and the chain continues.
9. **Criterion Sampling:** Here, a criterion is set and all cases that meet that criterion are picked. For example, all ladies six feet tall, all white cars, or all farmers who have planted onions. This method of sampling is very strong in quality assurance.
10. **Theory-based or Operational Constructs Sampling:** This involves finding manifestations of a theoretical construct of interest so as to elaborate and examine the construct.
11. **Confirming and Disconfirming Cases:** This involves elaborating and deepening initial analysis, for example, if a study has already started and the researcher is seeking further information or confirming some emerging issues that are not clear, seeking exceptions, and testing variations.
12. **Opportunistic Sampling:** This involves following new leads during field work, taking advantage of the unexpected flexibility.
13. **Random Purposeful Sampling:** This adds credibility when the purposeful sample is larger than one can handle. It reduces judgment within a purposeful category. However, it is not for generalizations or representativeness.
14. **Sampling Politically Important Cases:** This type of sampling attracts attention or avoids undesired attention or purposefully eliminates the samples from political cases. These may be individuals or may be localities for conducting the particular study.
15. **Convenience Sampling:** It is useful in getting general ideas about the phenomenon of interest. For example, a researcher decides to interview the first ten people he/she meets the next day morning. It saves time, money, and effort. It is the poorest way of getting samples, has the lowest credibility, and yields information-poor cases.
16. **Combination or Mixed Purposeful Sampling:** This combines various sampling strategies to achieve the desired sample. This helps in triangulation, allows for flexibility, and meets multiple interests and needs.

According to Lincoln and Guba, the most useful strategy for the qualitative approach is maximum variation sampling. This strategy aims at capturing and describing the central themes or principal outcomes that cut across a great deal of participant or program variation. For small samples, a great deal of heterogeneity can be a problem because individual cases are so different from each other. The maximum variation sampling strategy turns that apparent weakness into strength by applying the following logic: Any common patterns that emerge from great variation are of particular interest and value in capturing the core experiences and central, shared aspects or impacts of a program.

Sampling Error

As Patton (1990) has also highlighted, there are different types of sampling errors that can arise in qualitative research.

1. Error due to inappropriate sampling strategy
2. Error caused by inadequate number of samples
3. Error caused by inadequate information from each sample
4. Error caused by frequent changes or modifications as the study progresses

Selecting samples for qualitative studies is difficult and requires a lot of patience. However, it is essential that the researcher select a sampling strategy and samples that fulfil the purpose of the study while overcoming the various constraints of resources that may be present.

Advantages and Disadvantages of Purposive Sampling

Whilst each of the different types of purposive sampling has its own advantages and disadvantages, there are some broad advantages and disadvantages to using purposive sampling, which are discussed here.

Advantages of purposive sampling

1. Qualitative researches involve a lot of flexibility, which can be provided only by the various types of purposive sampling strategies. Furthermore, the wide range of dimensions that qualitative studies tend to cover can be studied only through different types of purposive sampling such as critical case sampling and maximum variation sampling.
2. Whilst the various purposive sampling techniques each have different goals, they can provide researchers with the justification to make *generalizations* from the sample that is being studied, whether such generalizations are *theoretical*, *analytical*, and/or *logical* in nature.

Disadvantages of Purposive Sampling

1. The main disadvantage of purposive sampling is *researcher's biasness* in the selection of samples. This is an issue usually argued upon by most of the researchers; however, this is inherent in qualitative research design.
2. On account of the researcher's judgment in selection of the samples, *generalization* of the findings is a constraint in qualitative studies using purposive sampling strategy. It is at times difficult to convince others regarding the criteria or judgment one has used for sampling.

Deciding When to Stop Sampling

The basic criterion that helps to decide to stop sampling is the point of data saturation or redundancy of information.

CONCLUSION

Although quantitative research designs continue to be the mainstay of research arena, qualitative research designs are a recent trend because researchers have found that the information that cannot be obtained by quantitative methods is possible only by qualitative methods. Furthermore, the upcoming drift from purely quantitative or qualitative research designs to a combination of the two (triangulation) urges a basic understanding of the qualitative research designs on the part of all researchers.

KEY POINTS

- Qualitative methods can be used to understand better any phenomenon about which little is yet known. They can also be used to gain new perspectives on things about which much is already known or to gain more in-depth information that may be difficult to convey quantitatively.
- The aim of most qualitative studies is to discover the meaning and to uncover multiple realities; therefore, *generalizability* is *not* the guiding criterion in *qualitative researches*.
- In quantitative enquiry, the dominant sampling strategy is probability sampling, which depends on the selection of a random and representative sample from the larger population. The purpose of probability sampling is subsequent generalization of the research findings to the population. In contrast, *purposeful sampling* is the dominant strategy in qualitative research. Purposeful sampling seeks information-rich cases, which can be studied in depth.
- In qualitative research, the sample size should be determined on the basis of informational needs. Hence, a guiding principle in sampling is data saturation and redundancy.

QUESTIONS

I. Essay-type Questions

1. Discuss the differences between the sampling strategies used for qualitative and quantitative studies.
2. Describe the various types of purposeful sampling in qualitative researches along with suitable examples for each type.

II. Short Notes

1. Distinct features of qualitative research
2. Sampling error in qualitative researches
3. Advantages and disadvantages of purposive sampling

III. Multiple-choice Questions

Circle the alphabet before the best answer

1. The sample size in qualitative researches should be
   (a) not less than 50
   (b) not less than 100
   (c) can be any number that adequately answers the research question
   (d) none of these
2. The type of purposeful sampling for qualitative research in which the researcher identifies samples who themselves can be a good source for finding more samples is
   (a) intensity sampling
   (b) typical case sampling
   (c) critical case sampling
   (d) snowball or chain sampling

3. In qualitative researches, the basic criterion to stop sampling is when
   (a) one does not get more samples
   (b) data saturation is achieved
   (c) researcher is exhausted
   (d) no such criterion is required
4. In qualitative researches, which type of cases that can be studied in depth is sought by purposeful sampling?
   (a) Information-rich
   (b) Random
   (c) Rare
   (d) Atypical
5. The type of sampling in which the researcher purposefully chooses a heterogeneous group of samples so that a wide array of aspects of the phenomenon can be studied is
   (a) maximum variation sampling or heterogeneous sampling
   (b) intensity sampling
   (c) criterion sampling
   (d) homogeneous sampling

Answer Keys

1. (c) 2. (d) 3. (a) 4. (b) 5. (a)

FURTHER READING

Lincoln, Y. S., Guba, E. G. 1985. *Naturalistic Inquiry*. Beverly Hills, CA: Sage Publications, Inc.

Marie C. Hoepfl. 1997. 'Choosing Qualitative Research: A Primer for Technology Education Researchers', *Journal of Education And Technology*, 9(1).

Patton, M. Q. 1990. *Qualitative Evaluation and Research Methods*. Second edition. Newbury Park, CA: Sage Publications, Inc.

Polit D. F, Hungler B. P. 2004. *Nursing Research: Principles and Methods*. Seventh edition. Philadelphia: Lippincott.

Stallings, W. M. 1995. 'Confessions of a Quantitative Educational Researcher Trying to Teach Qualitative Research'. *Educational Researcher*, 24(3): 31–32.

Strauss, A., Corbin, J. 1990. *Basics of Qualitative Research: Grounded Theory Procedures and Techniques*. Newbury Park, CA: Sage Publications, Inc.

www.socialresearchmethods.net/tutorial/Mugo/tutorial.htm.

chapter

9

Population and Sampling in Quantitative Studies

OBJECTIVES

Upon completion of this chapter the learner will be able to:

- Define the common terms used in sampling
- Describe various types of sampling
- Distinguish between probability and non-probability sampling
- Identify and describe several types of probability and non-probability sampling
- Describe the advantages and disadvantages of various types of sampling
- Critique the sampling design

INTRODUCTION

Sampling strategy is critical for ensuring the usefulness of a study. It helps to determine whether the results of a study can be applied as evidence. It contributes to the trustworthiness of results and is vital for drawing the logical conclusions from a study. In order to apply the findings of a study to other people, settings, or time periods, it is critical to carefully select the sample. Samples in research are drawn to represent the population under study as it is not always necessary or even possible to study the entire population. So, the researcher studies a subset of population called sample. For example, if a researcher is interested in testing the efficacy of an alternative nursing intervention in patients with asthma, then the researcher will reach conclusion without administering the intervention to all the asthma patients. However, the researcher cannot afford to draw conclusion about the effectiveness of the intervention or the validity of the relationship based on a sample or only a few subsets, may be, 4, 5, 10, 20, and so on.

Qualitative and quantitative researchers have different approaches to sampling. Quantitative researchers seek to select samples that will allow them to achieve statistical conclusion and validity and to generalize their results. Thus, they develop a sampling plan that indicates in advance how study participants or subsets are to be selected and how they need to be included. Qualitative researchers are more interested in ensuring that they develop a rich, holistic understanding of the phenomenon of interest. They make sampling decisions during the course of data collection based on information and theoretical needs and typically do not develop a formal sampling plan in advance. This chapter will focus on sampling in quantitative research.

BASIC TERMS USED IN SAMPLING

For quantitative studies, sampling is an important step in the research process. To begin with, we shall consider some important terms associated with sampling, which will enable the reader to understand the sampling process as a whole.

Population

Population is the entire set of subjects or aggregation of cases that are of interest to the researcher and that meet the specified set of criteria. For example, if a researcher is interested in studying the postgraduate critical care nurses, the population could be defined as all the nurses (RNRM) with postgraduate qualification working in critical care settings. Other examples could be all the lung cancer patients hospitalized in a selected hospital during 2010; all the children with low birth weight admitted in neonatal nursery during 2011; and all the women with breast cancer currently under treatment in Delhi (India).

The examples given here are related to human subjects only. However, the population may also be related to objects, places, and situations; for example, the population might consist of all the nursing records on nurse's notes in a hospital, all dispensaries, all antibiotics or drugs, or all nursing institutions offering postgraduate nursing degree programme.

Thus, it can be said that the population may involve thousands of individuals or sometimes include only several hundred people.

A population consists of all elements—individuals, items, or objects—whose characteristics are being studied.

Target and Accessible Population

Target population is the aggregate of cases about which a researcher would like to generalize, for example, all hypertensive patients or diabetic people. Accessible or source population is the aggregate of cases that conform to designated criteria and are accessible as subjects for a study.

If all diabetic population of New Delhi (India) will be the target population, then the diabetic patients attending the diabetic clinics will be the accessible population. Researchers usually take sample from an accessible population and try to generalize to a target population.

The population that is being studied is also called the target population. The accessible population is the aggregate of cases that conform to designated criteria and are accessible for a study.

Eligibility Criteria

A researcher needs to specify the criteria that define who is to be included or not to be included in the population. For example, if Indian nursing teachers is considered to be the population, then the researcher needs to answer the following questions: Does this population include all the teachers of various levels and qualifications teaching all types of nursing programmes such as ANM, GNM, B.Sc. M.Sc., and PhD? What about the qualifications of teachers—GNM with some diploma, B.Sc. Nursing, Post-basic Nursing, M.Sc. Nursing, PhD? How to consider the teachers who are on study leave, sabbatical leave, maternity leave, child care leave, and so on?. Therefore, a researcher must consider the exact criteria by which it can be decided whether an individual would or would not be included as a member of the population.

The criteria that specify population characteristics are referred to as eligibility criteria or inclusion criteria. Sometimes, population is defined in terms of characteristics that people must not possess, that is, specifying the exclusion criteria. For example, the population of nurse teachers as mentioned in the earlier example should exclude the teachers teaching ANM courses or teachers who have done GNM and some diploma course.

Sample and Sampling

Sampling is the process of selecting a portion of population to represent the entire population so that generalization about the population can be made.

A *sample* is a subset of the population, and if the sample is selected carefully it represents the population. When samples are selected using objective criteria, they help to control bias to a larger extent.

A portion of the population selected for study is referred to as a sample or it is a subset of population elements.

A representative sample is one whose key characteristics closely approximate those of the population. A representative sample can never be guaranteed, and it is not possible to make sure that a sample is representative without obtaining information from a population.

A sample that represents the characteristics of the population as closely as possible is called a representative sample.

Element

It is the most basic unit about which information is collected. In nursing research, humans usually represent the element.

An element or a member of a sample or population is a specific subject or object (for example, a person, firm, item, state, or country) about which information is collected. An element is the object about which or from which information is desired, for example, the respondent.

Strata

Population may consist of two or more subpopulations, which are referred to as strata. These are mutually exclusive segments of population based on specific characteristics. For example, suppose a researcher is studying the attitude of registered nurses (RNs) in India regarding nursing; here, the RNs are the population. This population of RNs can be divided into two strata based on gender, namely male nurses and female nurses. The population of RNs can also be divided into three or more strata based on age (25–30 years, 30–35 years, 35–40 years, and so on), social economic status, or income (high income, middle income, and low income groups).

Strata are often used in sample selection process to enhance sample representativeness.

Sample Size

It is the number of participants needed to achieve statistical conclusion validity. The number depends on the type of the problem investigated, precision required, and the resources available. In the absence of a power analysis, the safest procedure is to obtain data from as large a sample as is feasible.

Although there are no simple formulae that can tell how large a sample is needed in a given quantitative study, the usual way is that the researcher should select the largest sample possible. The larger the sample, the more representative of the population under study it is likely to be. Smaller samples tend to produce less accurate estimates than larger samples. Larger samples provide an opportunity to counterbalance atypical values. The safest procedure in most circumstances is to obtain data from as large a sample as is economically and practically feasible.

Power Analysis for Deciding Sample Size: Sample size can be estimated by using the technique of power analysis. The steps are as follows:

1. **Specifying the Power:** The experimenter specifies the power that he/she wishes to achieve. Then, the sample size needed for that level of power can be estimated. For example, suppose the

researcher is trying to find the choice of students in learning by discussion method and feels that 80 per cent of students like to be taught by discussion method. So, it can be said that the power is 80 per cent. Then, the data collected from 100 students will yield significant results 80 per cent of the time and non-significant results only 20 per cent of the time.

2. **Effect Size:** This is the actual size of the effect the researcher is looking for; it may be the effect of an independent variable on the dependent variable. For example, if the researcher says that 90 students should opt for learning by discussion, then 90 is the effect size the researcher is looking for.

Sample size is a function of a number of factors:

1. The research design being used
2. The variability of a key variable
3. The size of the difference when a hypothesis is being tested

The researcher tries to set a sample size that minimizes making two types of errors when drawing conclusion from the data.

The following is an approximate formula for determining the sample size:

$$n = \frac{(1 - n/N) \times t^2 (p \times q)}{d^2}$$

where

n = Sample size
N = Size of the eligible population
t^2 = Square value of the standard deviation score
p = Percentage category for which the sample size is being computed
$q = 1 - p$
d^2 = Square value of one half of the precision internal around the sample estimate

The formula states that the sample size is an expression of a finite population correction factor $(1 - n/N)$ times the probability level for the particular sample occurrence times the variable in population divided by the size of the confidence interval that the researcher wants for his/her estimate. This requires more of statistical calculations to achieve the exact sample size for a specific study.

There are a number of other factors that need to be considered when deciding the sample size; they are the nature of the study, resources available, sampling method used, homogeneity of the population, degree of the accuracy desired, degree of confidence, and effect size.

Sampling Bias

Sampling bias refers to the systematic over-representation or under-representation of some segments of population in terms of characteristics relevant to the research question.

As already discussed, a researcher would work with the samples and not the whole population, which is a time-consuming and expensive process. It is usually possible to draw or obtain accurate information from the samples. Despite this, sometimes the data obtained from a sample may not lead to logical conclusions because of under-representation or over-representation of the sample.

Inadequate sampling can also lead to sampling bias, which usually occurs unconsciously. Suppose the researcher plans to study nursing students and systematically interviews every tenth student who enters the school reading room. The sample will be biased in favour of the students going to the reading room even if the researcher is conscious about including every tenth student regardless of his/her appearance, gender, or other traits.

The result from a sample will never perfectly match the population values. Researchers use statistics to measure and account for this difference, which results in a value called sampling error.

Sampling Error

Sampling error is the key in hypothesis testing. It is a statistical value that indicates the differences in results found in the sample when compared to the population from which the sample was drawn. In other words, it is a statistical error described as the difference between a population parameter and a sample. It is difference between the population mean and sample mean.

Sampling error is sometimes referred to as chance or standard error. It is the criterion used to determine whether the statistical results are the result of real effects. Therefore, it is very important to use a sampling strategy that minimizes sampling error by maximizing the chance that the sample will represent the population well. Larger samples give smaller sampling errors.

Selection Bias

It is a condition that occurs when subjects are not selected for the study or assigned in groups in an impartial way. This may pose threat to the validity of the study.

Sampling Frame

This refers to the potential participants who meet the definition of the population and are accessible to the researcher. It is also called as available population. For example, the sampling frame for cardiac care nurses working in cardiac units could be on the membership roaster of Asian Cardiac Nurses Association.

Sample Selection Strategy

The use of objective selection criteria and sound sample recruitment methods are appropriate for all types of research. Objective selection criteria help minimize bias in both qualitative and quantitative studies.

Objective selection criteria may involve inclusion or exclusion criteria or both. The use of inclusion criteria provides guidelines for choosing subjects with a predetermined set of characteristics. These criteria define the major factors that are important to the research question. These may include clinical, temporal, demographic, and geographic criteria as appropriate. In other words, it can be said that inclusion criteria can help the researcher in objectively identifying who can be considered as subjects, thus helping to limit the sampling bias. Exclusion criteria are the characteristics that help the researcher to exclude a potential subset from the study. Some subjects or individuals are not suitable for the study even though they meet the inclusion criteria. These subjects might have clinical exclusion criteria (e.g., co-morbid conditions that might affect the study) or behavioural exclusion criteria (e.g., likelihood of being lost to follow up). The exclusion and inclusion criteria help to control extraneous variables.

Sampling Designs

The goal of quantitative studies is the representation of the population; the use of probability in sample selection or group assignment helps the researcher achieve this goal.

There are broadly two types of sampling designs:

1. Non-probability sampling design
2. Probability sampling design

Non-probability Sampling Design: In this, the elements are selected by using non-random methods. In this type of sampling, researchers cannot estimate the probability of including each element of population in the sample and each element may not have a chance of inclusion.

Probability Sampling Design: It involves random selection of elements. In this method, a researcher can specify the probability that each element of population will be included in the sample. Thus, a researcher can place greater confidence in the representativeness. Probability sampling is said to be the more respected approach of sampling among the two classifications.

CLASSIFICATION OF SAMPLING

Figure 9.1 shows the classification of sampling techniques.

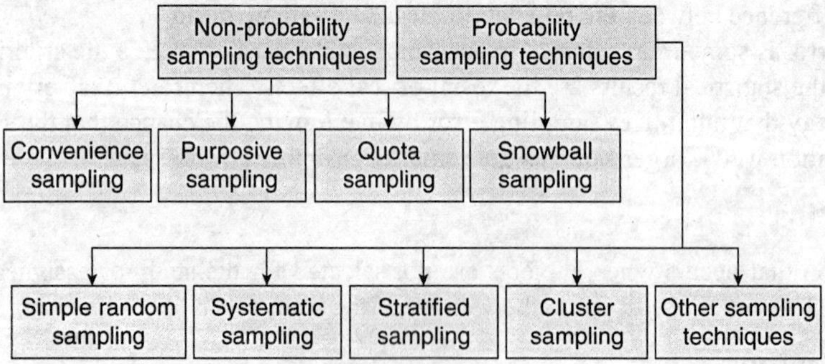

FIGURE 9.1 *Classification of Sampling Techniques*

We shall now discuss the different types of non-probability and probability sampling techniques.

Non-probability Sampling

The following are the four primary methods of non-probability sampling:

1. Convenience sampling
2. Snowball sampling
3. Quota sampling
4. Purposive sampling

Convenience Sampling

This is a non-probability method of selecting a sample that includes subjects who are available in a convenient way to the researcher. Convenience sampling (also called as accidental sampling) entails using the most conveniently available people as study participants.

If a researcher distributes the questionnaire related to his/her study to the nursing students in the classroom, it is an example of convenient sample. A nurse conducting an observation study of women having breech delivery in a maternity hospital is also an example of convenient sampling. Contacting people at a railway station or in a street corner to conduct an interview is another example of convenient sampling. Convenient samples do not necessarily comprise individuals known to the researchers.

Advantages: The following are the advantages of using convenience sampling technique:

1. It saves time and cost.
2. It has easy accessibility.

Disadvantages: The following are the disadvantages of this method:

1. There is difficulty in determining how much of the effect (dependent variable) results from the cause (independent variable).
2. The risk of sampling bias is greater.

Snowball Sampling

This sampling technique is also called as network sampling, chain sampling, or referred sampling. It is a non-probability sampling method that relies on referrals from initial subjects to recruit additional subjects.

In snowball type of sampling, each subject is asked to recruit other subjects as this may be the only way to reach the other subjects. Snowballing is used as a method of sampling when it is otherwise difficult to identify the population or sample (with certain characteristics). It is used when the samples possess sensitive characteristics such as the Indian migrant nurses in countries such as the USA or the UK, alcoholics, drug addicts, or teens.

The generalization of result may be limited, because the samples are not randomly selected and hence are not truly representative of the population.

With the snowball approach, early sample members (called seeds) are asked to refer other people who meet the eligibility criteria. Snowballing begins with a few eligible study participants and then continues on the basis of participant referrals.

Quota Sampling

This is a sampling method in which a researcher identifies the population strata and determines how many participants are needed from each stratum. By using the information about the composition of population, the researcher can ensure that diverse segments are represented. Let us consider an example. When a researcher is interested in studying the attitude of staff members towards working with HIV or AIDS patients admitted in the hospitals, the accessible population is the hospitals with, say, 2000 nurses and a sample size of 400 is desired. If the researcher uses convenience sampling, he/she will simply distribute the questionnaire to the staff nurses in the hospital. However, if the researcher suspects that male and female staff nurses as well as nurses with varied experience have different attitudes towards working with AIDS victims, then he/she uses quota sampling. In a quota sample, the researcher can guide the selection of subjects so that the sample includes an appropriate number of cases from each stratum. Quota sampling is relatively the easiest way to enhance the representation of a non-probability sample (Box 9.1).

Box 9.1

The following are the features of quota sampling:

1. Quota sampling is the process whereby a researcher gathers data from individuals possessing identified characteristics (quotas) and determines how many participants are needed from each stratum.
2. Researchers can ensure that diverse segments are represented in the sample, preferably in the proportion in which they occur in the population.
3. It is possible to establish *quotas* so that the sample includes the appropriate number of cases from both strata.

Advantages: The following are the advantages of quota sampling technique:

1. Quota sampling does not require sophisticated skills or a lot of effort.
2. Many researchers who use a convenience sample could profitably use quota sampling.

Disadvantages: The disadvantages in using this technique are as follows:

1. People who are less accessible (more difficult to contact, more reluctant to participate) are under-represented.

2. Quota sampling shares many of the same weaknesses as convenience sampling such as under- or over-representation.

Purposive Sampling

This is the process whereby the researcher selects a sample based on experience or knowledge of the group to be sampled. In this method, the researcher hand picks the sample based on knowledge about population, that is, the researcher purposely decides to select subjects who are typical of the population (Box 9.2).

Box 9.2

Purposive sampling has the following characteristics:

1. Sampling is done in a subjective manner.
2. Subjects who are judged to be a typical population and are knowledgeable about the issues under the study are selected purposely.

Examples are home care of diabetes mellitus and case studies.

Advantages: The advantages of using purposive sampling in research are as follows:

1. Nature of research requires small sample.
2. Small samples, less than 30, are not large enough for power of probability sampling.
3. It is also a good approach in two-staged sampling.

Disadvantages: The following are the disadvantages of purposive sampling:

1. It is difficult to choose subjects with appropriate variability in what is being studied.
2. The population is hard to get and cannot be found through screening general population.
3. Purposive sampling restricts the generalizability.

Probability Sampling

Probability sampling is also called as random sampling. It is a sampling process in which each member of the accessible population has an equal chance of being selected for the sample. A sample that is drawn randomly will represent the characteristics of the population and can be used to draw conclusion about the larger group even when the entire population cannot be included.

The various types of probability sampling are shown in Fig. 9.2.

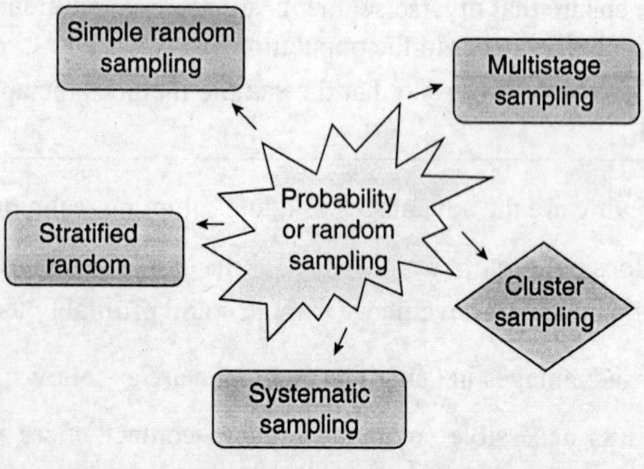

FIGURE 9.2 *Types of Probability Sampling*

Simple Random Sampling

It is the most basic probability sampling design. In simple random sampling, the researcher establishes a sampling frame. The sampling frame includes the entire population that is eligible for the study.

Suppose a researcher wants to study the health habits of a community in a selected area, then he/she has to prepare a list of all the individuals of the community, which will be a sampling frame.

To draw a simple random sample from the population, a researcher must make access to the list of all eligible individuals who are in the population and meet the selection criteria. The subjects are then numbered consecutively and among the list random numbers are drawn by using a table of random numbers to get a sample of desired size.

Steps in Random Sampling: The following are the steps to be following in random sampling:

1. Identify and define the population.
2. Determine the desired sample size.
3. List all members of the population.
4. Select a suitable sampling frame.
5. Assign each element a number from 1 to *N* consecutively (population size).
6. Select an arbitrary number in the table of random numbers.
7. For the selected number, look only at the number of digits assigned to each population member.
8. The numbers generated denote the elements that should be included in the sample.
9. Go to the next number in the column and repeat step 7 as given until the desired number of individuals has been selected for the sample.

Advantages: The advantages of this method are as follows:

1. It is easy to conduct.
2. The strategy requires minimum knowledge of the population to be sampled.
3. A sample selected randomly is not subject to bias.
4. Although there is no guarantee that a random sample will be representative, random selection ensures that differences in the attributes of the sample and the population are purely a function of chance.
5. The probability of selecting a deviant sample decreases as the size of the sample increases.

Disadvantages: The following are the disadvantages of using this method:

1. It needs the names of all population members.
2. There is difficulty in reaching all members selected in the sample.
3. It may over-represent or under-represent sample members.
4. It tends to be laborious.
5. Developing a sampling frame, numbering all elements, and selecting elements are time-consuming tasks, particularly if the population is large.
6. It is not always possible to get a list of every element in the population.

Systematic Random Sampling

In this type of sampling, the first subject is drawn randomly and the remaining subjects are selected at predetermined intervals. It involves selecting every *K*th case from a list such as every tenth person from patient list or every hundredth person from the telephone directory. For example, if a researcher needs 20 per cent of random sample from the patients visiting a cardiac clinic over a one-year period (12 months), the researcher may take a table of random numbers and then select one of the numbers randomly, say number eight in the table. Once the study begins the researcher may invite the eighth patient to the cardiac clinic and after that he/she may select every tenth patient as mentioned earlier. Systematic random sampling is useful when the researcher is unsure of how many individuals will eventually be in the population or if there is indefinite sampling frame.

Let us see how the sample can be selected in systematic sampling. Establish a decided sample size at some number (n). Estimate or know the size of the population (N). Dividing N by n, it is possible to establish the sampling interval (width) (K). So, the sampling interval or width is $K = N/n$

For example, if a researcher wants a sample of 100 from a population of 10,000 then the sampling interval would be as follows:

$$N = 10{,}000 \quad n = 10 \quad K = N/n$$

Therefore,

$$K = \frac{10{,}000}{100} = 100$$

That means every hundredth element on the list would be sampled. The first element is selected randomly using a table of random numbers. For example, if the randomly selected number from the table of random numbers is 75, then the people corresponding to the numbers 75, 175, 275, 375, and so on will be sampled, that is, every hundredth element is selected from the list.

Sampling interval = The standard distance between elements chosen for the sample

Systematic sampling conducted in this way yields the same result as simple random sampling but involves less work.

Steps in Systematic Sampling: The following are the steps to be followed in systematic sampling:

1. Identify and define the population.
2. Determine the desired sample size.
3. Obtain a list of the population.
4. Determine the sampling interval K by dividing the size of the population by the desired sample size, that is, $K = N/n$. If it is a fraction, round it to the nearest integer.
5. Start at some random place in the population list. Close your eyes and point your finger to a name.
6. Starting at that point, take every *K*th name on the list until the desired sample size is reached.
7. If the end of the list is reached before the desired sample is reached, go back to the top of the list.
8. If the ordering of the elements produces a cyclical pattern, systematic sampling may decrease the representativeness of the sample.

Advantage: The advantage is using this method is the sample selection is simple and unbiased if the sample is carefully selected.

Disadvantages: The following are the disadvantages of this method:

1. All members of the population do not have an equal chance of being selected.
2. The *K*th person may be related to a periodical order in the population list, producing unrepresentativeness in the sample.

Stratified Random Sampling

In this type of sampling, the population is first divided into two or more strata or subsets based on some characteristics, such as gender, ethnicity, caste, and diagnosis, from which elements are selected at random. Stratification based on some characteristics helps ensure that all subgroups are represented in proportion of their prevalence in population.

In this type of sampling, the researcher first divides the population into subgroups based on some characteristics and then picks up a representative sample from each group. Often, a population from each subgroup is predetermined. For example, suppose a researcher wants to conduct a study on hospital-acquired pneumonia and may like to ensure that smokers and non-smokers may be represented in the sample in the same way as they are in given population. This means if the general population has 15 per cent smoking rate, then the researcher will identify the smokers and non-smokers in the sampling frame (individual elements) and will randomly select the subjects from each group so that the sample will comprise 85 per cent non-smokers and 15 per cent smokers.

The researcher may sample either proportionately or disproportionately. Let us look at an example. If in a population of undergraduate nurses in a school of nursing, there are 20 per cent Hindu girls, 10 per cent Sikh girls, and 70 per cent Muslim girls. The proportionate sample of 100 undergraduate nursing students will consist of 20 Hindu girls, 10 Sikh girls, and 70 Muslim girls from the respective subpopulation. In this, the stratifying variable will be the religion, that is, Hindu, Sikh, and Muslim.

Stratified sampling can help a researcher to sharpen the precision and representativeness of the final sample. This may not be possible if the information on the stratifying variables is unavailable. For example, the roster of students may not include information related to religion. Moreover, this method is time consuming and requires more labour than simple random sampling.

Types of Stratified Sampling: The following are the two types of stratified sampling:

1. **Proportionate Stratified Sampling:** This involves the selection of subjects in proportion to the size of the stratum as discussed earlier.
2. **Disproportionate Stratified Sampling:** This involves the selection of sample between strata of unequal size.

Steps in Stratified Sampling: The steps involved in stratified sampling are as follows:

1. Identify and define the population.
2. Determine the desired sample size.
3. Identify the variable and subgroups (strata) for which you want to guarantee appropriate equal representation.
4. Classify all members of the population as members of one identified subgroup.
5. Randomly select, (using a table of random numbers) an appropriate number of individuals from each of the subgroups (appropriate meaning an equal number of individuals).

Advantages: The following are the advantages of the stratified sampling method:

1. The sample is more precise.
2. It can be used for both proportionate and stratification sampling.
3. The sample represents the desired strata.
4. It enables researchers to sharpen the representativeness of their samples.

When it is desirable to obtain reliable information about subpopulations whose memberships are small, stratification provides a means of including a sufficient number of cases in the sample by oversampling for that stratum.

Disadvantages: The following are the disadvantages of stratified sampling method:

1. It needs the names of all members in the population.
2. There is difficulty in reaching all members selected in the sample.
3. Stratifying attributes must be known in advance and may not be readily discernible.
4. It may be impossible if information on the critical variables is unavailable.
5. It requires even more labour and effort than simple random sampling because the sample must be drawn from multiple enumerated listings.

Cluster Sampling

This sampling is also called as *multistage sampling* because of successive stages. In cluster sampling, there is a successive random sampling of units. The first unit is large groupings or clusters. The researcher randomly selects entire groups and then randomly selects subsets only from those groups.

The usual procedure for selecting sampling from a general population involves successive sampling of units such as sampling of states, divisions, districts, blocks, and then households. The cluster can be selected by either simple or stratified method. For example, in selecting cluster of hospitals as described earlier, it may be possible to stratify on the basis of specialty area of the hospital.

Probability proportional to size sampling involves selecting broad groups (clusters) rather than selecting individuals. Cluster sampling is more economical and practical than any other type of probability sampling, particularly when the population is large and widely dispersed (Box 9.3).

Box 9.3

The following are the features of cluster sampling:

1. Cluster sampling is the process of randomly selecting intact groups, not individuals, within the defined population sharing similar characteristics.
2. The target population is first divided into mutually exclusive and collectively exhaustive subpopulations or clusters.
3. Then a random sample of clusters is selected, based on a probability sampling technique such as sample registration survey (SRS).
4. In multistage sampling, the whole country is divided into geographic clusters—metropolitan and rural areas.
5. Other areas are formed into strata of areas (e.g., middle-sized cities, rural counties); clusters are selected randomly from these strata.
6. Sample is selected from clusters in two or more separate stages; the approach is called multistage sampling.

Steps in Cluster Sampling: The following are the steps to be following in cluster sampling:

1. Identify and define the population.
2. Determine the desired sample size
3. Identify and define a logical cluster.
4. List all clusters (or obtain a list) that make up the population of clusters.
5. Estimate the average number of population members per cluster.
6. Determine the number of clusters needed by dividing the sample size by the estimated size of a cluster.
7. Randomly select the needed number of clusters by using a table of random numbers.
8. Include in the study all population members in each selected cluster.

The cluster selection and final selection of sample can be done by either simple or stratified random sampling method.

Advantages: The advantages in using cluster sampling are as follows:

1. It is efficient and saves time and money.
2. It is more practical than other types of probability sampling, particularly when the population is large and widely dispersed.
3. Arrangements are made with small number of sampling units.
4. The characteristics of clusters as well as those of population can be estimated.
5. Researcher does not need the names of all members of the population.
6. It is useful for educational research.

Disadvantages: The disadvantages in using cluster sampling are as follows:

1. Fewer sampling points make the sample less representative than the other methods.
2. The sampling errors are more than other probability samples.
3. It requires assignment of each member of population uniquely to a cluster.
4. Statistics are more complicated.
5. It tends to be less accurate than simple or stratified random sampling.

Figure 9.3 shows the various types of cluster sampling.

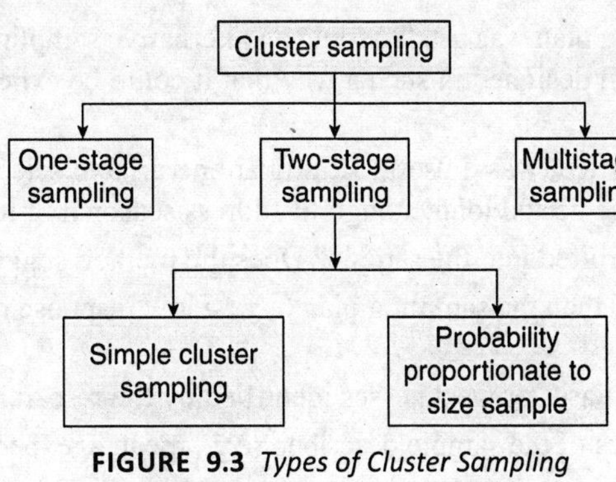

FIGURE 9.3 *Types of Cluster Sampling*

STEPS IN SAMPLING OF QUANTITATIVE STUDIES

Identify the Population

It is important to have a clear idea about the target population to which a researcher may generalize the results of the study. Researchers sometimes begin by identifying accessible population because it is not possible to access the entire or target population.

Specify the Eligibility Criteria

The next step is to spell out the eligibility criteria in the sample. The eligibility criteria should be as specific as possible.

Specify the Sampling Plan

Once the accessible population has been identified, the researcher has to decide the method of drawing the sample and the size of the sample.

The sample size can be selected by power analysis using probability sampling. Larger the sample, larger is the power. Sometimes, samples may be selected based on selected percentage basis, that is, 20 per cent, 30 per cent, or 40 per cent of the population depending upon the type of study. It is good to use as large a sample as possible to build the representativeness of population.

Recruit the Sample

Once sampling design has been specified, the next step is to recruit the prospective study participants according to the plan and ask for their cooperation. Sometimes, it may be necessary to develop a screening instrument, that is, a *form* or *brief interview schedule* that allows the researcher to determine whether the prospective subjects fulfil the eligibility criteria.

GUIDELINES FOR CRITIQUING THE SAMPLING DESIGNS

A researcher needs to follow the following guidelines while critiquing the sampling design:

1. Is the study population identified and described? Has the eligibility criterion been specified? Are the sample selection procedures clearly delineated?
2. Do the sample and population specifications support an inference of construct validity with regard to the population construct?
3. What type of sampling plan was used? Would an alternative sampling plan have been preferable? Was the sampling plan designed in such a way that it could be expected to yield a representative sample?
4. If sampling was stratified, was a useful stratification variable selected? If a consecutive sample was used, was the time period long enough to address seasonal or temporal variation?
5. How were people recruited into the sample? Does the method suggest potential biases?
6. Did some factor other than the sampling plan (e.g., a low response rate) affect the representativeness of the sample?
7. Are possible sample biases or weaknesses identified by the researchers themselves?
8. Are key characteristics of the sample described (e.g., mean age, percentage of male or female)?

9. Is the sample size sufficiently large to support statistical conclusion validity? Was the sample size justified on the basis of a power analysis or other rationale?
10. Does the sample support inferences about external validity? To whom can the study results reasonably be generalized?

KEY POINTS

- Qualitative methods can be used to understand better any phenomenon about which little is yet known. They can also be used to gain new perspectives on things about which much is already known or to gain more in-depth information that may be difficult to convey quantitatively.
- The aim of most qualitative studies is to discover the meaning and to uncover multiple realities; therefore, *generalizability* is *not* the guiding criterion in *qualitative researches*.
- In quantitative enquiry, the dominant sampling strategy is probability sampling, which depends on the selection of a random and representative sample from the larger population. The purpose of probability sampling is subsequent generalization of the research findings to the population. In contrast, *purposeful sampling* is the dominant strategy in qualitative research. Purposeful sampling seeks information-rich cases, which can be studied in depth.
- In qualitative research, the sample size should be determined on the basis of informational needs. Hence, a guiding principle in sampling is data saturation and redundancy.

QUESTIONS

I. Essay-type Questions

1. Describe the various types of non-probability sampling.
2. Differentiate between simple random sampling and systematic random sampling.
3. Write the advantages and disadvantages of cluster sampling.

II. Short Notes

1. Population
2. Sample and sampling
3. Strata
4. Sampling error and sampling bias

III Multiple-choice Questions

Circle the alphabet before the best answer

1. The most basic unit about which the information is collected is
   (a) sampling frame
   (b) strata
   (c) sampling error
   (d) element
2. A type of sampling in which each element of the population has the chance to be included in the sample is called
   (a) non-probability sampling
   (b) stratified random sampling
   (c) simple random sampling
   (d) probability sampling

3. A sampling method that relies on referrals is called as
   (a) network sampling
   (b) chain sampling
   (c) snowball sampling
   (d) judgemental sampling
4. A sampling method in which the researcher hand picks the sample is called as
   (a) convenient sampling
   (b) purposive sampling
   (c) quota sampling
   (d) cluster sampling
5. A type of sampling in which the population is first divided into two or more subsets based on some characteristics is called as
   (a) simple random sampling
   (b) systematic random sampling
   (c) stratified random sampling
   (d) non-probability sampling

Answer Keys

1. (d) 2. (a) 3. (c) 4. (b) 5. (c)

FURTHER READING

Cohen, J. 1988. *Statistical Power Analysis for the Behavioural Sciences*. Second edition. Mahwah, NJ: Lawrence Erlbaum Associates.

Levey, P. S., Lemeshow, S. 1980. *Sampling for Health Professionals*. New York: Life-time Learning.

Morse, J. M. 1991. 'Strategies for Sampling'. In J. M. Morse (ed.), *Qualitative Nursing Research: A Contemporary Dialogue*. Newbury Park, CA: Sage.

Patton, M. Q. 1990. *Qualitative Evaluation and Research Methods*. Second edition. Newbury Park, CA: Sage.

Polit D. F., Beck, C. T., Hungler, B. P. 2001. *Essentials of Nursing Research: Methods, Appraisal, and Utilization*. Fifth edition. Lippincott: Philadelphia.

Sharma, Suresh K. 2011. *Nursing Research and Statistics*. Elsevier: India.

chapter 10

Development of Research Tool

OBJECTIVES

Upon completion of this chapter the learner will be able to:

- Discuss the concept of measurements in research and the need for research tool
- Conceptualize the levels of measurements
- Explain the factors affecting data collection strategies
- List the types of instruments used in data collection and explain them
- Explain the steps in developing a data collection tool
- Differentiate between questionnaire, interview schedule, and observation
- Develop rating scales
- Describe reliability and validity and the different aspects of reliability and validity of a research tool
- Develop a data collection instrument for a study

INTRODUCTION

While conducting a research, any concept or set of concepts under investigation should be studied in depth, and the information generated therein needs to be transferred into data that can be analysed. Without high quality data collection methods, the accuracy and authenticity of the conclusions of a research can become questionable.

Developing or selecting a research tool is one of the essential steps in the research process, because whatever information the researcher plans to collect in the topic of his/her interest will be gathered with the help of some structured or standardized tool. Without high quality data collection methods, the accuracy and robustness of the conclusions are always subject to challenge.

DATA COLLECTION

Concept

Information about any topic of interest to the researcher may already exist in the form of literature, government reports, hospital reports, and so on or it may have to be generated. Depending upon the need for collecting data for a particular project, the researcher may explore the existing records and fruitfully exploit the existing data to find the answer to the research question. For example, suppose a nurse researcher is interested in knowing about the prevalence of tuberculosis in his/her district because of the feeling that the disease is rampant in that district; he/she also wishes to plan an awareness campaign to teach the people about the control of this disease. The researcher can explore the Internet and find all the needed information available at the website.

The purpose of a research is to collect information on the selected topic. The aim is to yield accurate, valid, and meaningful data. It requires considerable time and effort leading to thoughtful action to develop or select the appropriate tool for collecting the needed pieces of information.

The researcher must find answers to the following questions before planning the data collection: What type of data needs to be collected? How will the data be collected? Who will collect the data? Where will the data be collected? When will the data be collected?

Data collection methods are governed by the following factors:

1. Research question or hypothesis
2. Research design
3. Amount of knowledge available about the concepts or variables under study

Data Collection Instruments

There are a number of data collection instruments that can be used to collect data depending on the type of study and the variables to be explored or assessed. Data collection instruments, also called as tools, are devices used to collect data. These include *self-report questionnaire*, *interview schedule*, *attitude scales and opinionnaires*, *bio-physiological measure scales*, and *observation checklists*. Great care should be taken to select the most appropriate instrument for a particular study. An ideal instrument is one that results in measures that are relevant, accurate, objective, sensitive, and efficient. Measures that are physical and physiological have higher chance of success in attaining these goals than measures that are psychological and behavioural.

In survey type of explorative research, self-report questionnaires or interview schedules are appropriate. To assess the practices, an observation checklist would be most appropriate. Sometimes, the researcher employs more than one type of data collection methods. For example, a nurse researcher plans to assess the knowledge as well as skill of nurses working in the labour ward regarding 'new-born assessment'. He/She will use a self-report questionnaire for assessing the knowledge and an observation checklist for assessing the skill and will also measure the bio-physiological variables of the new-born baby.

Steps in Developing a Research Tool

The following are the steps involved in developing a research tool:

1. Develop the concept. Select sound concepts relevant to the study. Specify various dimensions of the concepts, thoroughly conceptualize the construct to be measured, and define the research question or problem.
2. Select the variables to be assessed and define them.
3. Develop hypothesis(es).
4. Decide the sample characteristics that need to be assessed.
5. Decide the research approach to be used—experimental or explorative.
6. Select the types of measurement to be included, indicators, and data collection method.
7. Adopt a theoretical model or develop a conceptual model. Once the basic decision regarding the study topic of interest has been arrived at and the concepts and variables to be studied are also agreed upon, the researcher formulates the conceptual model or decides to use an existing theoretical model relevant to the study. Use of a theoretical model or self-prepared conceptual model will provide a mapped relationship among the concepts under study. This will provide a direction

to the researcher to explore each concept and variable carefully and fully so that the objectives of the study are met, hypothesis is tested, and conclusions are drawn.

8. Select and develop the tool. This is the final step for data collection. The researcher may develop a tool, use one of the existing standardized tools, or use both self-structured and standardized tools appropriate to the study.

Standardized Tools Used in Nursing Studies

Measurement of nursing phenomena involves locating and obtaining instruments that are reliable, valid, and feasible for use with an intended sample. Beginning with a clear conceptualization of the problem and delineation of the measurement framework, the process of finding, legally obtaining, and using appropriate instruments can proceed. Resources for instruments are so numerous today that it is especially important to ensure that valuable resources are not overlooked. Standardized tools are existing instruments that a researcher may discover while conducting a review of literature. Use of an already tested instrument helps connect the present study with the existing body of knowledge on the variables. However, the instrument selected should be appropriate to measure the study variables to meet the objectives of the study.

Computerized resources offer comprehensive and efficient searches at low cost. An experienced nurse researcher who is aware of how to find and use the many resources available can select from among the numerous alternatives to measure nursing phenomena. The U.S. Copyright Act of 1976 has been shaped over the years by court cases and committee work to protect original work, including nursing research instruments. Knowledge of the provisions of copyright law may minimize the danger of unintentional violation while obtaining standardized instruments.

National League for Nurses (NLN) on its website has given a number of instruments, which after obtaining permission from the author can be used for collecting data in similar situations and among similar populations. Janice M. Bell has an organization called Family Health and Healing. At her website, www.janicembell.com, she has also given a list of family nursing instruments that she and her colleagues have developed, applied, and tested. One such instrument developed by this team is the Feetham Family Functioning Survey (FFFS). This can be requested by writing an email to stfeetham@earthlink.net. All such information about structured instruments can also be obtained from the website http:/nursing.unc.edu/research. Stanford Patient Education Research Center has developed a sample questionnaire for conducting survey on chronic diseases; it is simple yet adequate to get relevant information from people living with chronic diseases. This sample questionnaire is downloadable from the website http://patienteducation.stanford.edu. It is free of cost and no permission is required to use all or parts of the questionnaire. These are only some of the examples; there are many standardized tools available in social sciences such as sociology, psychology, psychiatry, and education.

We will now discuss the commonly used research tools, namely self-report or questionnaire, interview schedule, and observation checklist.

SELF-REPORT SCHEDULE OR QUESTIONNAIRE

A questionnaire is a printed self-report form designed to collect information from the respondents mostly in written form. Questionnaires are mostly used in descriptive studies in order to gather a broad spectrum of information from subjects. It is also called a paper-and-pencil self-report instrument. A questionnaire consists of a number of questions printed or typed in a definite order on a form or a set of forms. The questionnaire is either mailed or handed over to the respondents who are expected to read and understand the questions and write down the reply in the space provided in the form. Although development of a reliable and valid questionnaire is a difficult task, many literature resources are available for use in the construction of questionnaires. Help should also be obtained from the experts in the area of specialty in preparing a questionnaire. Researchers can use a questionnaire to measure knowledge levels, opinions, attitudes, ideas, beliefs, perceptions, and feelings and to gather factual information about persons, events, and other objects of interest.

Questionnaires should be neat in appearance and grammatically correct and should contain no typing or spelling mistakes. Proper spacing between sections and questions will make the questionnaire easy to understand. A questionnaire should be written in the respondent's preferred language and should be appropriate for the knowledge, reading, and understanding level of the least educated respondent. When constructing a questionnaire, the questions should be made as simple, clear, and specific as possible. The length of the questionnaire may influence the respondent's willingness to participate in the research. A lengthy questionnaire sent by mail may get poor response as compared with a reasonably short one.

The questionnaire should be constructed very carefully because quite often it is considered as the heart of a survey operation. Various aspects, such as the general form or sections, question sequence, question formulation, and wording, should be considered while constructing a particular questionnaire.

General Form and Sections

Questionnaires may be *structured* or *unstructured* or may be a combination of both. Structured questionnaires are those that contain definite, concrete, and predetermined questions. Structured questions are mostly closed ended, that is, of 'yes' or 'no' type. Unstructured questions are usually open ended, that is, inviting free response. Structured questions usually have fixed alternative answers from which the respondent is required to select one response. In an unstructured questionnaire, the interviewer is provided with a general guide on the type of information to be obtained, but the exact question formation is largely his/her own responsibility and the replies are to be taken in the respondent's own words to the extent possible. In some situations, tape recorder may be used with the permission of the respondent. Unstructured questionnaires are mostly used in qualitative studies.

Sequence of Questions

The question sequence must be clear and smoothly moving, with questions that are easier to answer being provided at the beginning. The first few questions are particularly important because they are likely to influence the attitude of the respondent while seeking his/her desired cooperation. Questions that put too great a strain on the memory or intellect and those of a personal character and related to personal wealth should be avoided as opening questions. Questions that are vital to the research problem should be placed following the opening questions and a connecting thread should run through successive questions. Relatively difficult questions must be put towards the end so that even if the respondent decides not to answer such questions, considerable information would have already been obtained.

Language and Question Formation

In general, all questions should meet the following standards:

1. Be easily understood.
2. Be simple, that is, convey only one thought at a time.
3. Be concrete and conform as much as possible to the respondent's way of thinking.

Closed- and Open-ended Questions

In a questionnaire, there are usually two types of questions—closed ended (multiple choice) and open ended. In the former, the respondent selects one of the alternatives or possible answers given in the questionnaire, whereas in the latter he/she has to supply the answer in his/her own words. Dichotomous questions, with only two possible answers (usually 'yes' and 'no'), can be taken as a special case of the multiple choice question or can be named as a *closed question*. Other multiple choice questions are those with more than two options, usually three to four, out of which the respondent is asked to encircle or tick mark the most suitable answer (usually one). Multiple choice or closed questions have the advantages of easy handling and being simple to answer, quick, and most amenable to statistical analysis. Although the provision of alternative replies helps to make clear the meaning of the question, the main drawback of such questions is that of putting the answers into people's brains; that is, such questions may force a statement of opinion on an issue about which the respondent does not in fact have any opinion or knowledge. Closed-ended questions are not suitable for studies that are meant to explore complex issues. In such studies, open-ended questions give the respondents the freedom to express their opinion in their own words. However, open-ended questions are more difficult to handle, raising problems of interpretation, interviewer's bias, and difficulty in establishing comparability.

Types of Closed-ended Questions

Dichotomous Questions: In this type of questions, the respondent is required to choose between two answers, such as 'yes' and 'no', 'male' and 'female', or 'boy' and girl'. This type is found most suitable for obtaining factual data.

Multiple-choice Questions (MCQ): In this type of questions, the respondent is given the option of selecting the best possible answer among three to seven alternate answers. Here, the respondent has more freedom to express his opinion on a wider area of alternatives. Opinions and attitudes can be measured more appropriately by MCQ type of closed-ended questions.

Rank-order Questions: In this type, the respondent is asked to 'rank the concept' given in the questionnaire on a continuum, such as 'most important to least important' or 'most liked to least liked' (items of food). The respondent is asked to give rank 1, 2, and so on, based upon a specific attribute or characteristic. There can be any number of items, preferably five to ten; this number is easily manageable for computation.

Rating Questions: In this type of question, the respondent is asked to rate his/her opinion, experience, or feelings on a scale of 0–10. For example, a patient after being given an intervention with specific therapy for pain relief is asked to mark on a 0–10 scale how much relief he/she got.

Checklists—Visual Analogue Scales (VAS): VAS are used to measure subjective experiences, such as pain, dyspnoea, fatigue, and comfort level. The scale is usually a horizontal line; one end of the scale is marked as extreme discomfort and the other end as most comfortable or in similar terms depending on the attribute in question.

There are a number of ways in which closed-ended questions can be formed. These various types of questions can be intermixed within a structured instrument.

Qualities of a Good Questionnaire

A good questionnaire has the following qualities:

1. It is short and simple.
2. Questions proceed in a logical sequence.

3. Technical terms are included to the minimum.
4. Adequate instructions or directions are given in the beginning about how to complete the questionnaire.
5. Language used is appropriate to the level of respondent's understanding.
6. Personal and intimate questions are avoided.
7. Adequate space is provided for open-ended questions.
8. Physical appearance of the questionnaire is attractive.

The following is an example of structured knowledge questionnaire.

***Knowledge of Mothers Regarding Care of Low Birth Weight Babies* by Harshita Ashline**

Instructions: Please tick one correct response from each question.

1. Low birth weight babies are those babies whose weight is
   (a) 2500 g at birth (b) <2500 g at birth (c) >2500 g at birth
2. A common problem in low birth weight babies is
   (a) inability to maintain temperature
   (b) breathing and feeding problems
   (c) both (a) and (b)
3. In low birth weight babies, heat loss occurs due to
   (a) decreased subcutaneous fat and brown fat
   (b) increased subcutaneous fat and brown fat
   (c) giving bath with warm water
4. Heat loss can be prevented in low birth weight babies by
   (a) skin to skin contact with appropriate clothing
   (b) nursing the baby in cradle
   (c) keeping the baby in sunlight
5. Warmth of the baby can be assessed by the mother by touching baby's abdomen using
   (a) palm of hand (b) dorsum of hand (c) fingers
6. Stimulation is essential in low birth weight babies, as it helps to
   (a) promote physical and mental growth
   (b) make the baby sleep
   (c) prevent infection
7. Stimulation is given to low birth weight babies by
   (a) massaging the body
   (b) talking, holding, and cuddling the baby
   (c) both (a) and (b)
8. Low birth weight babies should be bathed
   (a) daily (b) on alternate days (c) once a week

(*Continued*)

(*Continued*)

9. Kangaroo mother care (KMC) is given to the babies whose weight is
   (a) >1.5 kg but baby is stable
   (b) >2.5 kg and stable baby
   (c) >1.5 kg with any problem
10. In KMC, the baby is placed
   (a) against mother's shoulder with appropriate clothing
   (b) between mothers breasts
   (c) in mother's lap with appropriate clothing
11. In KMC, the baby will be in
   (a) a comfortable position with hands and legs flexed
   (b) a curved position
   (c) a position in which both hands and legs are extended
12. Duration of KMC per day should be
   (a) 30 minutes (b) 2 hours (c) as long as possible
13. The clothes used for the low birth weight babies should be of
   (a) nylon (b) smooth cotton (c) other synthetic fibres
14. Low birth weight babies should be fed preferably by
   (a) cow milk (b) formula milk (c) expressed breast milk
15. *Katori* and spoon should be boiled for
   (a) 10 minutes after boiling starts
   (b) 20 minutes after boiling starts
   (c) 30 minutes after boiling starts
16. The spoon used for feeding should be
   (a) round and smooth edged without designs
   (b) any type of spoon with long hand
   (c) sharp edged with design
17. During *katori* and spoon feeding, the position of the baby should be
   (a) supine (b) upright (c) lying down
18. While giving milk feeding, place the spoon filled with milk at the
   (a) lip of the baby in the corner of mouth
   (b) back of teeth
   (c) middle of the tongue

Scoring: 1–6: Below average knowledge; 7–12: Average knowledge; 13–18: Good knowledge

The following is an example of a self-report questionnaire.

Exercise Behaviours in Chronic Diseases

Important Instructions: During the past week (even if it was not a typical week for you), how much total time (for the entire week) did you spend on each of the following? Please circle one number for each question.

How Much Time During the Past Week	None	Less than 30 Minutes/ Week	30–60 Minutes/ Week	1–3 Hours/ Week	More than 3 Hours/ Week
1. Stretching or strengthening exercises (range of motion, weights, etc.)	0	1	2	3	4
2. Walk for exercise	0	1	2	3	4
3. Swimming or aquatic exercise	0	1	2	3	4
4. Bicycling (including stationary exercise bikes)	0	1	2	3	4
5. Other aerobic exercise equipment (StairMaster, rowing, skiing machine, etc.)	0	1	2	3	4
6. Other aerobic exercise (specify:_______)	0	1	2	3	4

Scoring: Code each item as the number circled, then covert as follows. If two consecutive numbers are circled, code the lower number (less exercise). If two non-consecutive numbers are circled, do not score the item. For 'Other aerobic exercise', try to fit the type of exercise into the existing aerobic categories (e.g., treadmill as 'other aerobic exercise equipment'); otherwise, leave as 'Other aerobic exercise' (e.g., dancing). However, if exercise is *not* aerobic, such as yoga or weight training, do not score as aerobic. Yoga, weight training, tai chi, and so on should be scored as 'Stretching or strengthening'.

Each category is converted to the number of minutes. Time spent in stretching or strengthening is the value for item 1. Time spent in aerobic exercise is the sum of the values for items 2 through 6.

None	Less than 30 Minutes/Week	30–60 Minutes/ Week	1–3 Hours/ Week	More than 3 Hours/Week
0	15	45	120	180

Source: Stanford Chronic Disease Self-management Study; http://patienteducation.stanford.edu. Reproduced with permission.

INTERVIEW SCHEDULE

Data collection with the help of interview schedule is a unique process. Therefore, before adopting it as a method for collection of information, the researcher must ascertain its appropriateness to the topic and the purpose of the study. In interview, the interviewer obtains responses from a subject in a face-to-face encounter or through a telephone call. Interview method of data collection is mainly used in qualitative studies. However, this method is also used in quantitative studies that are descriptive in nature. Interviews are used to obtain factual data about people as well as to measure their opinions, attitudes, and beliefs about certain issues. In study of phenomena that are complex in nature and where the subjects are unable to read or write, use of interview schedule is the most suitable one.

Types of Interview Schedules

The following are the various types of interview schedules:

1. Unstructured
2. Structured
3. Semi-structured

Unstructured Interviews: Unstructured interviews are started just like normal conversation. Slowly, the interviewer introduces the topic of investigation or research. Unstructured interviews are mainly appropriate for qualitative research studies.

Structured Interviews: Structured interviews are more appropriate when straightforward factual information is desired. The same questions on the given topic, in the same order and in the same manner, are asked to all the subjects. The interviewer uses a structured interview schedule that has been planned in detail for the purpose of collecting data on a topic from a number of subjects. Responses obtained are later compared across the respondents. The interviewer should try to remain very objective during the interview, avoid unnecessary interaction with the respondents, and try to spend equal time with each respondent.

Semi-structured Interviews: In semi-structured interviews, both types of questions are included. The tool is divided into sections. Some sections will have definite questions. However, usually at the end of the schedule, the respondents are asked to repeat whatever has been said before and they are free to add anything else that has come to their mind that could throw more light on the subject.

The information received through interview is usually recorded with the use of a tape recorder after obtaining the permission of the respondent. In case recording with tape recorder is not feasible, an assistant can write down what is being said, while the investigator is conducting the interview.

Telephonic Interview: This method is commonly used to gather data on some topic of interest when the subjects are at different places and it is difficult and uneconomic to contact them personally. Nowadays, the Internet is also used for such purpose.

Differences Between Questionnaire and Interview Schedule

Before the researcher proceeds to collect data, especially when it is going to be a descriptive design, he/she must consider the appropriateness of the data collection method. If the respondent does not have the problem of language or the understanding of what is expected of him and what type of information is sought, he/she can be given the self-report questionnaire to fill. In case the respondent is unable to read or write, the same questionnaire can be used as an interview schedule and the data can entered into the questionnaire after conducting an interview. As far as the choice between interview schedule and questionnaire as data collection method is concerned, the researcher needs to first understand the difference between the two. Therefore, we will see the advantages and disadvantages of both methods, which will make it easy for the researcher to determine which of the two methods will be more appropriate for the particular study he/she is planning to undertake.

Advantages of Interviews

Firstly, in interviews, it is not possible to maintain anonymity of the subjects and there is the risk of interviewer's bias. Secondly, interviews are expensive. Nevertheless, interviews are considered superior to questionnaires because of the following reasons:

1. **Provide Clarity:** Confusing and ambiguous questions are clarified by the interviewer according to each respondent's need and understanding. This prevents wrong responses as sometimes may happen in case of getting information through a questionnaire.
2. **Provide Better Response Rate:** In face-to-face interviews, the response rates tend to be high. A well-designed interview schedule and properly conducted interview normally achieves 80–90 per cent response as compared to questionnaires that are either posted or sent by email. However, questionnaires that are distributed personally and collected back have better response rate than those sent by mail.
3. **Only Choice for Certain Respondents:** For certain types of subjects such as children, blind people, and very old people who are not able to read or write with ease and those who are uneducated, interview method of collection of data is the most suitable mode.
4. **Allow 'In-depth' Questioning:** This is the main advantage of interviews. Where the concepts are complex and the respondent's personal experience needs to be explored, interview method is the most appropriate option. Open-ended questions are avoided in questionnaires; such questions are best probed through face-to-face interviews.
5. **Minimize Missing Information:** It is less likely for the respondents to leave a question unanswered, which usually happens in questionnaires. The interviewer will probe more deeply and the number of responses of 'I don't know' can be reduced.
6. **Acquire Additional Data:** In face-to-face interviews, the interviewer can add additional data through observation of lifestyle and body language and also through probing questions, which is not possible when a questionnaire is used as the data collection tool.

Moreover, in case of questionnaires, the respondent can skip some questions, go to next sections, attempt other questions, get some clues, and then respond to previous questions by getting exposed to leading answers. This can be avoided if the required information is gathered through interview method instead of a questionnaire.

Tips for Developing a Questionnaire or Interview Schedule

1. The investigator must be clear about the problem he/she is going to study. The concept, variables, and terms used in the study should be operationally defined. The aims, objectives, and hypotheses if any should also be clearly stated before preparing the questionnaire.

2. A rough draft (a one page outline) should be prepared, giving thought to sections to be included, sequence of questions, closed- and open-ended questions, and any rating scale to be included.
3. The investigator should try to find out whether any standardized tool is available on this topic; if available, some guidance can be obtained from it.
4. The questionnaire should contain clear guidelines or instructions for the respondent to gain direction and help in completion of the questionnaire.
5. Questions should be simple and of appropriate size; one question should carry only one idea to make it possible to get an unambiguous response from the subjects.
6. A statistician should be consulted at the time of structuring the questionnaire to get an expert's view on the feasibility of the questionnaire for statistical analysis later on.
7. Pilot study should be conducted, which will assess the suitability, applicability, and effectiveness of the questionnaire for gathering data on the specific topic. The questions can be redesigned in the light of the results of the pilot study.

OBSERVATION AS A METHOD OF DATA COLLECTION

Observation is universal. We continuously observe things happening around us. Although observations can be made by using all the senses, namely hearing, smelling, tasting, touching, and seeing, in research the investigator mainly uses visual observation as a tool for data collection. Sometimes, we observe certain phenomena more attentively and when we observe a particular phenomenon repeatedly we form some conclusion about it. It can be called a crude form of scientific enquiry. However, to give it a scientific tag we need to plan our observations more systematically, decide the purpose, make a conceptual framework about the concepts we are going to observe (this guides us in studying the concepts), formulate an observation checklist, and finally conduct the observation. The conclusions drawn based on the observation would be reasonably true and their generalizability will be less questionable. We can also call it structured observation. Such observation becomes a scientific tool and a method of data collection for the researcher, when it serves a formulated research purpose, is systematically planned and recorded, and is subjected to checks and controls on validity and reliability.

Observation method of data collection is used in situations where certain practices or behaviours need to be assessed. This method uses formal instruments and protocols, which dictate what to observe, how long to observe, and how to record the observations. The researcher must decide what behaviours will be observed, who will observe the behaviours, what observation procedures will be used, and what type of relation will exist between the observer and the subjects.

Types of Observations

Observations are of various types:

1. Structured and unstructured
2. Participant and non-participant

Structured and Unstructured

Depending upon the plan of action, the observations could be structured or unstructured.

Structured Observation: This is used when the researcher wants to find the answers to questions such as the following: How are the subjects carrying out an action? Are they practising the protocols or standards prescribed? Are they conducting the activities completely or partially? How much time is spent on a particular activity? Structured observation involves careful definition of units or concepts to be observed, a given style of recording the observed phenomenon, standardized conditions of observation, and selection of pertinent data of observation. In quantitative studies, structured observation is mostly used.

Unstructured Observation: Unstructured observation is mostly used in qualitative studies, when the researcher wants to observe the behaviours of the subjects in a natural setting as they go about doing their activities. The researcher does not have any preconceived idea of what will be seen and makes no formal plan about the observations he/she is going to make.

Nowadays, in nursing research, both quantitative and qualitative studies are being conducted. There are also instances of conducting mixed type of studies in which structured as well as unstructured observation may be combined. Nursing is a social science; people's social behaviour, cultural influence, traditions, beliefs, emotions, attitudes, and many such traits affect their health-seeking and treatment-receiving behaviours. Therefore, planned and structured instruments cannot always gather the desired information.

Participant and Non-participant Observation

When the observer conducts the observation by becoming more or less a member of the group that is being observed so that it is possible to experience what the members of the group experience, the observation is called participant observation. On the other hand, if the observant is observing the subjects without being a part of the group, it is non-participant observation. However, in the latter case, the subjects being observed should not know that they are being observed; otherwise, they will become conscious of being watched. Their behaviour may no longer remain natural and this will affect the findings of the study. Thus, the observer should observe the subject (or subjects) without their knowledge. This observation will yield uncontaminated desired information.

Merits and Demerits of Participant Observation

Merits: The following are the merits of participant observation:

1. The researcher records the natural behaviour of the group.
2. The researcher can verify the statement made by the informants in the questionnaire.
3. The researcher can gather information that could not easily be obtained if he/she would observe from a distance because the subjects should not know that they are being observed.

Demerits: The following are the demerits of participant observation:

1. The researcher may not be able to maintain objectivity.

Event and Time Sampling

During observation, a researcher may observe the entire procedure (event). For example, a researcher would like to observe how staff nurses are giving intramuscular injection. Here, he/she will make a checklist and observe the nurses doing the entire procedure. This is an *event* observation. In another study, the researcher may need to assess the activities of nurses during morning shift, evening shift, and night shift. For collecting data, the researcher plans to observe the activities for a specific period of time during each shift, for example, making a schedule for half an hour, at a specified time during each shift. He/she makes a specified number of observations (5–10) covering the total eight hours of each shift in the week. Records are then analysed and conclusions drawn. This is an example of *time* sampling.

Drawbacks of Observation Method

Data collection with the help of an observation checklist is most appropriate particularly for systematically recording aspects of people's behaviour or practices when they are not capable of describing them through self-reports or may not give true report. Yet, observation method, because it is subjective, is prone to bias.

The bias can be because of *halo effect*, *error of leniency*, or *error of severity*.

Halo effect is the tendency of the investigator to be influenced by one characteristic while judging another unrelated characteristic. For example, if someone is good in communication, that person may be rated as intelligent, loyal, or dependable, whereas these characteristics are different from communication. Similarly, someone may be too lenient to consider minor or even major shortcomings in a person as acceptable. The investigator may be too lenient, because of some previous experience or his/her personality is such and this can cause error of leniency, where he/she rates the subjects or the events very positively. On the other hand, another investigator engaged in a similar or same study may be too strict and may rate the situation or subjects strictly causing error of severity.

Another drawback of the observation method is that if the subjects know that they are being observed, their behaviour or practices will not be natural; they will work or behave in the ideal way, based on the code of conduct of a profession or the right practice as expected or desired of them. Therefore, if an investigator is using observation as a method of data collection, he/she should devise ways to avoid bias of all kinds while collecting data.

Methods to Prepare an Observation Checklist

The most common approach for organizing structured observation involves the construction of a category system to classify the observed phenomena. A category system represents an attempt to designate in a systematic way the qualitative behaviours and quantitative practices and the events occurring in the observational setting. Putting the concepts under study in assigned categories makes it easy to record the observation and it also helps in statistical analysis.

Category system forms the basis for constructing a checklist for observing a phenomenon of interest. Checklist is the tool observers use to record the observed phenomena. It is usually formatted with the list of behaviours, practices, or events on the left and a space for tallying the frequency or duration of occurrences of the behaviours, practices, or events on the right. The following is an example of a checklist, which was used by a researcher to assess the care received by critically ill patients from different categories of nursing skill mix and from informal caregivers.

Observation Checklist

Observational Schedule
(For selected needs of critically ill patients)
Part I—Patient's Baseline Data

Name
Diagnosis
Occupation
State of Consciousness
Level of Dependency
Family Caregiver

Date of Admission
Unit Number
Education
Marital Status

Key

1. Sister Incharge
2. Staff Nurse
3. ANM
4. Nursing Student
5. Ward Helper
6. Informal Caregivers

First Day

First observation	5.30 a.m.–7.30 a.m.	Fourth observation	6.00 p.m.–8.00 p.m.
Second observation	8.30 a.m.–10.30 a.m.	Fifth observation	9.00 p.m.–11.00 p.m.
Third observation	3.00 p.m.–5.00 p.m.		

Part II—Observation Checklist

S. No.	Care Domain	Care Indicated	Frequency Indicated	First						Second	Third	Fourth	Fifth
				1	2	3	4	5	6				
1.	Assessment of patient's needs (a) Physical (b) Psychological												
2.	Positioning for airway maintenance (a) Oxygen (b) Oral suctioning (c) Endotracheal tube care (d) Steam inhalation												

(*Continued*)

(*Continued*)

S. No.	Care Domain	Care Indicated	Frequency Indicated	First						Second	Third	Fourth	Fifth
				1	2	3	4	5	6				
3.	Observational needs (a) Level of consciousness (b) Temperature, pulse, respiration., B.P. (c) C.V.P. (d) Skin (e) General												
4.	Nutritional needs (a) Oral feeding (b) N.G. feeding (c) Intravenous (d) Changing of N.G. tube												
5.	Hygienic needs (a) Daily sponge bath (b) Care of hair (c) Care of nails (d) Eye care (e) Mouth care (f) Changing of clothes												
6.	Therapeutic environment (a) Reducing noise (b) Adjusting light or others												
7.	Elimination needs (a) Assisting in voiding (b) Care of external drainage (c) Care of urethral catheter												

(*Continued*)

(*Continued*)

S. No.	Care Domain	Care Indicated	Frequency Indicated	First						Second	Third	Fourth	Fifth
				1	2	3	4	5	6				
	(d) Emptying drainage bag (e) Assisting and cleaning or bowel management (f) Enema or bowel wash												
8.	Musculo-skeletal and skin maintenance needs (a) Care of pressure points (b) Changing of position (c) Maintenance of clean and dry bed (d) Use of pillows between the knees (e) Active or passive exercises (f) Prevention of foot and wrist drop												
9.	Prevention of chest complications (a) Deep breathing exercises (b) Encouraging to cough (c) Chest percussion												

(*Continued*)

(*Continued*)

S. No.	Care Domain	Care Indicated	Frequency Indicated	First						Second	Third	Fourth	Fifth
				1	2	3	4	5	6				
10.	Medication and treatment (a) Oral or N.G. medication (b) Parenteral medication (c) Dressings (d) Urine testing												
11.	Diagnostic needs (a) Assistance in diagnostic procedures (b) Arranging to send for investigation												
12.	Safety needs (a) General safety measures (b) Restraint or bed railings												
13.	Psychological needs (a) Explanation to patients or relatives (b) Conversation with patients or relatives												

In the observation check list given above, the researcher/observer puts a (✓) mark if the care is indicated, e.g. if assistance in diagnostic procedure was needed, if not needed an 'x' is marked. Similarly, in the second column 'frequency' indicated is marked as to how often the care is indicated/needed in a day. In the next column the observer puts a (✓) mark on who did the activity 1,2,3,4,5,6 stand for sister-in-charge, staff nurse, ANM, nursing student, ward helper, informal care giver respectively. If the indicated nursing care is not done by anybody, the observer puts an 'x' mark against it.

RATING SCALES

In research, scaling describes the procedure of assigning numbers to various degrees of opinions, attitudes, and other such abstract concepts. This is done in two ways: (a) Making a judgment about some characteristics of an individual and then placing him directly on a scale that has been defined in terms of that characteristic. (b) Constructing the questionnaire in such a way that the score of an individual's responses assign him a place on a scale.

In rating scale, the researcher observes the phenomenon of interest and rates it on the given scale. For example, a rating scale can be prepared and used to check certain prescribed steps in a standardized procedure. The aim can be to see whether the performer is doing it completely based on the standard guidelines, is doing the steps partially, or does not follow the given steps at all. In another case, the researcher may be interested to know how much pain is experienced by the subject before and after an intervention used for pain relief. In the former case the rating scale used is called *itemized rating scale*, and in the latter case it is called a *graphic rating scale*. The pain experienced by an individual can also be observed from the facial expression and body language of the subject by the investigator and rated on an itemized rating scale as shown in the following example. This can then be compared with the VAS (graphic scale) that the subject is asked to fill.

Effectiveness of Abdominal Effleurage on Labour Pain Intensity during First Stage of Labour among Parturient Mothers Admitted in the Labour Room

Rating Scale Based on Fordyce Pain Behaviour Scale (Fordyce 1976) for Assessing Pain Intensity

This is a rating that consists of observation scale for assessing labour pain intensity. The researcher observes the behavioural pattern of the mother carefully and puts a tick (✓) mark on the most appropriate number on the rating scale.

Pain Behaviour	Scoring
1. Grimacing	1
2. Taking deep breath	1
3. Sighing	1
4. Moaning	1
5. Clenching teeth	1
6. Rolling head from one side to another	1
7. Shutting eyes	1
8. Clenching fists	1
9. Guarding the site lumber or abdomen	1
10. Holding tight anything near	1
11. Rubbing the area or asking to rub lumber or abdomen	1
12. Crying	1
13. Screaming	1

Pain Intensity Interpretation:

A. 1–3 Mild pain
B. 3–6 Moderate pain
C. 6–9 Severe pain

(*Continued*)

(*Continued*)

D.	9–11	Very severe (intense) pain
E.	11–13	Unbearable pain

Visual Analogue Scale developed by Pitres. Huskisson EC., Measurement of Pain. Lancet 1974 Nov. 9;21127.37

Numerical Pain Assessment Scale

Instruction: Researcher will ask the parturient mothers to rate her intensity of labour pain on the scale between 0–10.

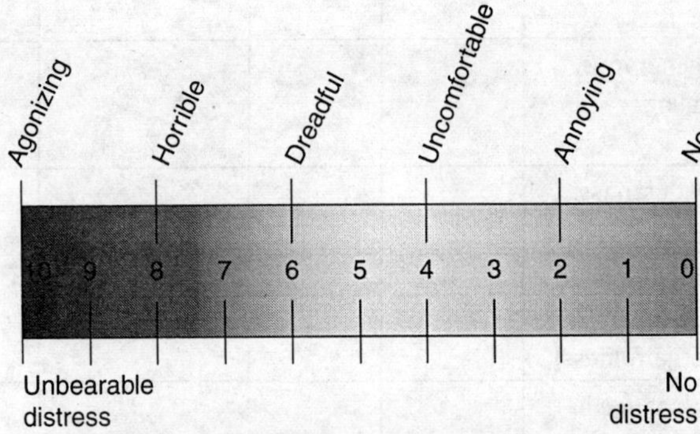

***The Severity of Menopausal Symptoms and the Life Satisfaction Levels among Menopausal Women* by Smitha Joel**

Based on Menopause rating Scale developed by Berlin center for Epidemiology & Health Research (ZEG) 1990

This is a based on rating scale, which is ordinal in nature and is also subjective. It has 11 items, which measure the severity of menopausal symptoms covering 4 areas of symptoms, namely psychological, somatic, urogenital, and sexual.

S. No.	Symptoms	None 0	Mild 1	Moderate 2	Severe 3	Very Severe 4
1.	Hot flushes (sweating or episodes of sweating)					
2.	Heart discomfort (unusual awareness of heartbeat, heart skipping, heart racing, tightness)					

(*Continued*)

(*Continued*)

S. No.	Symptoms	None 0	Mild 1	Moderate 2	Severe 3	Very Severe 4
3.	Sleep problems (difficulty in falling asleep, difficulty in sleeping through, waking up early)					
4.	Depressive mood (feeling down, sad, on the verge of tears, lack of drive, mood swings)					
5.	Irritability (feeling nervous, inner tension, feeling aggressive)					
6.	Anxiety (inner restlessness, feeling panicky)					
7.	Mental exhaustion (impaired memory, decrease in concentration, forgetfulness)					
8.	Sexual problems (change in sexual desire, sexual activity, and satisfaction)					
9.	Bladder problems (difficulty in urinating, increased need to urinate, bladder incontinence)					
10.	Dryness of vagina (sensation of dryness or burning in the vagina, difficulty with sexual intercourse)					
11.	Joint and muscular discomfort (pain in the joints)					
12.	Physical exhaustion (general decrease in performance)					

Scoring

Total items 12 Total scores 48

<12 Mild menopausal symptoms
13-24 Moderate menopausal symptoms
25-36 Severe menopausal symptoms
>36 Very severe menopausal symptoms
Interpretation to be completed

Based on Rating Scale to Measure Life Satisfaction; developed by Ed Diener and Diener, Emmones, Larsen 1985.

This is a rating that measure the life satisfaction on one global and six specific areas.

S. No.	Items	Very Satisfied 5	Satisfied 4	Neutral Score 3	Dissatisfied 2	Very Dissatisfied 1
1.	Life in general					
2.	Self-care activities of daily living					
3.	Leisure					
4.	Togetherness with friends					
5.	Togetherness with family					
6.	Marriage					
7.	Sexuality					
8.	Relationship with husband					

There are also a number of socio-psychological scales that are prepared and used by nurse scientists to find out the attitudes, opinions, and views of respondents on some topic of interest. A socio-psychological scale is used as a self-report instrument that is filled by the respondent. A scale provides a numeric score to place respondents on a continuum consisting of the highest point (in terms of some characteristic, e.g., preference, favourableness) and the lowest point along with several intermediate points between these two extreme points. Scales are used to discriminate quantitatively traits such as attitudes, fears, perceptions, and needs among people. Many sophisticated scaling techniques have been developed such as Likert scale, Thurstone scale, Guttman scale, magnitude estimation scale, and ratio scale. Most of the scales are named after the scientist who developed that scale.

Likert Scale: Likert scale has been named after the social psychologist, Rensis Likert, who developed it. This scale is also called the summated scale. Likert scales are developed by utilizing the item analysis approach wherein a particular item is evaluated on the basis of how well it discriminates between those persons whose total score is high and those whose total score is low.

Summated scales consist of a number of statements, which express either a favourable or unfavourable attitude towards the given object to which the respondent is asked to react. In a Likert scale, the respondent is asked to respond to each of the statements in terms of degrees, usually five degrees (in some cases there could be three to seven points or degrees) of agreement or disagreement. The respondent indicates his/her agreement or disagreement with each statement in the instrument. Each response is given a numerical score, indicating its favourableness or unfavourableness, and the scores are totalled to measure the respondent's attitude towards an issue.

The following is an example of Likert scale.

***Effectiveness of Educational Program on Husband Support during Labour among Husbands of Parturient in First Stage of Labour* by Sonia Samuel**

Based on Multidimensional Scale of Perceived Social Support

1. ***Very strongly disagree***
2. ***Strongly disagree***
3. ***Mildly disagree***
4. ***Neutral***
5. ***Mildly agree***
6. ***Strongly agree***
7. ***Very strongly agree***

The social support is perceived for the husband of the delivering mother in this study.

S. No.	Statements	1	2	3	4	5	6	7
1.	The person is a special person whom I need during labour.							
2.	The person is the one with whom I share my joys and sorrows.							
3.	The person really tried to help me and made me confident.							
4.	I got good emotional support, which helped me to look forward to the labour proceeding positively.							
5.	The person is a real source of comfort to me.							
6.	The person is a special person in my life; he cared about my feelings and accepted what I said and did so without judgment.							
7.	The person is the one who helped me to concentrate on an object in the room to distract myself.							
8.	I felt relaxed.							
9.	I kept myself in control.							
10.	I felt helpful.							
11.	I felt that I was treated with respect.							
12.	Most of my questions were answered truthfully.							
13.	I was concentrated on thinking about the baby positively, staying on top of each contraction.							
14.	I was able to keep myself in control and calmly think about relaxing.							
15.	I got good support, which helped me to bear the labour pain in my previous childbirth and to give birth to a healthy baby.							

RELIABILITY AND VALIDITY OF RESEARCH TOOLS

Reliability of Measurement Instruments

Reliability is defined as the ability of an instrument to create reproducible results, because without the ability to reproduce results no truth can be known. An instrument's reliability is the consistency with which it measures the target attribute. The less variation an instrument produces in repeated measurements, the higher its reliability. Therefore, reliability can be a measure's stability, accuracy, consistency, comparability, or dependability. An instrument that measures accurately and gives similar values on repeated application is considered to be accurate and consistent. This instrument is also expected to be stable, comparable, and dependable. The three essential aspects of a reliable instrument, namely stability, homogeneity (internal consistency), and equivalence, are discussed here.

Stability

Stability of an instrument is the extent to which similar results or responses are obtained on two or more separate occasions. The assessment of an instrument's stability involves a procedure that evaluates its *test-retest reliability*. Investigators administer the same measure to a sample twice and then compare the scores. Usually, an interval of two weeks is kept between the two assessments, because too short a period (less than two weeks) would influence the second scorings and too far apart in time would result in loss of subjects or unexpected change in the variable under study. The statistical test *coefficient of correlation* is computed to confirm the test's reliability. The possible values for a correlation coefficient range from −1.00 to +1.00.

A reliability coefficient above 0.80 is usually considered good; however, a score of 0.70 can be considered acceptable.

There are a number of statistical formulae that are used to compute reliability.

1. Stability (Test-retest) method

   Pearson's correlation coefficient formula for estimation of reliability

$$r = \frac{\sum XY - \dfrac{\Sigma X \Sigma Y}{n}}{\sqrt{\left[\Sigma X^2 - \dfrac{(\Sigma X)^2}{n}\right]\left[\Sigma Y^2 - \dfrac{(\Sigma Y)^2}{n}\right]}}$$

2. Equivalence (Inter-rater or inter-observer reliability)

Because all measurement techniques contain some error, reliability exists in degrees and is usually expressed as a form of correlation coefficient, with 1.00 indicating perfect reliability and 0.00 indicating no reliability. A *positive correlation* is denoted when the value of *r* is between 0.00 and +1 and *inverse* or *negative correlation* is denoted when the value of *r* is between 0.00 and −1. Certain physiological attributes have a positive correlation such as weight and height in children, that is, along with the weight, height also increases. Similarly, as a behavioural attribute, it is assumed that when knowledge increases, the behaviour or practice will improve. In health sciences, health care professionals including nurses educate the community regarding prevention of communicable diseases, imparting health information about the causes, characteristics, and prevention of specific communicable diseases. As a result of such health awareness campaigns, it is expected that people's practices will improve and the incidence of communicable diseases will decrease. Survey is conducted to find the expected results; if an inverse correlation between knowledge and incidence of communicable diseases is found, the campaign can be said to be successful.

Homogeneity (Internal Consistency)

Scales that are designed to measure an attribute are ideally composed of items that measure that attribute and nothing else. On a scale to measure married women's attitude towards family planning, it would be inappropriate to include few items that measure their attitude towards breast feeding. An instrument may be said to be internally consistent or homogeneous to the extent that its items measure the same trait. The most widely used method for evaluating internal consistency is coefficient alpha (Cronbach's alpha). By using *split-half* method, the internal consistency of a tool can be calculated with the help of Spearman–Brown correlation formula. Most statistical software can be used to calculate alpha. Coefficient alpha can be interpreted like other reliability coefficients. The normal range is between 0.00 and +1.00 and higher values reflect higher internal consistency. A high value would mean that all the items in the instrument will consistently measure the construct.

$$\text{(a) } r = \frac{\Sigma(x-\bar{x})(y-\bar{y})}{\sqrt{\Sigma(x-\bar{x})^2 \times \Sigma(y-\bar{y})^2}} \qquad \text{(b) } r = \frac{k}{k-1}\left(1-\frac{\Sigma\sigma_1^2}{\sigma y^2}\right)$$

The following is an example of determining reliability by split-half method.

Effectiveness of Educational Program on Husband Support during Labour among Husbands of Parturient in First Stage of Labour **by Sonia Samuel**

> The reliability of the tool was tested on six samples by split-half method. The scores obtained were then used to obtain a percentage of agreement. Reliability was established by Karl Pearson's correlation coefficient formula. It was found that for Response of Husband $r = 0.817$and for Perceived Husband Support $r = 0.996$, which proved the reliability of the tool for final data collection.

Equivalence

This form of reliability is also called *inter-rater* or *inter-observer reliability*. In the equivalence context of reliability, the primary concern of the researcher is to find the degree to which two or more independent observers or coders agree about the scoring of an instrument. A higher degree of agreement shows that the measurement errors have been minimized. Two or more trained raters are asked to independently rate the same object or event at the same time using the same instrument or plan. The scores obtained by them should be comparable if the instrument is reliable. This method is used by nurses mainly in observational studies. *Intra-rater* method can also be used instead of inter-rater, where the same person makes observations at different occasions and a comparison is made between the two observations. If the data obtained during two different observations are comparable, the instrument is considered reliable.

Significance of Reliability Coefficients in Research

Unreliable measures reduce statistical power and hence affect the statistical conclusion of the study. If the data fail to support a hypothesis, the reason might be that the instruments were unreliable and not necessarily that the expected relationships do not exist. Therefore, an instrument that has a reliability coefficient of less than 0.70 should not be accepted for collection of data. Because reliability coefficients are important for an instrument's quality, reliability should be briefly explained without elaborating on the technical details. Even if an investigator chooses an instrument that was previously demonstrated to be reliable, there is no guarantee of its high quality in the new situation. An instrument's reliability is not a fixed entity. The reliability of an instrument is a property not of the instrument but rather of the instrument when administered to a certain sample under certain conditions. Therefore, if a researcher finds an already existing instrument and wishes to use it for a new study, either the population, sample, setting and other such conditions should be similar or the instrument should be modified to make it suitable for the present conditions.

Validity of the Research Instrument

Validity of an instrument is the truthfulness of the measure in assessing the phenomenon of interest in a given sample or population. A valid instrument should actually measure what it is supposed to measure. Validity is the second important criterion for evaluating an instrument in quantitative research. An instrument should be both reliable and valid. Reliability and validity are not independent qualities of an instrument. An instrument that is not reliable cannot be valid, because if the instrument contains too many errors how can it be a valid indicator of the target variable? At the same time, the instrument may be accurate and sensitive to check certain attributes of the sample, but are those the attributes that the researcher intends to study? Unlike reliability, an instrument's validity is difficult to establish. There are no equations that can be easily applied to assess how good a job the scale is doing in validating the critical variable. Validation efforts should be viewed as evidence-gathering enterprises, in which the goal is to assemble sufficient evidence from which validity can be inferred.

Similar to reliability, there are different aspects of validity assessment, such as *face validity*, *content validity*, *criterion-related validity*, and *construct validity*.

Face Validity

It is the weakest, but also the first and easiest, method of declaring an instrument to be valid. Face validity at first glance declares whether the tool will measure the concepts that the study intends to explore. If just one look at the instrument conveys that it is fine, it is easier to persuade people to participate in the study.

Content Validity

Content validity is confirmed from the experts before the instrument is used to collect data from the sample. This is concerned with the degree to which an instrument has an appropriate sample of items for the construct being measured and adequately covers the construct's domain. In other words, content validity is done to determine whether the concepts that the researcher intends to explore through this instrument will be explored completely and adequately. Content validity is relevant for both affective measures (i.e., measures relating to feelings, emotions, and psychological traits) and cognitive measures. A researcher designing a new instrument should include all the questions on the topic under study, starting with the conceptualization of the construct, in order that the instrument captures the full content domain. For this, the researcher must use a variety of resources including rich first-hand knowledge, an exhaustive review of literature, consultation with experts, and findings from qualitative enquiry.

There are no completely objective methods of ensuring the adequate content coverage of an instrument. However, the instrument is usually sent to the experts to opine on the adequacy of the contents and the style of the question preparation. *Content validity index* (CVI) can be calculated by asking the experts to evaluate the individual items on the given measure as well as the overall instrument. The experts are asked to evaluate each item as relevant and appropriate in terms of construct and whether the items adequately measure all the dimensions of the concept under study. At the item level, the expert is asked to rate the items on a four-point scale of relevance: 1—not relevant, 2—somewhat relevant, 3—quite relevant, and 4—highly relevant. Then, for each item, the number of raters giving a score of three or four divided by the number of experts will give the proportion in agreement about relevance. For example, an item that is rated as quite relevant or highly relevant by four out of five experts would have a CVI of .80, which can be considered an acceptable value.

$$r = \frac{\text{Number of agreements}}{\text{Number of agreements} + \text{Number of disagreements}}$$

The following is an example of content validity and modified CVI format, which is sent to the experts. The tool is a standardized pain behavior scale used for assessing the intensity of labour pain as experienced by parturient during the first stage of labour.

***Effectiveness of Abdominal Effleurage on Labour Pain Intensity during First Stage of Labour among Parturient Mothers* by Nissy Mathew**

A request to the experts: *Kindly go through the items in the observation schedule, questionnaire, and pain behaviour scale and give your suggestions regarding the accuracy, relevance, and appropriateness of the contents. There are two response columns—agree and disagree. Kindly mark a tick against the specific column. If any suggestions are there, please mention them in the remarks column.*

SECTION A

Questionnaire to Collect Socio-demographic Variables

Instruction: The questions will be verbally asked by the researcher to the study participants. Based on the participant's response to the individual questions, the researcher would (✓) the appropriate option.

1. Age in years
   (a) Below 20 [ ]
   (b) 21–25 [ ]
   (c) 26–30 [ ]
   (d) 31 and above [ ]
2. Educational status
   (a) Illiterate [ ]
   (b) Primary school [ ]
   (c) Middle school [ ]
   (d) Higher secondary [ ]

(Continued)

(*Continued*)

(e) Graduate [ ]
(f) Postgraduate and above [ ]

3. Job status
   (a) Working [ ]
   (b) Not working [ ]
4. Parity:
   (a) Primipara [ ]
   (b) Multipara [ ]
5. (a) Were family members present during first stage?
      (i) Yes [ ]
      (ii) No [ ]
   (b) If yes, then which family member was present was?
      (i) Mother [ ]
      (ii) Husband [ ]
      (iii) Mother-in-law [ ]
      (iv) Others [ ]

SECTION B

Structured Observational Schedule

Section B consists of the items which the researcher observed at the time of intervention; the researcher would (✓) the appropriate option.

1. Duration of contractions
   (a) 30–45 s [ ]
   (b) 46–60 s [ ]
   (c) More than 60 s [ ]
2. Dilatation of cervix
   (a) 4–5 cm [ ]
   (b) 6–7 cm [ ]
   (c) 8–10 cm [ ]
3. Interval of contractions
   (a) 1–2 min [ ]
   (b) 3–4 min [ ]
   (c) 4–5 min [ ]
4. Rupture of membranes
   (a) Yes [ ]
   (b) No [ ]

SECTION C

Modified Fordyce Pain Behaviour Scale for Assessing Pain Intensity

This is a rating that consists of observation scale for assessing labour pain intensity the researcher observe the behavioural pattern of mother carefully and tick (✓) the most appropriate answer on the rating scale.

Pain Behavior	Rating Scale
1. Grimacing	1
2. Taking deep breath	2
3. Sighing	3
4. Moaning	4
5. Clenching teeth	5
6. Rolling head from one side to another	6
7. Shutting eyes	7
8. Clenching fists	8
9. Guarding the site lumber or abdomen	9
10. Holding tight anything near	10
11. Rubbing the area or asking to rub lumber or abdomen	11
12. Crying	12
13. Screaming	13

Pain Intensity Interpretation:

A. 1–3 Mild pain
B. 3–6 Moderate pain
C. 6–9 Severe pain
D. 9–11 Very severe (intense) pain
E. 11–13 Unbearable pain

A. Criteria Checklist for Socio-demographic Variables

Items	Accuracy		Relevance		Appropriateness		Remarks
	Agree	Disagree	Agree	Disagree	Agree	Disagree	
1.							
2.							
3.							

(*Continued*)

(*Continued*)

Items	Accuracy		Relevance		Appropriateness		Remarks
	Agree	Disagree	Agree	Disagree	Agree	Disagree	
4.							
5. (a) (b)							

B. Criteria Checklist for Baseline Data at the Time of Intervention

Items	Accuracy		Relevance		Appropriateness		Remarks
	Agree	Disagree	Agree	Disagree	Agree	Disagree	
1.							
2.							
3.							
4.							

C. Criteria Checklist for Modified Fordyce Pain Assessment Scale

Items	Accuracy		Relevance		Appropriateness		Remarks
	Agree	Disagree	Agree	Disagree	Agree	Disagree	
1.							
2.							
3.							
4.							
5.							
6.							
7.							
8.							
9.							
10.							
11.							
12.							
13.							

Content validation of an instrument should be done with a minimum of three experts. For postgraduate studies, a panel of six experts is considered adequate; however, the panel should include at least one statistician.

Criterion-Related Validation

Criterion validity is used when the researcher wants to predict a subject's present or future standing, related to the topic under study. It also concerns itself with the inclusion criteria of the sample. Therefore, criterion validity assesses the ability of the instrument to determine a subject's response at the present time or predict a subject's response in the future. Criterion validity is of two types, namely *concurrent* and *predictive*.

An instrument is said to be valid if its scores correlate highly with the scores on the criterion. For example, if a measure of attitude towards breast feeding correlates highly with subsequent breast feeding in a sample of newly married women (predictive), then the attitude scale would have good validity. A correlation coefficient is computed between the scores on the instrument and the criteria. This will require a longitudinal study to actually find the validity of the instrument; therefore, in cross-sectional studies that nurses commonly undertake, criterion validity is not usually established.

Construct Validity

Construct is an abstraction or concept that the researcher has deliberately invented or constructed for a scientific purpose. Construct validity refers to the validity of inferences from observed persons, events, settings, and interventions in a study to the constructs that these instances might represent; with an instrument, it refers to the degree to which it measures the construct under investigation. It is a determination of the extent to which the instrument actually reflects the abstract construct (or concept) under examination. It involves inferences from the particulars of the study to the higher-order constructs that they are intended to represent. Construct validity is important because constructs are the means for linking the operations used in a study to a relevant conceptualization and to mechanisms for translating the resulting evidence into practice.

Construct validity is in fact a hypothesis-testing endeavour, typically linked to a theoretical perspective regarding the concept. Construct validation can be approached in different ways, but it always involves logical analysis and hypothesis tests. One way is to administer the tool to a known group, which is called *known group technique*; the other methods are *hypothesized relationship* and *factor analysis*. These areas are not explored in this section of the book. This is because at undergraduate and even at postgraduate levels of research studies in India, construct validity is not normally indicated to be formally established.

How is the validity of an instrument established? The answer to this question is that an instrument does not possess or lack validity; it is a question of degree. An instrument's validity is not proved, established, or verified but rather is supported to a greater or lesser extent by evidence. Researchers do not validate an instrument but rather they validate an application of it. The more evidence that can be gathered that an instrument is measuring what it is supposed to be measuring, the more confidence researchers will have in its validity. However, it may be noted that if the investigator has taken strong steps to enhance the content validity of the instrument, construct validity will also be strengthened.

PROCEDURE FOR DATA COLLECTION

Sources of Data

Data collection procedure includes planning for collection of data, selecting or developing the instrument identification of the subjects and setting(s), obtaining permission from the concerning authorities, obtaining informed consent of the subjects participating in the study, and precise and systematic gathering of information.

Data for the research can be collected from primary sources or secondary sources. Primary data are collected by the investigator directly from the subjects or events. The secondary data are compiled from the existing data that are available in pre-existing reports, records, and published and unpublished documents.

Collection of Data

The procedure for primary data collection will depend on the research approach, which may be experimental or explorative. It will also depend upon the method selected for gathering data, whether it is with the use of a questionnaire, an interview schedule, or an observation technique. Many other factors, such as the proximity and number of setting(s) and samples, also affect the data collection procedure. If the sample is large and the settings are more than one, time schedule will have to be prepared to reach them. Availability of subjects will also have to be considered. In the case of explorative study, for the self-report, the questionnaire will be distributed and collected directly from the respondents or will be sent by mail, or the data will be collected through email. The procedure will be different for each of these methods.

There are five tasks involved in data collection—selecting the subject; collecting the data in a consistent way; maintaining research controls as indicated in the research design; protecting the integrity of the study; and solving the problems that threaten to disrupt the study. The researcher should describe the data collection process in the published study. The strategies used to approach potential subjects who meet the sampling criteria should be made clear. The approach used to perform measurements and the timings and setting(s) need to be described. A step-by-step narration of exactly how the data were collected should be given; it will create a vivid picture of the scene of data collection.

The following is an example of procedure of data collection with the use of an observation checklist.

An Observational Study to Assess the Care Provided by Skill Mix and Informal Caregivers to the Critically Ill Patients in Selected Hospitals of Ludhiana, Punjab

Data Collection Procedure: Data collection for the study was carried out from December 1994 to February 1995. Before commencing the task of data collection, prior permission from the competent authorities was obtained. Care provided to 30 critically ill patients was observed. Observations were done by the investigator herself for two consecutive days on each patient starting at 5.30 a.m. until 11 p.m. according to time segments selected earlier, that is, 5.30 a.m. to 7.30 a.m., 8.30 a.m. to 10.30 a.m., 3.00 p.m. to 5.00 p.m., 6.00 p.m. to 8.00 p.m., and 9.00 p.m. to 11.00 p.m. A total of 10 observations on each patient were done. The observer stayed at a convenient distance and observed the care provided by the nursing personnel (skill mix) and informal caregivers. Ward staff and patients' relatives were told about the study being conducted but were not given details about the nature of the study to ensure objectivity. Observations were simultaneously entered in the observation checklist for analysis later on. For a few items, patient's charts were consulted such as to find out the diagnosis and some of the care being indicated by the doctors. (Observation checklist of this study is given on page …)

Sometimes, during the collection of data, accidental discovery of something useful or valuable may happen. Such discoveries should not be ignored; these could be used as additional findings of the study and should be included in the study while writing the final report. These would enrich the study. This may even open doors for further research concerning the issue at hand. The term used for this kind of findings is *serendipity*.

Despite improvement in instrument development, a prospective instrument user still needs to read widely and think critically and creatively to select or develop an instrument for the specific study under consideration.

KEY POINTS

- In quantitative research, the concepts under study are given numerical values in order to measure them.
- The purpose of measurement is to produce trustworthy evidence that can be used in evaluating the outcomes of the research.
- The purpose of the research is to collect information on the selected topic. An instrument in a research study is a device used to measure the concept of interest in a research project. The instrument should yield accurate, valid, and meaningful data. It requires considerable time and effort leading to thoughtful action to develop or select the appropriate tool for collecting the needed pieces of information.
- The instruments of data collection are self-report schedules or questionnaires, interview schedules, observation checklists, and rating scales.
- A questionnaire is a printed self-report form designed to elicit information that can be obtained through written responses of the subjects.
- Interviews involve verbal communication between the researcher and the subject, during which information is gathered by the researcher.
- Observational measurement may be structured or unstructured, and participatory or non-participatory. Practices and behaviours are measured with the help of observation checklists.
- Rating scales are used to measure the behaviours, attitudes, and opinions of the subjects.
- Reliability and validity are two statistical properties used to evaluate the quality of a research instrument.
- It is important that the instrument possesses both validity and reliability.
- The reliability of an instrument reflects its stability, homogeneity (internal consistency), and equivalence.
- The validity of an instrument is a determination of the extent to which the instrument actually reflects the abstract concept being examined. Validity, similar to reliability, is not an all-or-nothing phenomenon but rather a matter of degree. No instrument is totally valid.
- Four types of validity are used to judge the accuracy of an instrument. They are face validity, content validity, criterion-related validity, and construct validity.
- Data collection procedure and process requires five tasks: obtaining subjects, collecting data in a consistent way, maintaining research controls; protecting the integrity of the study, and solving the problems that threaten to disrupt the study.

QUESTIONS

I. Essay-type Questions

1. Discuss the factors governing data collection.
2. Enlist the methods of data collection
3. Describe the steps in development of research tool.
4. Explain the points to be kept in mind while constructing a questionnaire.

5. Describe the drawbacks of observational method.
6. Explain the significance of validation of research instrument.
7. Explain how reliability of an instrument can be achieved.
8. Discuss the characteristics of reliability.
9. Prepare an observation checklist to assess the steps taken by midwives in conducting antenatal examination of pregnant women in a selected district hospital.

II. Short Notes

1. Differentiate between the following with examples:
   (a) Structured and semi-structured interview schedule
   (b) Questionnaire and interview schedule
   (c) Questionnaire and observation checklist
   (d) Validity and reliability
   (e) Participant and non-participant observation
   (f) Graphic rating scale and itemized rating scale
   (g) Face validity and content validity
   (h) Open-ended and closed-ended questions

III. Multiple-choice Questions

Circle the alphabet before the best answer

1. Instruments or devices used for data collection are
   (a) self-report questionnaire and interview schedule
   (b) dichotomous and nominal scales
   (c) only (b)
   (d) both (a) and (b)
2. Data collection methods are governed by
   (a) research question or hypothesis
   (b) research design
   (c) variables under study
   (d) all of these
3. The types of interview schedules are
   (a) structured and unstructured
   (b) semi-structured and telephonic
   (c) both (a) and (b)
   (d) none of these
4. The drawbacks of observational method are
   (a) halo effect, error of leniency, and error of severity
   (b) sunflower effect and Hawthorne effect
   (c) both (a) and (b)
   (d) none of these
5. The essential aspects of reliable instruments are
   (a) stability
   (b) homogeneity
   (c) equivalence
   (d) all of these
6. Validity assessments are done by
   (a) face validity and content validity
   (b) criterion validity and construct validity
   (c) both (a) and (b)
   (d) only (b)

Answer Keys

1. (a) 2. (d) 3. (c) 4. (a) 5. (d) 6. (c)

FURTHER READING

Ashline, Harshita Prabhakaran. 2010. *Knowledge of Mother Regarding Care of Low Birth Weight Babies*. M.Sc. Thesis. Choithram College of Nursing, Indore, DAVV.

Burns, Nancy, Grove. Susan K. 1999. *Understanding Nursing Research*. Saunders, pp. 257–279.

Christ J Main, 2008, *Pain Management. Practical applications of the Biophysical Perspective: Churchill Livingstone*. Elsevier. P.182

George, Julia B. 2011. *Nursing Theories: The Base for Professional Nursing Practice*. New Delhi: Pearson, p. 8.

https//www.workcover.com

Joel, Smitha. 2009. *Severity of Menopausal Symptoms and the Life Satisfaction Level among Menopausal Women*. M.Sc. Thesis. Choithram College of Nursing, Indore, DAVV.

Kothari, C. R. 1985. *Research Methodology Methods and Techniques*. New Delhi: New Age International Publishers, pp. 71–75.

Mathew, Nissy. 2010. *Effectiveness of Abdominal Effleurage on Labour Pain Intensity during 1st Stage of Labour among Parturient Mothers Admitted in the Labour Room*. M.Sc. Thesis. Choithram College of Nursing, Indore, DAVV.

Nieswiadomy, Rose Marie 2008. *Foundations of Nursing Research*. Fifth edition. New Delhi: Pearson Education, p. 240.

Polit, Denise F., Hungler. Bernadette P. 1999. *Nursing Research: Principles and Methods*. Philadelphia: Lippincott, pp. 310–313.

Polit. Denise F., Beck. Cheryl Tatano. 2008. *Nursing Research: Generating and Assessing Evidence for Nursing Practice*. Philadelphia: Lippincott, pp. 407–409. Sharma. K. Suresh. 2011. *Nursing Research and Statistics*. Elsevier, Haryana Rajkamal Press, p. 126.

Samuel, Sonia. 2012. *Effectiveness of Educational Program on Husband Support during Labour among Husbands of Parturient in First Stage of Labour*. M.Sc. Thesis. Choithram College of Nursing, Indore, DAVV.

Stanford Patient Education Research Centre. Stanford University School of Medicine. http://patienteducation.stanford.edu.August 2007.

Ukande, Usha. 1995. *A Study to Assess the Care Provided by Skill Mix and Informal Care Givers to the Critically Ill Patients*. M.Sc. Thesis. Christian Medical College, Ludhiana, Punjab.

www.janicembell.com. NLN- National League for Nurses.

Young, A., Taylor, S. G., Renpenning, K. 2001. *Connections: Nursing Research, Theory and Practice*. Saint Louis: Mosby, pp. 80–89.

chapter 11

Data Analysis and Interpretation

OBJECTIVES

Upon completion of this chapter the learner will be able to:

- Describe the key terms used for data analysis
- Explain the various aspects of data analysis
- Elaborate on the details of descriptive statistics with illustrations
- Give details of inferential statistics and its applications
- Define meta-analysis
- State the usage of advanced statistical methods
- Portray the outline of qualitative data analysis
- Explain the generalization of research findings
- Illustrate the methods of presenting the analysed data

RESEARCH DATA ANALYSIS

In our day-to-day life, many questions arise—some out of mere curiosity, some looking for solution to problems. There are some queries that seek ways to get to the truth of the matter, leading to discoveries and inventions. The key to all answers lie in the sources of information, obtained through valid methods and reliable instruments. When such information is obtained through a systematic research process, it is called *data*. Data may be in any form—documented facts, figures, observations, objects, images, and so on. Moreover, they may be from past events, ongoing current incidences, or about evidence-based future predictions. Concrete forms of data are collected by using one or more of our sensory organs. Some data are abstract, such as perceptions, attitude, behaviour, opinion, experiences, and attributes. Data may be presented in diverse ways, depending on the purpose of the research study. However, to get the precise answer to the research question, the obtained data have to be organized, processed, and analysed.

Let us recollect and make ourselves clear about a few terms that are essentially innate to the activity of research data analysis:

1. Variables
2. Unit of analysis
3. Types of data

Variables

The characteristics of items, events, behaviour, and so forth on which observations are made and whose values are likely to vary or change by deliberate manipulation or accidental cause are called as variables. There are three basic categories of variables, which are explained using the following research report.

The clinical competencies for subcutaneous insulin administration and professional behaviour of the first, second, and third year undergraduate degree nursing students were compared. The findings showed that the clinical competency mean score of third year students was significantly higher than that of the second year students, inferring that repeated and extended clinical exposure and academic maturity might have had positive influence on the students' clinical competency. However, the students' professional behaviour was found to be independent of the above influences.

Now, let us analyse the three categories of variables using the variables in this report.

Dependent or Target Variable

This is a variable whose value may change when another variable in the study is manipulated by the researcher. Sometimes, it is also referred to as the *criterion variable*. In the given research project, *clinical competency* is the dependent variable.

Independent or Predictor Variable

This is a variable whose value is manipulated by the researcher to predict and change the value of the dependent variable. Hence, this is also referred to as the *manipulated variable*. In the given research project, *repeated and extended clinical exposure* and *academic maturity* are the independent variables.

Confounding Variable

This is a variable that the researcher fails to control, or eliminate, thus affecting the internal validity of an experiment. It may influence the relationship between the independent and dependent variables. As a result, the outcome does not reflect the actual relationship between the variables under investigation. Confounding variables are of two kinds, namely *extraneous and intervening*.

Extraneous Variable: This is a variable other than the independent variable that could cause a change in the dependent variable, such as gender, ethnicity, social class, genetics, intelligence, and age. Extraneous variable in an experimental design is controlled and conditioned. It correlates with both dependent and independent variables. In the given research project, *age*, *gender*, *social class*, *ethnicity*, *reason for preference of profession*, and *academic performance score* are the extraneous variables. These were in predetermined ranges for both experimental and control groups of students.

Intervening Variable: This variable refers mostly to intangible attributes and is much more difficult to control or condition. Intervening variables include emotional status, motivation, tiredness, life experiences and any such factor that arises during the course of research. In the given research project, *any* or *all* of these might have influenced the students' professional behaviour, because they could not be controlled or conditioned. A thorough review of literature could help to avoid these lacunae.

In statistical calculations, variables are either *continuous* or *categorical*.

Continuous Variable: A continuous variable has numeric values such as 1, 2, 3, and so on. The relative magnitude of the values is significant (for example, a value of 2 indicates twice the magnitude of the value 1). Blood pressure, height, weight, income, age, and so on are continuous variables. These are also referred to as *ordered* or *monotonic* variables.

Categorical Variable: A categorical variable has values that function as labels rather than as numbers but can be coded with numbers. For example, male (code 1) and female (code 2). The actual magnitude of the value is not significant (2 is not twice 1). In computer programs, non-numeric *string values* (sequence of words) may also be used for categorical variables, such as the strings *Male* and *Female* or *M* and *F* for a categorical gender variable. Because categorical values are stored and compared as string values, a categorical value of 001 is different from a value of 1. In contrast, the values of 001 and 1 would be equal for continuous variables. Categorical variables are also referred to as *nominal* variables.

Unit of Analysis

It is the core component around whom or which the whole process of data analysis unfolds. The individual subject or object upon whom or which information is collected is known as the *statistical unit*. Any of the following could be a unit of analysis:

1. Individuals
2. Groups (children, adult, men, women, etc.)
3. Objects or artefacts (books, photos, newspapers, etc.)
4. Geographical units (rural, urban, etc., settings)
5. Behavioural units (addiction, personality traits, etc.)
6. Social interactions (relationships)
7. Physical or physiological parameters (height, weight, Haemoglobin (Hb) level, blood pressure, etc.)

Types of Data

Data are the units of information about the issue or matter under study. It may be individuals, families, houses, villages, attitude, knowledge, skills, facts, figures, material attributes, and so on. The data collected may be called as *observations*. The items or characteristics on which the observations are made are known as *variables*. Data are commonly classified as *categorical*, *quantitative*, and *qualitative* data.

Categorical Data

These are defined groups with specific characteristics. Examples of categorical data are gender, age group, and educational level. When the data size is large, it is always better to categorize variables into a relatively small number of groups.

Analysis of categorical data generally uses data tables. A *two-way table* presents categorical data by counting the number of observations that fall into each group for two variables, one divided into rows and the other divided into columns. For example, in a survey, 20 selected children of classes I, II, III, and IV were asked to identify the colour of the pencils given to them. The two-way table presenting the results is shown in Table 11.1.

TABLE 11.1 *Two-way Table*

Pencil Colour					
Class	**Blue**	**Green**	**Red**	**Black**	**Total**
I	2	1	2	1	6
II	1	1	2	0	4
III	1	0	4	2	7
IV	1	0	2	0	3
Total	5	2	10	3	20

The total of each category, also known as *marginal distribution*, provides the number of individuals in each row or column, without accounting for the effect of the other variable (in the example given, the total number of children with blue pencils, regardless of the class, is five).

Two-way tables are often converted into percentages. In this example, there are four children (20%) in class II. Calculating percentages within a given category for these four children, two (50%) have red pencils, one (25%) has a blue pencil, and one (25%) has a green pencil. Categorical data can be also presented using graphs or diagrams, as shown in Fig. 11.1.

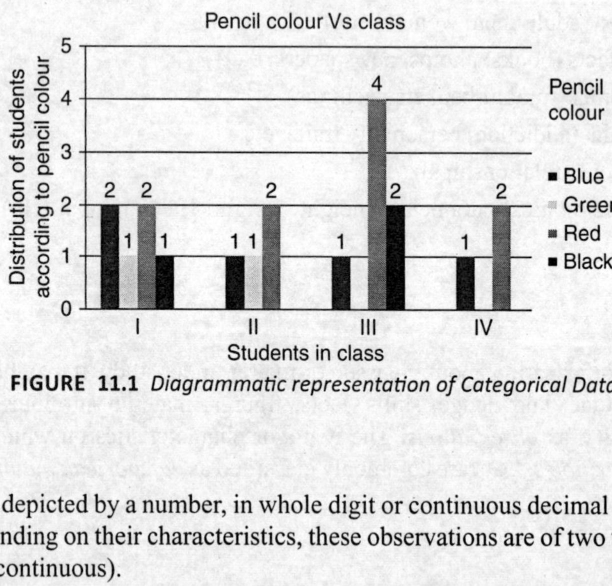

FIGURE 11.1 *Diagrammatic representation of Categorical Data*

Quantitative Data

The observations are depicted by a number, in whole digit or continuous decimal numbers, for example, 1, 2, 3, 3.5, 4.2. Depending on their characteristics, these observations are of two types, namely continuous and discrete (discontinuous).

Continuous observations can take any value within a continuous range, can be divided into smaller units, and use measuring devices, for example, height, weight, age, temperature, and serum cholesterol.

Discrete observations contain distinct whole number values, which cannot be divided internally. For example, goals in a football game can be 1, 2, and so on, but the goal count cannot be 1.5 or 2.7.

Qualitative Data

Vague estimates of subjective observations, abstract opinions, emotions, perceptions, and so on are known as qualitative data. These are data that describe but do not measure the attributes. Qualitative data can be quantified for ensuring objectivity of the research findings and quantitative data may be described on the basis of qualitative characteristics of the research unit. When qualitative and quantitative methods are used sequentially and simultaneously, it is called *triangulation*. In this method, the qualitative method may be used initially, until the emergence of the hypotheses. Then, the hypotheses may be tested using a quantitative method.

WHAT IS DATA ANALYSIS?

Data analysis has been defined and explained in many ways. It is a body of method that helps to describe facts, detect patterns, develop explanations, and test hypotheses. Analysis of data is a process of inspecting, cleaning, transforming, and modelling data or observations with the goal of highlighting useful information, suggesting conclusions, and supporting decision-making. It is a process of evaluating information using analytical and logical reasoning to inspect each part of the data provided. Data analysis is a practice in which raw data are prepared and organized so that useful information can be taken out from it. The process of organizing and thinking about data is most important to identify what the data contain and what more is to be done.

In short, data analysis is the step-by-step process of dissecting, scrutinizing, cleaning, and transforming raw data into clear information, which can answer the research questions presented as study hypotheses, suggest conclusions, and support decision-making.

DATA MEASUREMENT

The collected data must be appropriate and dependable for attaining the goals of any research study. This is possible if suitable methods and tools are used for measuring the data or information. For example, the knowledge of students can be measured by asking questions in written examination or viva voce, whereas their professional behaviour can be measured only by an observation checklist and not by a written examination.

Measurement is the process of assigning numbers to variables and may be *direct* or *indirect*. Examples of *direct measurements* are height, weight, vital signs, and physiological parameters. In the case of variables such as pain, stress, coping, self-esteem, and perception, concrete measurement is not possible, because the levels are not always consistent. At any given time, only some elements can be measured using the indicators for the purpose of analysis. These are *indirect measurements*.

Error is natural in any measurement approach. For example, while measuring a medicine for injection, the upper meniscus of the liquid must be at the graduated level marked on the syringe and the syringe has to be held at the eye level to see the mark correctly. In this step of procedure, human error is natural. Validity and reliability are the two essential safeguards to avoid these errors. In standardized tools, these errors are corrected by specific statistical methods.

Selecting the appropriate method for data analysis requires the understanding of the *levels of measurement*.

Levels of Measurement

There are four levels of measurement, which are also known as *measurement scales*. The mathematical calculations that can be done with the data depend on them. The level of measurement refers to the relationship among the values that are assigned to the attributes for a variable. In the research study mentioned earlier, the clinical competency of first, second, and third year undergraduate nursing students are compared. For purposes of analyses, the numbers 1, 2, and 3 are arbitrarily assigned to these three groups. The level of measurement describes the relationship among these three groups. There are typically four levels of measurement, namely *nominal*, *ordinal*, *interval*, and *ratio*.

Nominal

In nominal measurement, the numerical values are just *name* or *category*, which cannot be compared. In the given illustration, the numbers are simply assigned as symbols or code numbers to categories that are exhaustive in nature and have no quantitative meaning. Number 2 does not mean that second year students have more clinical competency than first year students (number 1), nor does it mean that they have less clinical competency than third year students (number 3). Moreover, the group members in the first, second, and third year classes are not more or less in number than the others. Data such as gender, marital status, religion, clinical diagnosis, and academic level are examples of *nominal level of measurement*, which shows distinct qualitative differences among the groups. These data are presented in a research report as *frequencies* and *percentages*; they cannot be added or subtracted. The nominal measurements are considered as the lowest or the least rigorous of the measurement levels.

Ordinal

In this measure, the data are assigned to categories that can be rank-ordered such as higher or lower, but the exact differences between the ranks cannot be specified. As with nominal measurement, the categories must be exhaustive and exclusive. Here, the distances between the attributes do not have any meaning. For example, in a survey, the education level of the subjects may be coded as follows:

0—No formal education

1—Less than higher secondary education

2—Higher secondary education

3—Less than college degree

4—College degree

5—Postgraduate education

In this measure, higher numbers mean *more* education. However, it can be seen that the distance from 0 to 1 is not the same as that from 3 to 4. The interval between values is not interpretable in an ordinal measure as the intervals are not equal. The arrangement in an ascending or descending order is made arbitrarily.

Interval Measurement

In *interval* measurement scales, there are equal numerical distances between the intervals. These scales have mutually exhaustive and exclusive categories or rank-ordering, consist of actual numbers, and represent a continuum of values, as in a thermometer. Therefore, the attributes can be more precisely defined. On measuring temperature (in Fahrenheit), the distance from 30 to 40 is the same as that from 70 to 80; hence, average reading is possible. The interval between the values is interpretable.

Ratio Scale

In a *ratio scale*, the numbers can be compared as multiples of one another. The name *ratio* indicates that measurements are in ratio. Thus, one person can be twice as tall as another person. Moreover, the number zero has a meaning. A person can also have an age of zero. Ratio data can be multiplied and divided because not only is the difference between 1 and 2 the same as that between 3 and 4, but also 4 is twice the magnitude of 2.

For more precision in data analysis, it is better to use higher levels of measurement, such as interval or ratio. It is all the more appropriate because the qualities of the lower levels of measurement are anyway built-in in the immediate higher level measurement.

For example, in a class, the aggregate maximum mark is 500. The obtained aggregate marks of students ranked as first, second, and third are 475, 402, and 390, respectively. This ranking order is designed following the ordinal level of measurement, as the difference in marks between the consecutive ranks is not the same. If the researcher wants to use the interval level of measurement in the same example, he/she has to define the actual and equal marks difference, may be 25, thus making them 475, 450, and 425, respectively. To ensure approximate accuracy, the ranking also can be done as 450–475, 425–450, and 400–425.

Nominal and ordinal data are classified under *categorical* or *discrete* type of variables. Continuous type of variables is classified as *interval* and *ratio* data. The measurement of these data follows the specific type. It is important to take the measurement levels of the variables into account for the analyses, as special statistical techniques are available for each level. See Fig. 11.2.

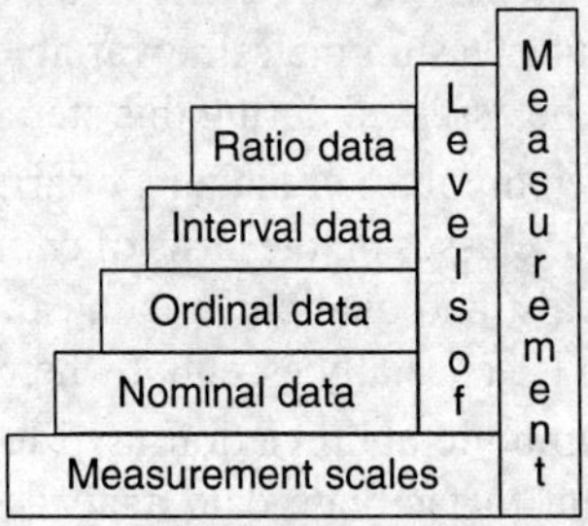

FIGURE 11.2 *Levels of Measurement for Various Data*

Exceptions

In some situations, the measurement scale is ordinal but the variable is treated as continuous. For example, a five-point Likert scale (strongly agree, agree, neutral, disagree, and strongly disagree) is ordinal. However, when a Likert scale contains seven or more values (strongly agree, moderately agree, agree, neutral, disagree, moderately disagree, and strongly disagree), the underlying scale is sometimes treated as continuous.

STEPS IN DATA ANALYSIS

The data analysis process aims at answering the research questions. In this, either an exploratory or confirmatory approach can be adopted, which is usually decided before data are collected. In an *exploratory analysis* no clear hypothesis is stated, and an effort is taken to explore or search for the data using a suitable tool. Established conceptual models may be used to provide direction and road map to search for the data and describe them. In a *confirmatory analysis*, clear hypotheses about the data are tested to determine the relationship between variables.

It is important to follow systematic steps for analysing data, as this phase is the central part of any research study. The main steps are as follows:

1. **Data Preparation:** Cleaning and organizing the data for analysis
2. **Describing the Data:** Using descriptive statistics
3. **Testing Hypotheses:** Using inferential statistics

Data Preparation

This involves checking or logging the data in, checking the data for accuracy, entering the data into the computer, transforming the data, and developing and documenting a database structure that integrates the various measures. It can be also done manually. Data preparation consists of the following steps:

1. **Data Cleaning:** Data cleaning is done at the stage of data entry. In this step, the data are inspected and flawed data are corrected. However, it is important not to throw information away during the cleaning phase; all information should be saved and should always be retrievable. Moreover, it should always be possible to undo any data set.
2. **Data Compilation:** This refers to arranging data in a meaningful order. While doing this, it is imperative to check the quality of data, missing data, and extreme observations to see if they disturb the distribution.
3. **Data Editing:** Checking all data for their accuracy, usefulness, and adequacy is made in this step. Incorrect data and those too far away from the mean value can influence the outcome of the study to a great extent. *Internal consistency* (homogeneity) must be taken care of to ensure that all items of the measurement instrument measure the same variable. Sample dropout, non-response, and treatment quality also need to be assessed during this step.
4. **Data Categorization:** This step involves organizing or arranging the data and dividing them into several homogeneous groups or classes on the basis of common characteristics. Quantitative data are categorized in class intervals, and qualitative data can be categorized according to different attributes. Data categorization is especially essential when there is a large volume of raw data.
5. **Data Coding:** A code is a symbolic abbreviation used to classify data. Coding is a method of categorizing and indexing data to facilitate data analysis and retrieval whenever necessary. It can be done before or after the data are collected. Manual coding can be done creatively by using colours, objects, numbers, letters of the alphabet, and so on. Computer language is used for computer-assisted data analysis. The appropriate method of coding is better decided while developing the research tools in order to avoid errors in data analysis. The important considerations for data coding are that data categories must be exhaustive, that is, all data are placed in one or other category, and the codes should be mutually exclusive, that is, each code should be specific to specific category of data.

Data Organization and Computerization

The decision about the type and amount of data to be collected depends on the research objectives, and appropriate methods of data organization help in accurate statistical data analysis. When the sample size is small and the aspects of the matter to be studies are limited, data organization is a simple task and can even be done manually. However, if the sample size is very large and the study aims at establishing multiple correlations of varieties of components, data organization must be done methodically, preferably by a computer.

In large studies, data management is relatively difficult and requires more people, time, money, and other such facilities. Data storage to keep track of the information and periodic review of the research progress are necessary steps in the process. This stored information is utilized by research studies, such as longitudinal retrospective or prospective studies. Two systems can be of use for data organization:

1. Maintaining a formatted register (spreadsheet), designed for entering relevant information from each record in a brief manner or as coded materials, for example, medical records.
2. Introducing a unit record system, where individual records are maintained for each unit, for example, the cumulative records of students from admission to course completion.

With the advent of computers, data management by either of these systems has become faster and easier. Computers are useful for data entry, data storing, data editing, data management and follow up, data monitoring, word processing, and preparing reports for presentations and manuscripts for publications. Internet facilities have enhanced the computer capacity in data analysis manifold.

Computer Hardware

Computers are electronic devices that can store large quantities of data and analyse them at high speed. There are three basic categories of computers, namely microcomputers, minicomputers, and mainframe computers. The most common type is the microcomputers, which in the form of compact desktop computers are used for office as well as personal purposes.

The following are the physical hardware units or components of a computer:

1. Central processing unit (CPU)
2. Monitor (visual display unit)
3. Keyboard (for data entry)
4. Magnetic storage devices (hard disk, compact disk, printing or plotting units)
5. Accessories, such as UPS (uninterrupted power supply), air conditioning, modems, storage facilities for records, and printers

The capacity of a computer is usually expressed in terms of *bytes* (measure of information it can store in memory).

8 bits = 1 byte
1024 bytes = 1 kilobyte or KB
1024 KB = 1 megabyte or MB
1024 MB = 1 gigabyte or GB

Computer Software

This includes a special kind of program called an *operating system*, which controls the flow of information between the different components. One such system commonly used is MS DOS (Microsoft Disk Operating System). One of the most important functions of an operating system is to make the hardware understand the instructions of the software. In addition, it manages all files on the disks and maintains a file directory. There are several kinds of user-friendly software available for each of these functions. The basic component of all these machines is the *microprocessor*, comprising thousands of transistors on a silicon chip.

Programming a computer requires knowledge of special computer languages. Some examples for such languages are COBOL (Common Business Oriented Language), FORTRAN (Formula Translation), BASIC (Beginners All-purpose Symbolic Instruction Code), Visual Basic, and JAVA. Other software commonly used includes MS Word and MS Excel. Moreover, statistical package programs, such as SAS, SPSS, STATA, MS Excel, Epi Info, Egret, and many other advanced ones are available in the market. These are used to summarize and analyse statistical data. The following are a few commonly used statistical packages.

MS Excel (Spreadsheets): Many varieties of worksheets are available, with cells formed by rows and columns, usually known as *spreadsheets*. The most common is Microsoft Excel or MS Excel. It is used for entering data and for performing mathematical calculations and statistical computations. It is also used for univariate statistical analysis, simple tabulation, keeping accounts, and drawing histograms, scatter diagrams, and so on.

SPSS (Statistical Package for Social Sciences): It contains all simple and advanced statistical procedures, such as multivariate analyses, non-parametric analyses, and survival analyses, and can export files. STATA is more specific than SPSS and occupies less memory space.

Epi Info: This epidemiological data management software was developed by Centers for Disease Control and Prevention (CDC), Atlanta, Georgia, USA. It is very useful for public health studies.

Data Tabulation

It is the process of arranging the categorized data in numerical form, manually or using computerized methods, usually in rows and columns. Tabulation helps in understanding the data more clearly and deciding suitable statistical tests for data analysis.

Describing the Data

This is done by using descriptive statistics, which are used to describe the basic features of the data in a study and provide summaries about the sample and the measures in simple terms. They form the basis of almost every quantitative analysis of data.

Testing Hypotheses

This is done by using inferential statistics. These are concerned with population and use the data to make *inference* about a population. Examples are finding differences, relationships, and association between two or more variables.

DESCRIPTIVE STATISTICS

This is a set of tools and techniques used to organize, describe, and summarize numerically the characteristics of samples, populations, or related collection of information; this collection is sometimes called as *data set* or just *data*.

In general, descriptive statistics is classified into the following *four* categories:

1. Measures to condense data
2. Measures of central tendency
3. Measures of variability
4. Measures of relationships

Measures to Condense Data

When the collected data size is very large, it is necessary to summarize and make it compact for easy understanding. Usually, quantitative data are condensed. The various measures used to condense data are as follows:

1. Frequency distribution
2. Graphic representation
3. Percentages

Before we discuss these measures in detail, let us recall the basics of *tabulation*.

Tabulation or *classification* is the process by which the data are systematically organized and recorded, to make it easy for analysis and interpretation. A set of categories is formed to classify data. It is important to remember that these categories should be selected in such a way that each one of the observations falls into any one of these categories; however, an observation should appear in only one category. All observations should be in either of these categories, and nothing should be left out. The following are the essential requirements to form a table:

1. Every category of observations included in a table must be related to the research problem.
2. The table must be clear and must have the total number of observations (N) written on the top of the table at the right side.
3. The title of the table must explain in specific terms what the data represent.
4. The numerical value of observations or figures in the body of the table must be arranged in a logical order; depending upon the point discussed in the text, it may be highest to lowest or lowest to highest.
5. When several points are to be highlighted using the same data, it would be preferable to present the data in many small tables, one to illustrate each point.

Frequency Distribution

It can be used for reporting all levels of data (nominal, ordinal, interval, and ratio). The scores are usually grouped into *class intervals* or *ranges* of numbers. A range is the difference between the highest and the lowest score values. The class interval may be arbitrarily chosen to represent the data and it has to be the same for all levels of frequencies. If the numerical value of the observation or score is small, that is, less than 20, each score may be listed individually.

Cumulative Frequency (Ogive): It is the *running total* of frequencies, that is, the total of a frequency and all frequencies below it in a frequency distribution. Cumulative frequency gives the total number of events that occurred up to some value and is used extensively in risk or reliability analysis to determine the chances for an event to occur. For example, in an objective test for a class of 50 students, the maximum score assigned is 100. The scores obtained by the students fall in the range of 0 to 98. The raw data arranged from lower to higher scores are shown in Fig. 11.3 and Table 11.2.

0	28	49	68	79
04	31	50	68	80
09	35	52	70	83
10	36	53	71	85
15	40	53	74	88
19	44	54	75	88
25	45	54	76	88
26	46	62	76	89
27	47	65	77	89
27	48	67	78	98

The range of raw data 0–98 is divided into nice groups, by selecting 11 as the class interval (CI). the number of raw data available in each group is entered against the respective CI, counting by using tallies. Cumulative frequencies are estimated by adding the successive frequencies. CI may be of any number by dividing the range of values. A frequency table is created by organizing all these in a systematic manner.

FIGURE 11.3 *Frequency Table*

TABLE 11.2 *Frequency Distribution of Students' Objective Test Score in a Range of 0–98*

$n = 50$			
Class Interval of Score	**Rate Tallies**	**Frequency (*f*)**	**Cummulative Frequency (*cf*)**
0–10	////	04	04
11–21	//	02	06
22–32	卌 /	06	12
33–43	///	03	15
44–54	卌 卌 //	12	27
55–65	//	02	29
66–76	卌 ////	09	38
77–87	卌 /	06	44
88–98	卌 /	06	50
Total	0 – 98	50	

The findings from Table 11.2 show that with a class interval of 11, the maximum number of students, 12, has scored in the range of 44–54. It may be inferred from the cumulative frequencies that there are chances of 15 students (30%) scoring below the pass marks (50%) in the forthcoming qualifying examination. It makes us think of ways and means to help these 15 students to score better in the qualifying examination.

The frequency table shown here is a visual representation of the observations by using tallies. In this method, there is a possible loss of information. In the given list of raw data, one student has got just 0, one has got 04, one has got 09, and one has scored 10. When these are grouped in a class interval and summarized, it shows that four students have scored in the range 0–10. Here, the true picture of students' performance is not seen.

Characteristics of a Frequency Distribution: After developing a frequency distribution, the next step is to calculate certain values that are used to describe the characteristics of that distribution. These values help to compare different kinds of observation. There are *four* major characteristics of a frequency distribution:

1. The measures of central tendency (location, position, average)
2. The degree of scatter of the observations around the measure of central tendency (variability, dispersion, spread)
3. The extent of symmetry in the shape of the distribution (skewness, asymmetry)
4. The fatness or peakness of the distribution (kurtosis)

Of these four, the first two are commonly used to describe a set of data.

Graphic Representation

Graphs are used to present data in an organized and concise manner. They must have a title and an index, and the scales must be appropriate. The graphs that are commonly used in research reporting are bar diagram, pie chart, frequency polygon, line graph, cumulative frequency curve, scatter diagram, pictogram, and maps. Figure 11.4 shows examples of a bar diagram, line graph, and pie chart.

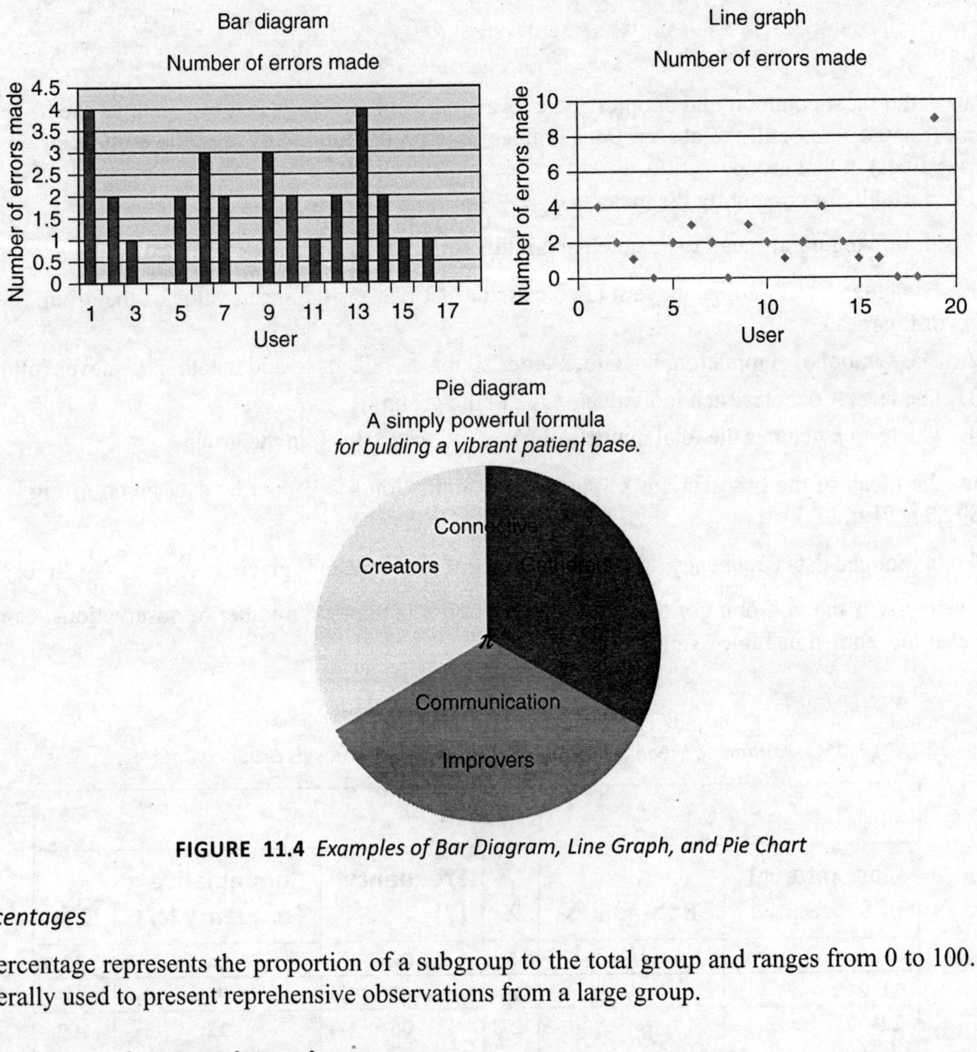

FIGURE 11.4 *Examples of Bar Diagram, Line Graph, and Pie Chart*

Percentages

A percentage represents the proportion of a subgroup to the total group and ranges from 0 to 100. It is generally used to present reprehensive observations from a large group.

Measures of Central Tendency

In any set of data, though the values of the observations are not equal, a general tendency of these observations to cluster around a particular point or level is noticed. In this situation, it may be necessary to distinguish each group of observations by such a level or point (value), which is referred to as the *central tendency* of that group. This single value for each group of observations serves as a representative of that group. This level or point may vary from group to group and is known as the *average*. For example, the average haemoglobin levels of people of two different age groups vary. Though individual values may overlap, the two distributions have different *central positions* and therefore differ in their characteristic of *location*.

Measures of central tendency can be calculated in several ways for a group of observations. The commonly used measures are *mode*, *median*, *mean*, and *percentile*. They may not have the same value and each provides a different type of information about a distribution score. Choosing the most appropriate measure for a particular distribution would depend upon the way the observations in the group cluster or gather around that central point or level.

Mean

Mean is the most common and simplest type of average computed. It is also called as the *arithmetic mean*. It is the sum of all the observations (values) in a group divided by the total number of observations (values) in that group.

The formula for computing the mean is $\bar{X} = \dfrac{\Sigma X}{n}$.

The following points need to be noted about this formula:

1. The letter X with a line above it (also called as 'X bar') is the mean value of the group of score or the mean.
2. The symbol of summation, the Greek letter sigma Σ, tells us to add together whatever follows it.
3. The term X denotes each individual value in the group.
4. The term n denotes the total number of observations (values) in the group.

Thus, the mean of the observations of students' examination scores as raw data given in Fig. 11.3 is 2580/50 = 51.6.

For a grouped data (frequency distribution), the arithmetic mean is given by $\bar{X} = \sum \dfrac{fx}{n}$ Here, f is the frequency, X is the mid-point of the class interval, and n is the total number of observations. Consider the example shown in Table 11.3.

TABLE 11.3 *Arithmetic Mean of Students' Objective Test Scores as Grouped Data*

$n = 50$					
Class Interval of Score	**Rate Tallies**	**X**	**Frequency (*f*)**	**Cummulative Frequency (*cf*)**	**Σfx**
0–10	////	5	04	04	20
11–21	//	16	02	06	32
22–32	𝍸 /	27	06	12	162
33–43	///	38	03	15	114
44–54	𝍸 𝍸 //	49	12	27	588
55–65	//	60	02	29	120
66–76	𝍸 ////	71	09	38	639
77–87	𝍸 /	82	06	44	492
88–98	𝍸 /	93	06	50	558
Total	**0–98**		**50**		**2725**

The mid-points of the given class intervals are

$$X = (0 + 10)/2, (11 + 21)/2, (22 + 32)/2, (33 + 43)/2, (44 + 54)/2,$$
$$(55 + 65)/2, (66 + 76)/2, (77 + 87)/2, (88 + 98)/2$$
$$\Sigma fx = (5 \times 4 = 20), (16 \times 2 = 32), (27 \times 6 = 162),$$
$$(38 \times 3 = 114), (49 \times 12 = 588), (60 \times 2 = 120),$$
$$(71 \times 9 = 639), (82 \times 6 = 492), (93 \times 6 = 558)$$
$$\text{Total: } 20 + 32 + 162 + 114 + 588 + 120 + 639 + 492 + 558 = 2725$$

So, now the calculated arithmetic mean of the students' score is $X = \sum \frac{fx}{n}$, that is, 2725/50= 54.5.

The arithmetic mean is also defined as the point at which the sum of the deviations from the mean is equal to zero. So, if we have scores such as 3, 4, and 5, where the mean is 4, the sum of the deviations (−1, 0, and +1) is zero.

Median

Median, which is sometimes abbreviated as *Md* or *Mdn*, is the middle score or value in a group of data. For interval and ratio data, the median divides the frequency distribution of the data in half. If the number of values is an odd number, the middle value is the median. If the number of values is an even number, the average of the two middle values will give the median.

For the data in Fig. 11.3, the number of values is an even number, 50. Therefore, the median is calculated as (53 + 54)/2 = 53.5.

Mode

The mode, which is abbreviated as *Mo*, is the most frequently occurring category or value in a set of data or a group of observations. It is the value around which the observations tend to be most heavily concentrated.

In Fig. 11.3, the score 88 is the mode. If the students' scores are 66, 68, 71, 77, 83, and so on, it is apparent that there is no mode. It should be noted that mode is the only measure of central tendency appropriate for nominal data, though it may also be used for ordinal, interval, and ratio data.

When the data are only categories, and not in number, the category with the greatest frequency is called the *modal class*. For example, if an observation consists of 30, 40, and 50 students of classes V, VI, and VIII, respectively, the modal class will be the 50 students of class VIII.

If the distribution of the observation is symmetrical in a frequency distribution, the mode has the same value as the median and mean. The set of observations is *unimodal* if there is only one value occurring most frequently. If two values have the same high frequency, the set of observations is called *bimodal*, and when there are more than two same frequency values, it is termed as *multimodal*. Mode is a crude estimation of the average value of observations, so its usage is comparatively less than the median and mean.

For a moderately asymmetric frequency distribution, the mode is calculated by the empirical relationship

$$\text{Mode} = 3 \text{ Median} - 2 \text{ Mean}$$

or using the formula $L_M + \frac{d_1 C}{d_1 + d_2}$,

where

L_M = Lower limit of the modal class
d_1 = Frequency in modal class *minus* frequency in the preceding class
d_2 = Frequency in modal class *minus* frequency in the succeeding class
C = Class interval of the modal class

For the data of Table 11.2,

Mode = 88 (most frequently repeated value)

For modal class, $\text{Mode} = 88 + \frac{44 \times 11}{50 \times 11} = 88 + \frac{484}{550} = 88.8$

Percentile

The value below which a given percentage of observations occurs is called a *centile* or *percentile*. The median is also called the fiftieth percentile because it divides a distribution into half. The twenty-fifth and seventy-fifth percentiles are known as *lower quartile* and *upper quartile*, respectively.

Measures of Variability or Dispersion

The deviation of values or observations from the average is known as *variation* or *dispersion.* The *degree of variation* is calculated by the measures of variation or measures of dispersion. It helps to characterize the observations. The haemoglobin values of the following two groups of children have the same central tendency (12.5), but the degree of variation of observations from the mean greatly differs, which differentiates the groups from each other.

Group I:	12.1,	12.2,	12.8,	12.9,	12.3,	12.4,	12.7,	12.6,	12.5
Group II:	12.1,	12.3,	11.7,	11.9,	13.1,	13.3,	12.5,	12.9,	12.7

The following are the common measures of variability:

1. Range
2. Interquartile range
3. Standard deviation
4. *z*-Score
5. Coefficient of variation

Range: It is the interval between the highest and lowest values of the observations (highest – lowest). The occurrence of rare observations in a group greatly influences the range and so this is not an ideal measure of variation.

Interquartile Range: It is the difference between the upper and lower quartiles and, hence, covers the middle 50 per cent of the observations in the group. Unlike the range, this measure is not affected by the occurrence of rare values. When the extreme values are not very accurate, the median and interquartile range can be adopted to measure the central tendency and dispersion, respectively.

Standard Deviation: It is the most commonly used measure of variability for interval and ratio data. The word *standard* here means *average*. It indicates the measure of how the values are spread out and their distance from the mean, that is, the *average deviation* of all the values from the mean value of the observations. Similar to arithmetic mean, it includes all the values in a distribution.

The formula for calculating standard deviation is SD or $= \sqrt{\dfrac{\Sigma(X-\bar{X})^2}{n}}$

where SD or s denotes the standard deviation, X denotes the value, and n denotes the number of values.

Because a sample may be a biased estimation of a population, $n - 1$ should be used while estimating a population standard deviation from a sample data.

Figure 11.5 shows the calculation of standard deviation for various occurrences.

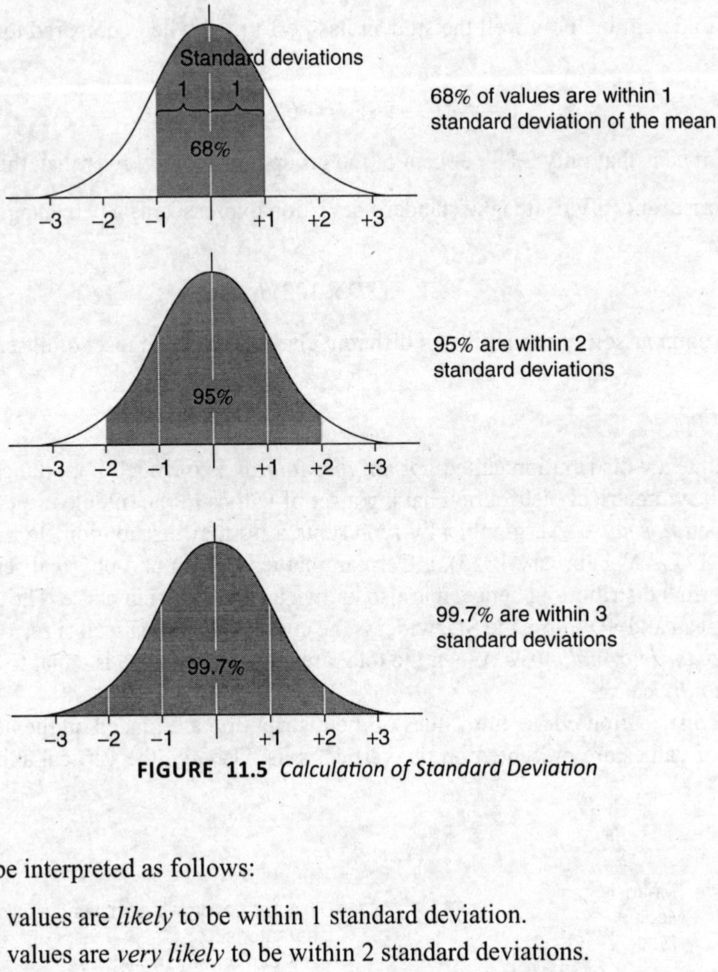

FIGURE 11.5 *Calculation of Standard Deviation*

The figure can be interpreted as follows:

1. 68 of 100 values are *likely* to be within 1 standard deviation.
2. 95 of 100 values are *very likely* to be within 2 standard deviations.
3. 99.7 of 100 values are *almost certainly* within 3 standard deviations.

The number of standard deviations from the mean is also called the *standard score*, *sigma*, or *z-score*.

***z*-Score:** This indicates the distance of a particular observation (value) from the mean in terms of standard deviation. It is also called a standard score, because it is interpreted in relation to the standard deviation units above and below the mean.

The formula for calculating z-score is $Z = \frac{X - \bar{X}}{SD}$
where

$Z = z$-Score
X = Raw score or observation (value) to be standardized
$\bar{X}$ = Mean raw score or value of the population
SD = Standard deviation of the population

The z-score is important for interpreting a particular value in comparison to the other values in a distribution. For example, a student has scored 92 in a class test with 110 objective type questions. The mean raw score is 98 and $SD = 3$.

It is possible to determine how well the student has performed when compared to other students by using the z-score.

$$(92 - 98)/3 = -6/3 = -2.0$$

The score '–2.0' means that only 2.28 per cent of the group had scored lower than this student.

Coefficient of Variation (CV): It is the standard deviation expressed as a percentage of the arithmetic mean, that is,

$$CV = (SD \times 100)/\text{Mean}.$$

It is used for the comparison of variability of different characteristics of a set of observations.

Normal Distribution

A theoretical frequency distribution called *normal distribution* is of much importance in research data estimation. It is a symmetrical distribution having a set of values in the middle or peak of the distribution. A bell-shaped *normal curve* graphically represents a normal distribution. Johann Carl Friedrich Gauss (30 April 1777–23 February 1855), a German mathematician and physical scientist, developed the concept of normal distribution; hence, it is also known as the Gaussian curve. The shape of the curve depends on the mean and SD; more the SD, wider is the curve. When the mean is zero and the SD is one, it is called as *standard normal curve*. When the total area under the curve is equal to unity, it is known as *normal probability curve*.

In the normal distribution curve, the values of the distribution are placed on the horizontal axis and the frequencies of values are presented on the vertical axis. Usually, the vertical axis is not displayed (Fig. 11.6).

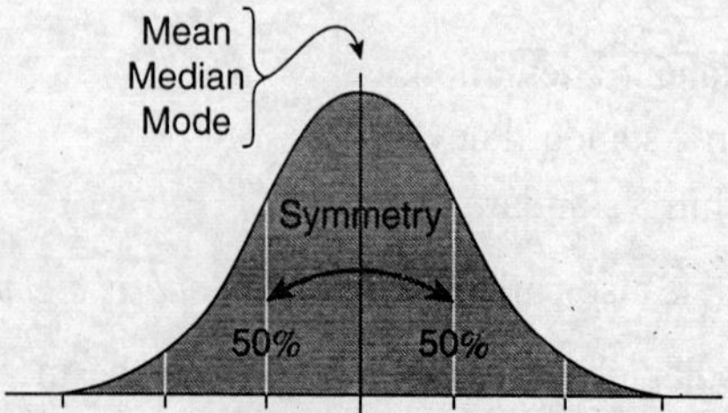

This normal distribution has the following characteristics:
- Mean = Median = Mode
- There is symmetry about the centre.
- Fifty per cent of the values are less than the mean and fifty per cent are greater than the mean.

FIGURE 11.6 *Normal Distribution*

Many human characteristics tend to follow a normal distribution. It includes biological measurements such as height, weight, and blood pressure. For example, in a random sample, the height of adults in India will measure between 120 cm and 200 cm. Only few heights will be measured outside this range. Normal distributions generally develop when the sample size or number of observations are very large.

Consider the weight of nine newly born babies given in kilograms as 3.2, 3.0, 2.9, 2.8, 3.0, 3.2, 3.1, 2.7, and 2.5. The mean, median, and mode of that data are approximately equal; mean = 2.93, median = 3, and mode = 3. In this case, the mean values are in the same spot at the middle of the normal curve. However, sometimes, some scores in a data set are not equal on both the sides. Moreover, these scores fall farther towards the tail of the curve.

Let us assume that there are two malnourished babies in the given example; so, we replace 3.2 and 3.0 by 1.0 and 1.1, respectively. In this case, mean = 2.47, median = 2.8, and mode = 1. Due to these two malnourished children, the mean weight of the babies gets shifted towards the negative end. When low scores pull the mean towards the left tail, the data are said to be *negatively skewed*. On the other hand, if some healthy babies are also part of this case, the mean shifts towards the positive side; such types of data are called *positively skewed data*.

The *probability curve* is symmetrical but only moderately. If it rises rapidly, reaches a maximum, and then falls slowly, it is a called a *positively skewed curve*. If it rises slowly, reaches a maximum, and then falls rapidly, it is called a *negatively skewed curve*. For these curves, the mean, the median, and the mode do not coincide (Fig. 11.7).

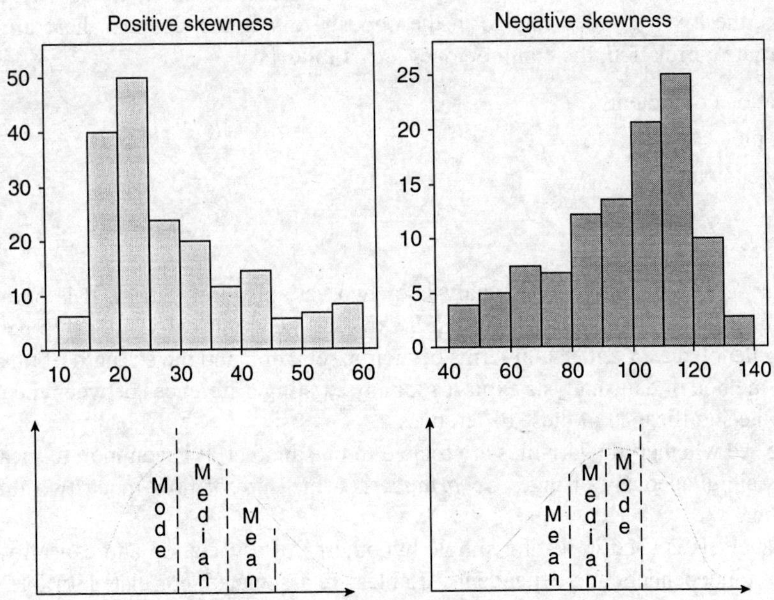

FIGURE 11.7 *Skewness and Normal Distributions*

However, there are many studies where the data tend to be around a central value with no bias to left or right; they get close to a normal distribution as shown in Fig. 11.8.

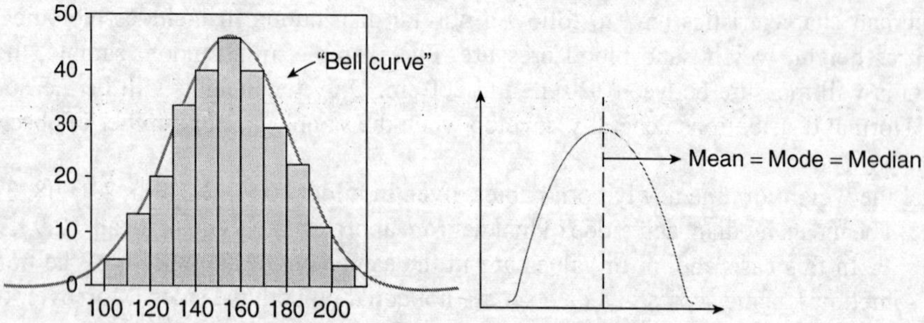

FIGURE 11.8 *Normal Distribution*

Measures of Relationship (Multivariate)

This is to find the *correlations between quantitative variables* of similar characteristics, for example, height, weight, and biological variables such as pressure and pain. *Correlational analysis* that is done to find the *direction* (positive or negative) and *magnitude* (strength) of the relationship between two variables is a *bivariate correlation*.

For example, as the pressure exerted on a body part increases, the intensity of pain also increases simultaneously due to nerve injury and vice versa. Both variables change in the same direction, either increasing or decreasing. This is a *positive correlation*.

A person's degree of dehydration affects his blood pressure reading. That is, as the degree of dehydration increases, the blood pressure reading falls below normal. This is a *negative* (*inverse*) *correlation*. In this, the two variables change in the opposite directions. Though there are many ways to measure bivariate correlation, the common ones are as follows:

1. Correlation coefficient
2. Scatter plot
3. Contingency table

Bivariate Analysis

Bivariate analysis is the simultaneous analysis of two variables (attributes). It is one of the simplest forms of the quantitative (statistical) analysis. It explores the empirical relationship between two variables (usually denoted as X and Y), in terms of their association and the strength of this association. In addition, this method of data analysis explores for any existing differences between the two variables in question and the significance of these differences.

In order to see whether the variables are related to one another, it is common to measure how these two variables simultaneously change. *Covariance* is a measure of how much two random variables change together.

Bivariate analysis is used in testing simple hypotheses of association and causality—checking the extent to which independent and dependent variables are associated, correlated, or one causes changes in the other.

Types of Bivariate Analysis: The common forms of bivariate analysis involve creating a *percentage table* and the computation of a simple *correlation coefficient, scatter plot graph*, and *contingency table* (Table 11.4).

TABLE 11.4 *Percentages of Men and Women in Categories of Earning*

n = 200		
Earnings	**Men**	**Women**
<₹20,00	47%	52%
₹20,000–50,000	45%	47%
>₹50,000	8%	1%
Valid cases: 200 Missing cases: 0		

A bivariate analysis is intended to investigate whether there is any significant difference in the earnings of men and women. A table of percentages of the population is created within various categories, based on gender and earnings.

- The data are described in percentages, not associated or correlated.
- The types of analysis that are suited to particular pairs of variables vary in accordance with the level of measurement of the variables (for example, nominal or categorical, ordinal, interval or ratio).

1. **Correlation Coefficient:** It can be seen that bivariate analysis is a simple (two variable) variant of multivariate analysis (where multiple relations among multiple variables are examined simultaneously). The degree of the relationship between these two variables is presented through a measurement called a *correlation coefficient*, which is represented by r. Hence, $r = +1$ symbolizes a perfect positive relationship, $r = -1$ symbolizes a perfect negative relationship, and $r = 0$ indicates the absence of any relationship. Therefore, r can vary between -1 and $+1$, the extremes of a perfect relationship. As the r value approaches 0, the strength of the relationship decreases. Biological variables generally do not show perfect correlations; there are only *moderately positive correlations*, $+0 < r < 1$, and *moderately negative correlations*, $-1 < r < 1$.

   The magnitude or strength of a relationship is indicated by its size. For example, $r = 0.8$ denotes a stronger relationship than a value less than 0.80, such as 0.70, 0.60, or 0.50. For positive correlation, the + sign is not always required. Similarly, $r = -0.50$ is stronger than $r = -0.40$. The sign indicates only the direction of relationship.

   Correlation can be measured between two different variables taken from a set of observations, such as height and weight of under-five children. Moreover, one variable taken from two sets of homogeneous or matched observations can be correlated, for example, weight of under-five children of high- and middle-income groups. Interval level data can best be correlated. Large samples with varied scores are better for correlational analysis, as the number of extreme values (+1 to −1) influences the result.

   Correlation coefficients may be used to measure the reliability of a research instrument by the test-retest method, where $r = 1.00$ indicates a perfect reliability, $r = 0.80$ is the lowest acceptable reliability measure of a well-developed measurement tool, and $r = 0.7$ is just acceptable to approve a research tool.

   The following is the Spearman–Brown prophecy formula for reliability testing:

$$r^1 = \frac{2r}{1+r}$$

If $r = 0.7402$,

$$r^1 = \frac{2 \times 0.7402}{1+0.7402} = \frac{1.4804}{1.7402} = 0.8499$$

Hence, the reliability of the research instrument is 0.8499.

There are no established criteria to evaluate the strength of a correlation coefficient. It depends on the nature of the variables. According to Polit, correlations between psychosocial variables rarely exceed 0.5.

The computation of correlation coefficients can be done in the following two methods:

(a) Karl Pearson's correlation coefficient

(b) Spearman's rank correlation coefficient

(a) **Karl Pearson's Correlation Coefficient:** This is also known as *Pearson product–moment correlation*. This bivariate correlation measures the extent of relationship between two variables. It is computed by using the formula:

$$r = \frac{\Sigma(x-\bar{x})(y-\bar{y})}{\sqrt{\Sigma(x-\bar{x})^2\,\Sigma(y-\bar{y})^2}}$$

where r = correlation coefficient, x = variable 1, and y = variable 2.

An easier version of the formula is as follows:

$$r = \frac{\Sigma\, dx \cdot dy}{\sqrt{\Sigma\, dx^2 \cdot \Sigma\, dy^2}}$$

$$dx = (x-\bar{x})$$

$$dy = (y-\bar{y})$$

$$dx^2 = (x-\bar{x})^2$$

$$dy^2 = (y-\bar{y})^2$$

Suppose $dx \cdot dy = 71.82$ and $dx^2 \cdot dy^2 = 86.2 \times 109.2$.

$$r = \frac{71.82}{\sqrt{86.2\ x\ 109.2}}$$

$$r = \frac{71.82}{97.02} = 0.7402$$

r^2 represents the percentage of variance shared by two variables, explained by the relationship.

(b) **Spearman's Rank Correlation Coefficient:** This is used to compute the correlation between two variables by their ranks. It is a non-parametric measure of correlation. Spearman's correlation coefficient, which is denoted by the symbol ρ and also signified by r_s, measures the strength of association between two ranked variables for ordinal, interval, and ratio data. It can take values from +1 to −1. An r_s value of +1 indicates a perfect association of ranks, zero indicates no association between ranks, and −1 indicates a perfect negative association of ranks. When r_s is very close to zero, it indicates weaker association between the ranks.

(i) **To Calculate a Spearman's Rank Order Correlation on Data *without any Ties*:** Suppose the marks obtained by some school students in subjects English and Maths are as follows:

English	56	75	45	71	62	64	58	80	76	61
Maths	66	70	40	60	65	56	59	77	67	63

Table 11.5 is computed from this data.

TABLE 11.5 *Correlation of Students' Marks (without Tie) Obtained in Two Subjects*

***n* = 10**					
Mark (English)	**Mark (Maths)**	**Rank (English)**	**Rank (Maths**	***d***	***d*²**
56	66	9	4	5	
75	70	3	2	1	
45	40	10	10	0	
71	60	4	7	3	
62	65	6.5	5	1	
64	56	5	9	4	
58	59	8	8	0	
80	77	1	1	0	
76	67	2	3	1	
61	63	6.5	6	1	

Here, d = difference between ranks and d^2 = difference squared.

$$\sum d_i^2 = 25+1+9+1+16+1+1=54$$

where d_i = difference in paired ranks, i = paired score, and n = number of values in a data set. The scores for Maths and English need to be ranked separately. The score with the highest value should be labelled '1' and the lowest score should be labelled '10', because there are 10 values for each subject. If the data set has more than 10 values, the lowest score will be the total number of values of the data set.

The following formula is used when there is *no tie* in the values of the given data set:

$$\rho = 1 - \frac{6\Sigma d_i^2}{n(n^2-1)}$$

$$\rho = 1 - \frac{6\times 54}{10(10^2+1)}$$

$$\rho = 1 - \frac{324}{990}$$

$$\rho = 1 - 0.33$$

$$\rho = 0.67$$

This indicates a strong positive relationship between the ranks, that is, the students who ranked high in Maths also had a higher rank in English and vice versa.

(ii) **To Calculate a Spearman's Rank Order Correlation on Data *with ties*:** Suppose the following are the marks obtained by some school students in subjects English and Maths:

English	56	75	45	71	61	64	58	80	76	61
Maths	66	70	40	60	65	56	59	77	67	63

The procedure for ranking these scores is as follows: First, a table with four columns is created and labelled as shown in Table 11.6.

TABLE 11.6 *Correlation of Students' Marks (with Tie) Obtained in Two Subjects*

$n = 10$			
Mark (English)	**Mark (Maths)**	**Rank (English)**	**Rank (Maths)**
56	66	9	4
75	70	3	2
45	40	10	10
71	60	4	7
61	65	6.5	5
64	56	5	9
58	59	8	8
80	77	1	1
76	67	2	3
61	63	6.5	6

The scores for Maths and English need to be ranked separately. The score with the highest value should be labelled '1' and the lowest score should be labelled '10', because there are 10 values for each subject. If the data set has more than 10 values, the lowest score will be the total number of values in the data set. In the given data sets, two students have scored 61 in the English exam (highlighted in bold). Their joint rank is 6.5. When there are two identical values in the data (called a *tie*), the average of the ranks $(6 + 7)/2 = 6.5$ is taken and assigned to each of these *tied* scores. This is because, in this example, there is no way of knowing which score should be ranked 6 and which should be ranked 7. The ranks of 6 and 7 do not exist for English.

The following formula is used when there is a *tie* in the values of the given data set:

$$\rho = \frac{\sum_i (x_i - \bar{x})(y_i - \bar{y})}{\sqrt{\sum_i (x_i - \bar{x})^2 (y_i - \bar{y})^2}}$$

where x = marks series of English, y = marks series of Maths, and i = paired score.

Spearman's correlation coefficient can be used when there is a *monotonic relationship* between the variables. A monotonic relationship is one that does one of the following: (a) As the value of one variable increases, the value of the other variable also increases. (b) As the value of one variable increases, the value of the other variable decreases. Examples of monotonic and non-monotonic relationships are presented in Fig. 11.9.

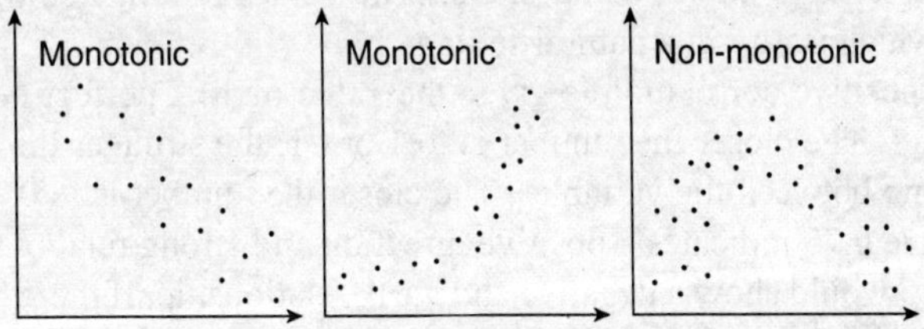

FIGURE 11.9 *Monotonic and Non-monotonic Relationships among Variables*

Spearman's correlation coefficient can be used when both dependent (outcome or response) and independent (predictor) variables are *ordinal numeric* or when one variable is an *ordinal numeric* and the other is a *continuous variable*. However, it can also be used when both variables are *continuous*.

2. **Scatter Plots:** These are the graphic presentations of the relationship between two *continuous variables*, including the direction and magnitude. Scatter plots are also called *scatter diagrams* or *scattergrams* and show how one variable is affected by the other. The *X* variables are plotted on the horizontal axis and *Y* variables on the vertical axis.

   Pairs of scores from two sets of observations are plotted on a graph by placing the dots to indicate where each pair of *X*s and *Y*s intersects. For a *positive correlation*, the lowest values of the *X* and *Y* variables fall at the lower left corner of the graph. As the higher values are plotted, they are seen going up the vertical axis, simultaneously moving towards the right side of the horizontal axis. In a *negative correlation*, the values are distributed from the upper left corner down towards the lower right corner. Figure 11.10 shows the scatter plot diagrams of a high positive and a high negative correlation.

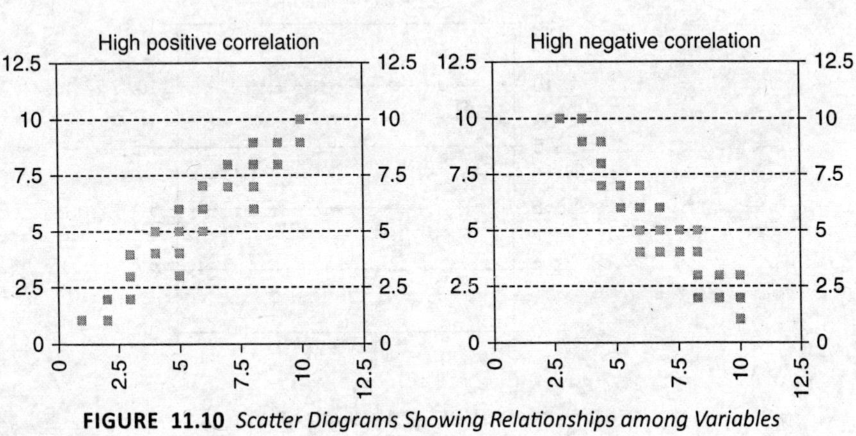

FIGURE 11.10 *Scatter Diagrams Showing Relationships among Variables*

Scatter plots usually consist of a large body of data. Closer the values plotted, when making a straight line, higher the correlation between the two variables and stronger the relationship, either positive or negative.

An example is finding relationships between the examination scores of individual students with an assumption that the scores obtained in the theory examination of community health nursing are correlated with the obtained scores of practical examination of the same subject. If the scores are the same (5 and 5, 6 and 6, etc.), the values fall on a straight line depicting a perfect correlation, which is rare in a natural setting.

A perfect positive correlation is given the value of 1. A perfect negative correlation is given the value of –1. The closer the number is to 1 or –1, the stronger the correlation, or the stronger the relationship between the variables. The closer the number is to 0, the weaker the correlation. Thus, the value 0.75 indicates a positive direction and strong relationship between the variables, whereas –0.15 would show a negative and weak relationship. If there is absolutely no correlation, the value would be zero. Figure 11.11 shows the scatter plot diagrams of a perfect positive correlation, a perfect negative correlation, and no correlation.

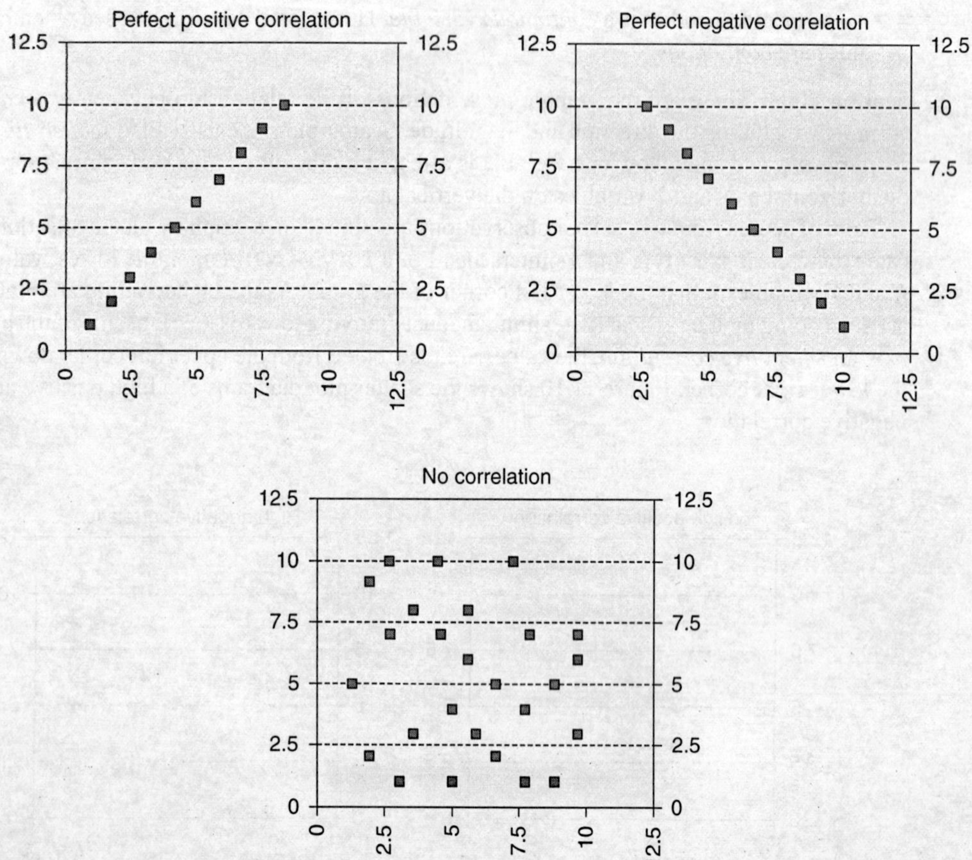

FIGURE 11.11 *Scatter Plots*

The following statistics are calculated for scatter plots:

Mean *X* and *Y*	The average of all the data points in the series
Maximum *X* and *Y*	The maximum value in the series
Minimum *X* and *Y*	The minimum value in the series
Sample Size	The number of values in the series
***X* Range and *Y* Range**	The maximum value minus the minimum value
Standard Deviations for *X* and *Y* values	Indicates how widely the data is spread around the mean
Line of Best Fit—Slope	The slope of the line that fits the data most closely (generally using the least squares method)
Line of Best Fit—*Y*-intercept	The point at which the line of best fit crosses the *y*-axis

In a scatter plot, the variables move together, whatever the distance may be between them, showing the possibility of a relationship. However, it cannot prove that one variable is causing the change in the other. It is important to keep this point in mind while choosing scatter plots for graphical representation of analysed data.

3. **Contingency Table:** For nominal or categorical data, relationships cannot be depicted on a scatter plot, as no actual scores are available and only the frequencies of the occurrences of the values are shown. A *contingency table*, also called a *cross-tabulation*, can display the relationships between sets of nominal data.

   The term *contingency table* was first used by the statistician Karl Pearson in 1904. Contingency tables will normally have as many rows as there are categories and will have an equal number of rows and columns.

   For example, Table 11.7 showing the relationship between gender and smoking behaviour data obtained from 50 males and 50 females.

TABLE 11.7 *Correlation between Gender and Smoking*

$n = 100$			
S. No.	**Smoke**	**Do Not Smoke**	**Total**
Male	40	10	50
Female	15	35	50
Total	55	45	100

The data from the table indicate that more number of male subjects smoke than the number of female subjects. Chi-square test may be used to determine the significance of this relationship. Even if the relationship is statistically significant, it cannot be concluded that the male gender is the cause of smoking behaviour.

This table is called a 2 × 2 contingency table, because there are two variables and each variable has two categories. This is the most common type. If one more response such as 'Smoke Occasionally' is placed in one more column, it would be called a 2 × 3 contingency table, and so on.

One of the meanings of the word contingency is unforeseen event. A categorical forecast is a forecast of the occurrence or non-occurrence of a specific event, which must be clearly defined. For example, in forecasting weather, this method may be employed.

Table 11.8 examines the differences between univariate and bivariate data.

TABLE 11.8 *Differences between Univariate and Bivariate Data*

Univariate Data	Bivariate Data
• Involves a *single variable*	• Involves *two variables*
• Does not deal with causes or relationships	• Deals with causes or relationships
• Major purpose of univariate analysis is to describe	• Major purpose of bivariate analysis is to explain
• Central tendency—mean, mode, median • Dispersion—range, variance, max, min, quartiles, standard deviation • Frequency distributions • Bar graph, histogram, pie chart, linegraph, box-and-whisker plot	• Analysis of two variables simultaneously • Correlations • Comparisons, relationships, causes,explanations • Tables where one variable is contingent on the value of the other variable • Independent and dependent variables
Sample question: How many of the students in the freshman class are female?	**Sample question:** Is there a relationship between the number of females in computer programming and their scores in maths?

INFERENTIAL STATISTICS

Descriptive statistics is all about the sample (a smaller representative group of a larger population), describing its central tendency and variability. Inferential statistics focuses on drawing conclusions and making statements about the population (larger group). It is the mathematics and logic of how this generalization from sample to population can be made.

For example, a nursing college has 600 students. To know these students' opinion about the curriculum, we need not ask all 600 students; instead, we randomly select 100 students and obtain their opinion. It is assumed that the sample of 100 represents the larger population of 600 in all characteristics. Therefore, the sample mean and population mean are more or less the same.

Inferential statistics is commonly used to test hypotheses based on random sampling. In this, *statistics* are the measures of the samples and *parameters* are the measures of the population.

To construct the reasoning for inferential statistics, some basic concepts of probability and probability-related distributions (mostly theoretical) need to be used. The word *chance* is used to explain probability. Other terms used interchangeably are *sampling error* and *random error*. All inferential statistics are based on the assumption that chance (sampling error and random error) is the only relationship possible in research studies, for example, the relationship between gender and smoking in Table 11.7. Moreover, research studies strive to establish that chance is NOT the reason for the relationships found by the research.

Inferential statistics are based on the assumption that the sample was randomly selected, as each member of the population has an equal chance of being selected; these samples called as *probability samples*. The methods of sample selection are known as *probability sampling techniques*. However, for some studies, random sampling is not possible due to constraints of time, money, manpower, materials, and ethical issues. Shott stated that it is appropriate to make inference from a non-random sample to the population as long as the researcher does not deliberately select a biased sample. Polit cautioned about interpreting such study findings. The findings involving non-random samples cannot be generalized unless the same study is repeated in different settings.

Purposes of Inferential Statistics

The following are the purposes of inferential statistics:

1. To estimate population parameters (values) from sample data, done after data collection
2. To test hypotheses, done before the data collection begins. The decision about acceptance of rejection of the hypotheses is made after data analysis.

Let us discuss these purposes in detail.

Estimating Population Parameters

To estimate the population parameters from a sample data, sampling error and sampling distribution are to be considered. *Sampling error* occurs when the sample does not accurately reflect or represent the population. The standard deviation of any sampling distribution is called a *standard error* (denoted by SE).

Sampling distribution is a theoretical distribution that is based on an infinite number of samples. It is derived from mathematical formulae and logic. Inferential statistics uses *sampling distribution of mean*. When the values of a set of observations are normally distributed, approximately 68 per cent of the values lie between ±1 SD and approximately 95 per cent lie between ±2 SD, precisely 1.96 SD from the mean (Fig. 11.5).

$$SE = \sqrt{\frac{(SD_1)^2}{n_1}} + \sqrt{\frac{(SD_2)^2}{n_2}}$$

where SD = Standard deviation and n = sample size.

The standard deviation of any sampling distribution of the mean is called the standard error of the mean ($SD\overline{x}$).

When the sample mean and population mean values are closer to each other, the standard error becomes smaller.

$$SD_{\overline{x}} = \frac{\sigma}{\sqrt{n}}$$

Still, questions remain: How to be sure that the sample mean and the population mean are more or less the same? Is it possible to say for sure that the sample characteristics are the same as the characteristics of the population from where they have been taken, when there are so many individual differences in characteristics?

To solve this issue, researchers established a range of values within which the population parameter is thought to fall or be present. This range of values is called as the *confidence interval* (denoted by C.I.), which, with a specific degree of probability, is thought to have the population value somewhere within the range. It contains a lower and an upper limit. The confidence interval gives us some confidence to state that the population parameter lies within those boundaries.

For example, the mean and standard error of a large sample of people's haemoglobin level are 11.4 g/100 ml and 0.7, respectively. Considering that the sample mean is the best estimation of the population mean, it is 11.4 g/100 ml. The interval with 1.96 times standard error below and above the mean is 11.4 ± 1.96(0.7) is 10.0 g to 12.8 g. This interval is the confidence interval. Now, we can confidently say that the population mean of haemoglobin level lies at some point between 10.0 g and 12.8 g.

The formula for calculating the confidence interval is $C.I = \overline{x} \pm m$.

Testing Hypothesis

Hypothesis is a statement about one or more parameters. Usually, it shows the relationship between two variables. Hypothesis testing is a procedure to determine whether the hypothesis is consistent with the sample data. (The sample data presumably represent the population data.) If it is not consistent, it is rejected. If it is consistent with the sample data, the hypothesis is accepted as a possible relationship between variables.

There are commonly two types of research process that need hypothesis testing:

1. Comparison of two or more populations, for example, patients with disease A and disease B
2. Relationship between two or more factors in a population, for example, smoking and lung cancer

Principles of Hypothesis Testing

The following are the principles of hypothesis testing:

1. Determining the sampling variation when the samples are drawn from statistically identical populations
2. Determining the correlation between factors in the population when they are not related

If the assumption is that there is no difference between population values or no relationship between factors in a population, it is a *null hypothesis* (H_0).

Before we proceed further about hypothesis testing, we need to understand the meaning of a few terms.

Level of Significance: It is the probability of rejecting a null hypothesis when it is true. It is represented by the Greek letter alpha (α) and the symbol of probability level is *p*. The value of *p* has been already set by scientists as .05 (no zero before the decimal). A significance level of .05 means that the researcher, when rejecting the null hypothesis, is willing to risk being wrong 5 times out of 100. If the decision needs to be much more accurate, such as whether the treatment is effective or not, the level of significance might be set at .01 or even .001. This means the risk of being wrong is 1 time out of 100 and 1 time out of 1000, respectively. If $p = <.05$, the null hypothesis is rejected. If $p = >.05$, the null hypothesis cannot be rejected.

The test of any hypothesis can have one of the four possible results mentioned in Table 11.9, based on the actual situation in the population and the researcher's decision.

TABLE 11.9 *Four Possible Outcomes of Hypothesis Testing*

<table>
<tr><th>Researcher's Decision</th><th>True Hypothesis</th><th>False Hypothesis</th><td rowspan="3">• Type I error is also called alpha (α) error and type II error is also known as beta (β) error.
• In any statistical test, there is the possibility of making only one type of error.
• In general, reducing the risk of one type of error increases the risk of other type of error.
• If type I error limit is fixed, then type II error can be decreased by increasing the size of the sample.</td></tr>
<tr><td>Accept</td><td>Correct</td><td>Type II error</td></tr>
<tr><td>Reject</td><td>Type I error</td><td>Correct</td></tr>
</table>

One- and Two-tailed Tests: A research hypothesis (H_1) may be stated in the *directional form*, wherein the degree of difference or type of correlation is predicted. It may be also in the *non-directional form*, wherein a difference or correlation is predicted, but the degree of difference or type of correlation is NOT indicated.

The directional hypothesis should be based on a sound theoretical or conceptual framework as the rational for the prediction. For the directional hypothesis, it is appropriate to use a *one-tailed test of significance*. In this, the differences of populations or correlations between factors are required in only one tail of the theoretical sampling distribution. A *two-tailed test of significance* is used to determine the differences of populations or correlations between factors in both ends of the sampling distribution.

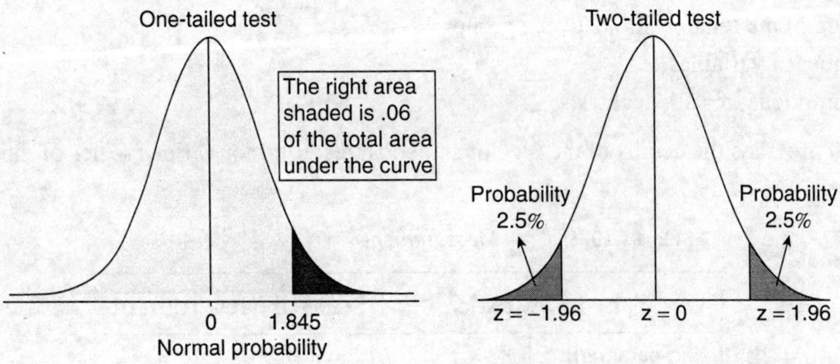

The z-score for one-tailed test is 1.65 and for two-tailed test is 1.96.
Significant values at (α) = .05

FIGURE 11.12 *One-tailed and Two-tails Tests*

It is easier to reject a null hypothesis for one-tailed test, as the entire area of rejection is only in one tail. In two-tailed test, .05 has to be divided into .025 in each tail of the distribution. However, one-tailed test is more powerful than the two-tailed test. Moreover, higher the level of significance, more powerful is the statistical test (.05 is higher than .01).

Degree of Freedom (df): It is the number of values in a set of observations that are free to vary. For example, if we need to pick a number between 1 and 10, we have 10 degrees of freedom, because we can pick up any number from the 10 numbers. Now, if we need to pick up three numbers that add up to 10, and we take any two numbers, say, 3 and 6, then the third number has to be 1 to make it 10. Here, we have only one degree of freedom.

Parametric and Non-parametric Statistical Tests: Classification of Inferential Statistics

Parametric tests deal with population parameters and make assumptions about the population from which the sample was drawn; data are normally distributed (following a classic bell-shaped curve). Moreover, they require interval scale for measurement. For example, 10 digital thermometers are standardized in the physics lab, and on random selection, 2 are used for a study about temperature variation in new-borns.

Non-parametric tests are used when the data are measured on nominal or ordinal scale, data distribution is markedly skewed, and sample size is very small, thus limiting generalization of findings. For example, from the population of 100 tuberculosis patients, 30 are selected by random sampling technique for a DOTS compliance study. It is found that 65 per cent had full compliance to DOTS, 10 per cent patients had partial compliance, and remaining 25 per cent had no compliance.

Choosing Correct Statistical Tests

The following five issues must be considered when choosing the statistical tests:

1. Scale of measurement
2. Number of samples or groups
3. Nature of the relationship between groups
4. Number of variables
5. Assumptions of statistical tests

Table 11.10 provides the details of the type of statistical test used for various scales of measurement.

TABLE 11.10 *Scale of Measurement*

Type of Statistic		Scale of Mesurement
Non-parametric	–	Nominal
Non-parametric	–	Ordinal
Non-parametric	Parametric	Approcimately Interval
–	Parametric	Interval
–	Parametric	Ratio

Table 11.11 shows the common non-parametric tests used for nominal and ordinal data.

TABLE 11.11 *Common Non-parametric Statistical Tests*

Nominal Data	Ordinal Data
Chi-square Goodness-of-Fit Test	Mann-Whitney *U* Test
Chi-square Test of Independence	Wilcoxon *T* Test
McNemar Test	Kruskal-Wallis *H* Test
	Friedman ANOVA by Ranks
	Spearman's r_s

Figure 11.13 shows the various statistical tests used for nominal data for one sample and two samples.

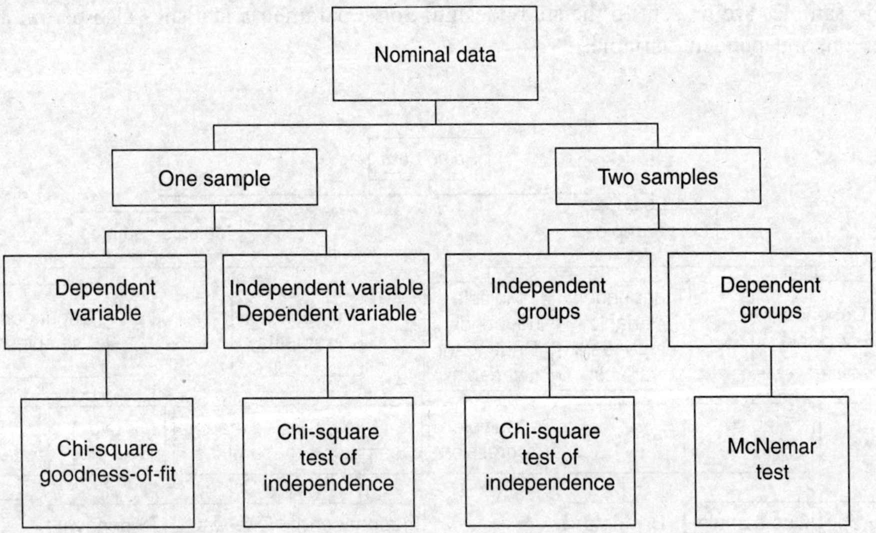

FIGURE 11.13 *Statistical Tests for Nominal Data with Sample Size*

Figure 11.14 shows the various statistical tests used for ordinal data for one sample and multiple samples.

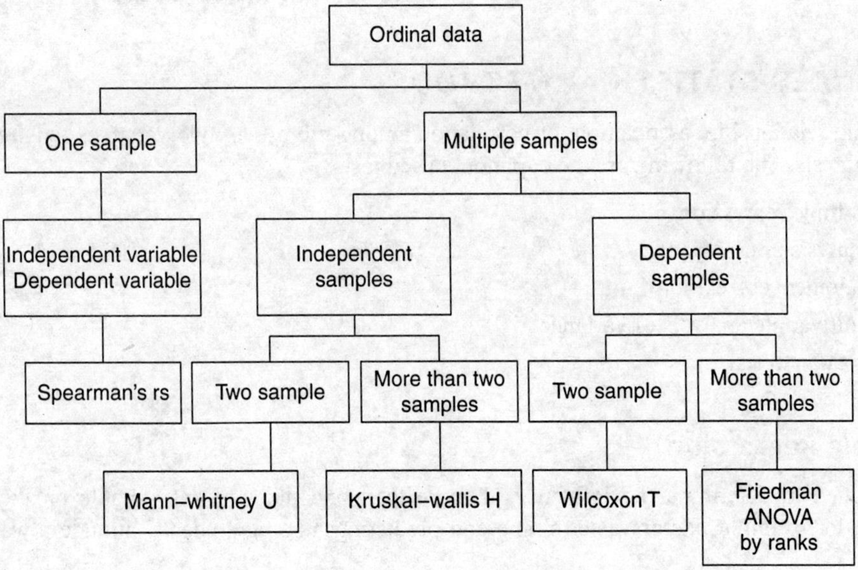

FIGURE 11.14 *Statistical Tests for Ordinal Data with Sample Size*

Figure 11.15 shows the tests that can be used with all types of scale data. Selection of the test is determined by the number of samples and whether a hypothesis is being tested about group differences or the association between independent and dependent variables. If we are testing a hypothesis about group differences, we also must consider whether the groups or samples are independent or dependent and how many samples are present in the study design. Some parametric statistics also permit analysis of more than one independent variable.

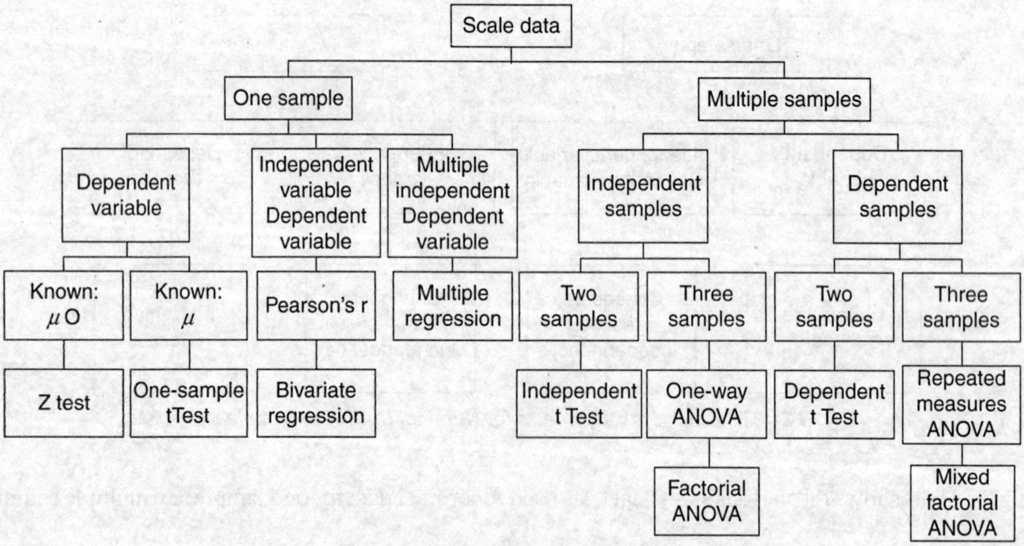

FIGURE 11.15 *Statistical Tests for Scale Data with Sample Size*

ADVANCED STATISTICAL METHODS

Measuring relationship, association, or correlation among more than two variables requires advanced statistical tests. The following are the commonly used tests:

1. Multiple regression
2. Analysis of covariance
3. Canonical correlation
4. Multivariate analysis of variance
5. Meta-analysis

Multiple Regression

It is applied to determine the influence of more than one independent variable on the dependent variable, for example, factors determining and predicting nursing students' attitude towards nursing profession.

Analysis of Covariance (ANCOVA)

It is a powerful statistical test and is used when some variables that might have an influence on the dependent variable are statistically controlled. It is important for true experimental study, wherein two groups are made statistically equal before the experimental treatment is administered. This is to control bias by controlling the confounding variables. For example, physiological parameters such as pulse, respiration, and blood pressure of both experimental and control groups are kept constant to determine peoples' reaction to aerobics.

Canonical Correlation

It examines the correlation between two or more independent variables and two or more dependent variables.

Multivariate Analysis of Variance (MANOVA)

It examines the difference between the mean scores of two or more groups on two or more dependent variables examined at the same time.

Meta-analysis

It is a statistical procedure for synthesizing research results in order to draw general conclusions. Studies that address a common subject or issue are compiled. The common measure for expressing the results across the studies is the *effect size* (ES). It is the standard score (*z*-score) of the mean of one group referenced in the distribution of another group.

Mixed Method Data Analysis

Conducting mixed methods research involves collecting, analysing, and interpreting quantitative and qualitative data in a single study or in a series of studies that investigate the same underlying phenomenon. It is a combination of two types of research. It is also called pluralistic research. It provides a bridge between the qualitative and quantitative paradigms. In qualitative research, a multi-method approach to data collection and data analysis is known as *methodological triangulation.* Combining of qualitative and quantitative research is becoming more and more common in nursing research. The barriers that hinder combination include philosophical differences, cost, inadequate training, and publication bias.

ANALYSIS OF QUALITATIVE DATA

Qualitative research is collecting, analysing, and interpreting data by observing what people do and say. Quantitative research refers to counts and measures of things. Qualitative research refers to the meanings, concepts, definitions, characteristics, metaphors, symbols, and descriptions of things. Qualitative data are words rather than numbers. Words describe and explain. Words suggest new perspectives. Conclusions expressed as words seem more convincing than pages of numbers. However, words are also ambiguous and difficult to compare objectively.

The nature of this type of research is exploratory and open-ended. It uses very different methods of collecting information, mainly individual in-depth interviews and focus groups. Participants are asked to respond to general questions. The interviewer probes and explores into their responses to identify and define people's perceptions, opinions, and feelings about the topic or idea being discussed and to determine the degree of agreement that exists in the group. The quality of the finding from qualitative research is directly dependent upon the skills, experience, and sensitivity of the interviewer.

In general, qualitative research generates rich, reliable, detailed, and valid data that contribute to in-depth understanding of the context. Qualitative data, if collected and analysed properly, can establish convincing cause-and-effect relationships. However, it is never clear how much of a verbal description of an incidence is perceived by the receiver of the message. The decision to choose a quantitative or a qualitative research will depend on the study focus, the type of information needed, the context of the study, and the availability of resources (time, money, and human).

Types of Qualitative Research

There are many types of qualitative research, such as ethnography, phenomenology, grounded theory, life history, and ethnomethodology. Three of the most commonly used approaches to qualitative research in nursing are phenomenology, ethnography, and grounded theory.

Phenomenology

The aim of a phenomenological approach to qualitative research is to describe accurately the lived experiences of people and not to generate theories or models of the phenomenon being studied. Examples are the lived experience of child birth and the experience of living with cancer. These studies help us to understand happiness and sorrow from other people's view point.

Ethnography

The goal of ethnography is to learn about a culture from the people who actually live in that culture. Holistic nursing takes into consideration the cultural aspects of health and illness.

Grounded Theory

The purpose of a grounded theory approach in qualitative research is to discover social–psychological processes. An example is a study of the change in nursing students' attitude towards nursing profession during the course of their education.

Qualitative research is much more subjective than quantitative research and hence uses methods such as in-depth interviews and focus group discussions for collecting information. A small number of people are interviewed in-depth and/or a relatively small number of focus group discussions are conducted as a combined method of data collection.

Some of the sampling strategies used in qualitative research are maximum variation sampling, stratified purposeful sampling, and snowball sampling. Purposive sampling decisions influence not only the selection of participants but also the settings, incidents, events, and activities for data collection. Sampling in qualitative research is flexible and often continues until no new themes emerge from the data; it is a point when no more information is available on the subject, and this phenomenon is called *data saturation*.

Forms of Data

Qualitative data is information gathered in a non-numeric form. The following are the common examples of such data:

1. Interview transcript
2. Field notes (notes taken in the field being studied)
3. Video recordings

4. Audio recordings
5. Images
6. Documents (reports, manuscripts, letters, books, etc.)

Qualitative data analysis is the range of processes and procedures to convert the collected data into some form of explanation, understanding, or interpretation of the people and situations under investigation. Data analysis helps us to understand the following:

1. What are the subjects' interpretations of the world?
2. Why do they have that point of view?
3. How did they come to that view?
4. What have they been doing about it?
5. How have they conveyed their views of their situation?
6. How do they identify or classify themselves and others in what they say?

The process of qualitative data analysis usually involves two things—writing and identification of themes.

Tools Used for Qualitative Data Collection and Method of Data Analysis

1. **Unstructured Tools:** These are open-ended items, which are commonly asked as questions, collected from a discussion, generated through counselling, gathered from write-ups, or obtained by listening to stories or incidents. The senses of smell, taste, and touch are also useful for qualitative data collection, but it is difficult to check their validity and reliability. However, the data are rich and wholesome when all components are included. It requires the researcher's communication skill, experience, and expertise to collect useful data. *Content analysis* method is used to analyse the data.
2. **Structured Tools:** These are very specific tools, guided by a script (health education programme, teaching module, etc.) often like a questionnaire, rating scale, or checklist. Validity and reliability may be established, and hence, it is replicable; but it may lack richness of information, as it is developed from the researcher's view point of the study matter. It can be administered by anyone, even someone other than the researcher. *Statistical methods* are available for data analysis.
3. **Semi-structured Tools:** These are guided by a specific script, but important issues and concerns can be explored in-depth by adding open-ended questions, discussions, or any other method of data collection. This way, there is a balance between the richness of qualitative data and replicability of the quantitative aspects of the data. As nursing profession takes care of the human health, semi-structured tools are most suitable for collecting all-encompassing data. *Statistical methods* and *content analysis* both are used relevantly for data analysis.

Qualitative Data Processing

The three key rules for preparing the data for analysis *are coding*, *memoing*, and *concept mapping*.

Coding is classifying or categorizing individual pieces of data, for example, views about self, family members, and others.

Memoing is writing memos or notes. It is appropriate at several stages of data processing to capture code meanings, theoretical ideas, preliminary conclusions, and other thoughts that would be useful during data analysis.

Concept mapping uses diagrams to graphically explore the relationships in the data.

Qualitative data analysis, unlike quantitative data analysis, is not concerned with statistical analysis but with the analysis of codes, themes, and patterns in the data. Computer software programs are used to assist in coding and analysis of data. These reports often contain direct quotes from participants that provide rich illustrations of the study themes. Qualitative research, unlike its quantitative counterpart, does not have an empirical conclusion, but it allows the generalization of the understanding of the experience being examined.

Steps in Qualitative Data Analysis

1. Taking in-depth interview or observing the situation on specific points
2. Data coding to specific themes—It is to group all data with similar words or phrases into some classifications or categories. The categories may or may not be predetermined, depending on the plan of the study.
3. Data interpretation—It is to explain the data from all dimensions, in the light of available sources of literature information. Content analysis method is commonly used.
4. Generalizing the findings
5. Proceeding until data saturation

WHAT IS GENERALIZATION

Generalization means to conclude that the research findings obtained by testing on the selected samples are applicable for the population of a particular setting. See Fig. 11.16

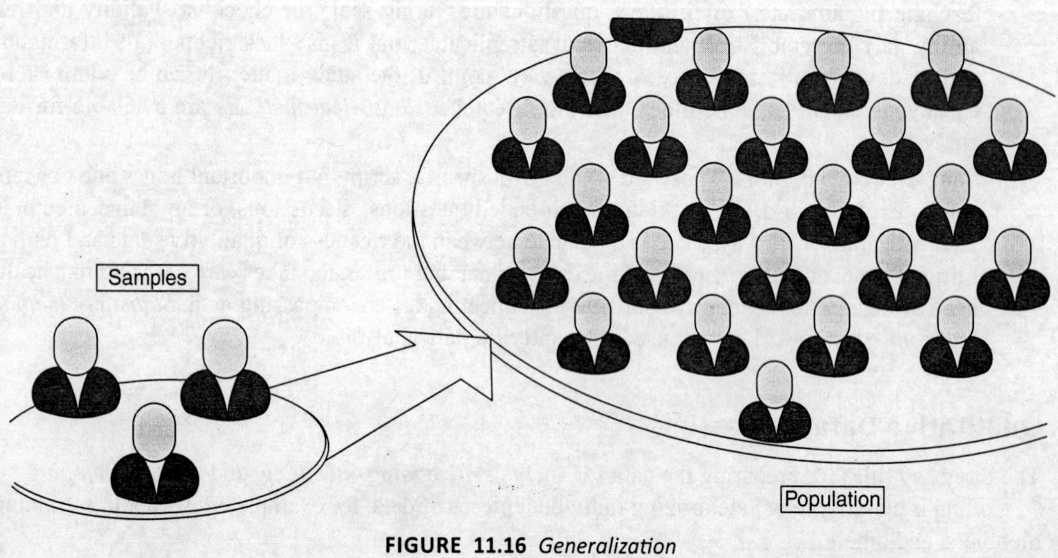

FIGURE 11.16 *Generalization*

For example, to find out the impact of a specially made iron-containing food on childhood anaemia, it is not always possible to experiment on 2000 anaemic children of a given population. There may be constraints of money, time, manpower, and so on. Hence, only 500 children are selected randomly out of 2000. After three months of making the children eat the specially prepared experimental food, it is estimated that their average haemoglobin (Hb) level has increased. Therefore, it is concluded that the same experimental food would have a similar impact on the remaining 1500 anaemic children in increasing their Hb level. This is called *generalization*. In this, the selected 500 anaemic children is the representative group, which is chosen to represent the whole population of 2000 children.

Following are the conditions to conclude generalization:

1. The sample group must be truly representative of the whole population.
2. The study period must be chosen with precision as the behaviours can change in the course of passing days, weeks, months, or years.
3. The size of the sample must be statistically proportionate and comparable with the target population.

For the perfect experiment, every single child must be given the experimental food and their Hb levels are compared against a control group. This may not be possible without a huge number of researchers and much time and money.

To solve this problem, a sample group can be selected from the target population, which would represent the population, in order to generalize the outcome of the experiment. However, the sample group must be large enough for possible generalization. The decision about the size of the sample group depends on the individual research study.

However, if the study result is applied or implemented to a similar setting and a similar sample group, it acquires external validity and thus can be fairly generalized, if not most perfectly.

Figure 11.7 depicts the entire process of generalization in research.

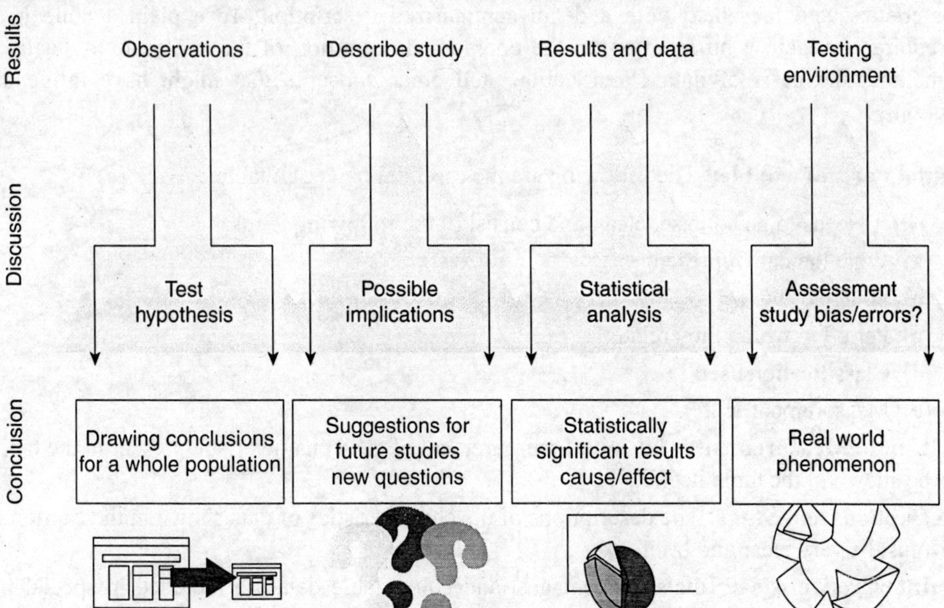

FIGURE 11.17 *Generalization in Research*

PRESENTATION OF DATA

Data are analysed and presented in records and reports, which are used for publications or as other means of communicating the research findings. More attractive the presentation is, more interesting it is for the reader or viewer.

Basic Principles of Data Presentation (ABCDE Principles)

1. *A*ccuracy of data ensures accurate communication of research outcome.
2. *B*rief and specific information is easy to understand and correlate.
3. *C*ompleteness of presentation gives overall idea about the research subject.
4. *D*irect approach to the method of presentation considers study focus.
5. *E*mpirical evidence reflected in data presentation makes it scientific.

Common Methods of Data Presentation

1. Tables
2. Graphs and diagrams
3. Pictorial figures or objects

Tables

To prepare a data table, data are broken down to possible aspects, classified according to common characteristics, and presented with a detail summarized description. To explain a table in detail, it is required to enclose information on the operational definition of the related terms, data collection method, the basis of data classification, and other concerns that might have influenced the tabulation.

Essential Parts of a Table: The following are the essential parts of a table:

1. **Title:** Needs to be concise, clear, and consist of the following items:
   (a) What the data represent
   (b) Source of the data
   (c) Period in which they relate
   (d) Classification used
   (e) Measurement unit
2. **Unit of Measurement:** The unit of measurement of each characteristic present in the table must be shown in the table itself.
3. **Captions and Stubs:** The descriptions of the characteristics of data shown in the caption or stub must be very clear and brief.
4. **Interpretive Aids:** Totals, percentages, and comparable data are included in special purpose tables.

Graphs and Diagrams

These provide a visual method of presenting research findings and may be used alone or along with tables. They should be relevant to the information, very specific, and attractive and should not be crowded with too many characters and colours and too much information.

Essential Parts of a Graph or Diagram: The following are the essential parts of a graph or diagram.

1. **Title:** Need to indicate what is being presented
2. **Labels:** For both the *x*-axis and the *y*-axis, labels should be provided indicating the unit of measurement.
3. **Categories:** Classification or categories of data must be presented on the axes.
4. **Legends or Keys:** The description of the data categories is presented in the legends or keys, instead of on the body of the graph or diagram.
5. **Interpretive Aids:** Totals, percentages, and comparable data are included in special purpose graphs or diagrams.

Differences Between Graphs and Diagrams

1. Graph paper is used in constructing a graph. It helps to study the mathematical relationship between two variables such as education and knowledge; time of the day and blood pressure; or family earning and anaemia. On the other hand, diagrams are generally constructed on a plain paper. A diagram is used for subjective comparison between two variables but not for studying the relationship objectively.
2. Graphs are more precise and accurate than diagrams. They are more helpful to a researcher for statistical analysis and interpretation. Diagrams are not of much use to a researcher for data analysis. As diagrams are attractive to look at, they are used for publicity and propaganda.
3. Graphs are used to present time series data and frequency distributions. Diagrams are useful in presenting geographical or spatial series. Presentation of data through graphs is easier than through diagrams.

Graphs: A graph is a visual representation of data by a continuous curve on a squared (graph) paper. Graphs can be made attractive and eye-catching, giving a bird's eye-view of the data and inter-relationships.

Commonly Used Graphs or Diagrams

1. Histogram
2. Bar—Simple bar representing only one variable and multiple bar depicting more than one variable in proportionate comparison
3. Pie
4. Line

Histogram: Figure 11.18 shows a histogram.

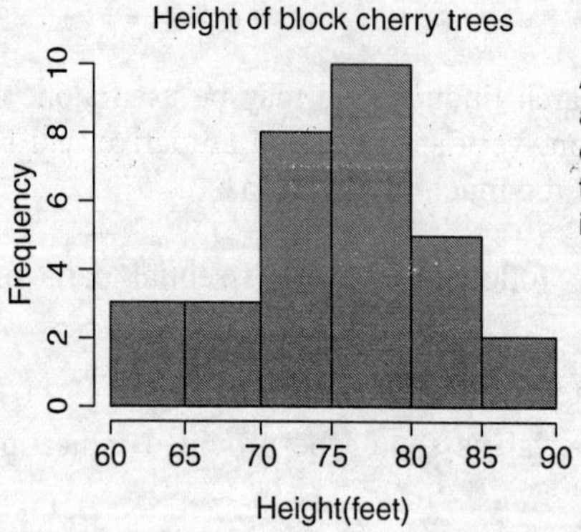

A histogram consists of tabular frequencies, arranged in adjacent rectangles, erected over discrete intervals. It has an area equal to the frequency of the observations in the interval.

FIGURE 11.18 *Histogram*

Simple Bar—One Variable: Figure 11.19 provides a simple bar diagram for the data provided in Table 11.12.

TABLE 11.12 *Birth Rate per Thousand of Different Countries over a Certain Period of Time*

Country	Birth Rate	Country	Birth Rate
India	33	China	40
Germany	15	New Zealand	30
U.K.	20	Sweden	15

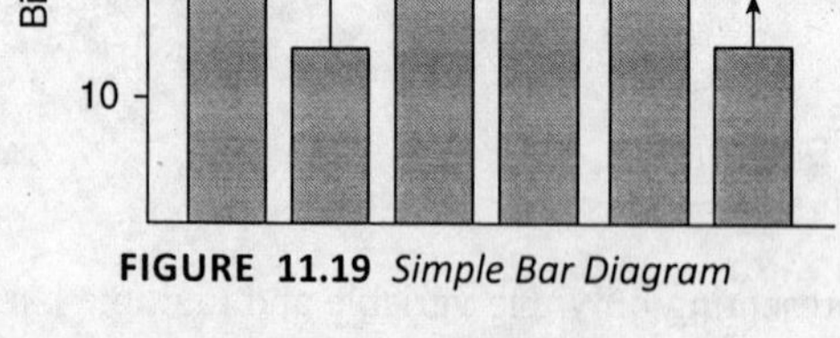

FIGURE 11.19 *Simple Bar Diagram*

Sub-divided Bar Diagram: In this bar diagram, more than one component of a variable is displayed for comparison. Each bar is presented in the order of magnitude with the largest component at the bottom and the smallest at the top. The components are shown with different shades or colours.

For example, during 1968–71, the number of students in University X was as shown in Table 11.13. This data are represented in a sub-divided bar diagram in Fig. 11.20.

TABLE 11.13 *Number of Students in Various Branches*

Year	Arts	Science	Law	Total
1968–69	20,000	10,000	5000	35,000
1969–70	26,000	9000	7000	42,000
1970–71	31,000	9500	7500	48,000

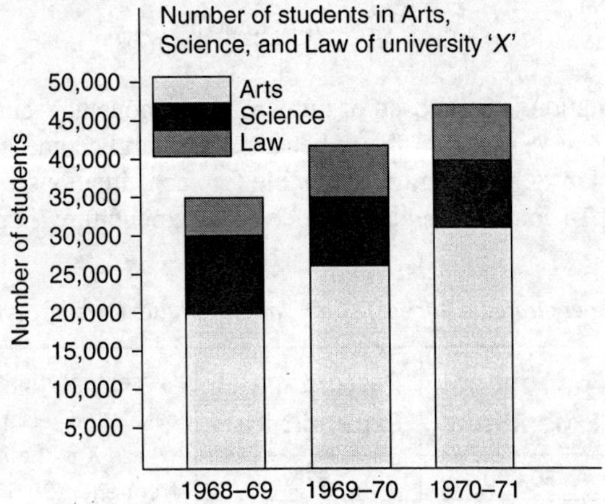

FIGURE 11.20 *Sub-divided Bar Diagram*

Multiple Bar Diagram: An example for multiple bar diagram is shown in Fig. 11.21.

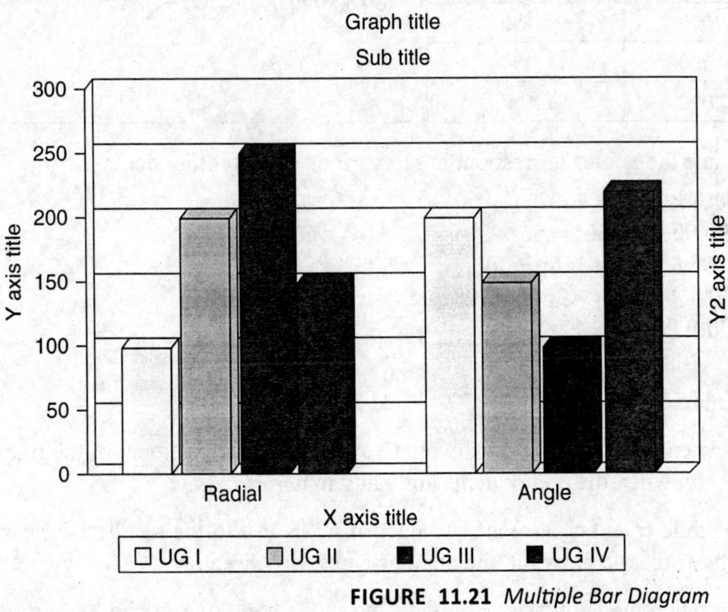

When the data comprise two or more variables in proportionate comparison, a multiple bar diagram can be used for their representation. The variables are depicted in adjoining bars and coloured in different shades.

The figure depicts the attitude of the undergraduate (UG) nursing students studying in two different nursing colleges towards preventive health care. The four shaded bars show the changes in their attitude scores from the first to fourth years of the UG nursing programme.

FIGURE 11.21 *Multiple Bar Diagram*

Another example of multiple bar diagram is Fig. 11.1, which shows pencil colour against class.

Pie Diagram: This diagram consists of a circle (pie), which is divided by the radii into various components (like slices of a cake or pie). Geometrically, it can be seen that the area of a component of a circle taken according to its radius is proportional to the angle at its centre. It is, therefore, sufficient to draw angles at the centre, proportional to the original figures. In total, 360° is completed.

For example, let the total be 1000 and one of the components be 200. Then the angle will be

$$\left(\frac{200}{1000}\right)\times 360° = 72°$$

In general, the angle of component at the centre corresponding to a component

$$= \left(\frac{\text{Component}}{\text{Total}}\right)\times 360^0$$

When a statistical computation is composed of numerous components (four or more components), bar charts are not suitable to represent them. This is because the chart becomes very complex and crowded, giving a peculiar impression. A pie diagram is suitable for such situations.

For example, Table 11.14 contains the data of the yearly expenditure (in rupees) of an undergraduate nursing student.

TABLE 11.14 *The Yearly Expenditure (in Rupees) of an Undergraduate Nursing Student*

Category	Amount of Expenditure	Percentage of Expenditure	Percentage for each of the category is calculated using the formula $(X/N)100$, where X is the frequency and N is the total frequency (90,000 for this table). For example, Tuition fees = 60,000 Percentage of tuition fees in total expenditure = (60,000/90,000) × 100 = 67%
Tuition fees	60,000	67%	
Hostel and food	14,000	16%	
Books and uniform	10,000	11%	
Co-curricular activities	3000	3%	
Miscellaneous	2000	2%	
Library charges	1000	1%	
Total expenditure	90,000	100%	

Now, as explained, let us calculate the angles corresponding to various items (components).

Tuition fees = (60,000/90,000) × 360° = 240°
Hostel and food = (14,000/90,000) × 360° = 56°
Books and uniform = (10,000/90,000) × 360° = 40°
Co-curricular activities = (3000/90,000) × 360° = 12°
Miscellaneous = (2000/90,000) × 360° = 8°
Library charge = (1,000/90,000) × 360° = 4°

The corresponding pie diagram in shown in Fig. 11.22

Uses: A pie diagram is useful when we want to show the relative positions (proportions) of the figures that make the total. It is also useful when the components are many in number.

Note: The components of the circle (pie diagram) are arranged from largest to the smallest for easier interpretation of the data and they must be drawn in the counter-clockwise direction.

Line Graph: This is preferred when the emphasis is on the time series trend over a chosen period in several intervals of time, rather than a comparison of the data in the series. A line graph is a way to summarize how two pieces of information are related and how they vary depending on one another. It allows comparison of multiple sets of data over time in the same graph.

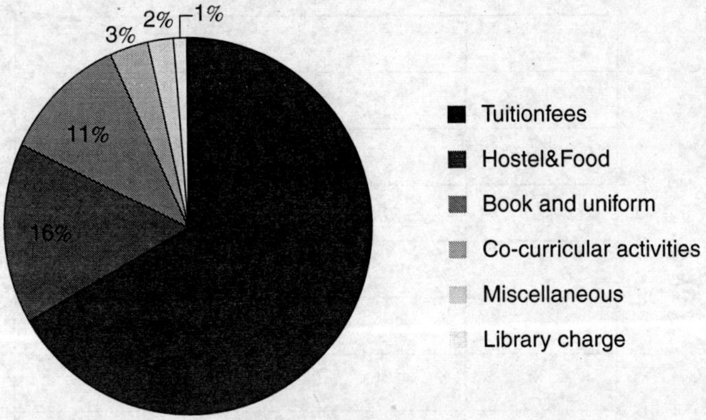

FIGURE 11.22 *Pie Diagram*

The numbers along a side of the line graph are called the scale. Each variable is plotted along an axis. A line graph has a vertical axis (y—dependent variable) and a horizontal axis (x—independent variable). It is created by connecting a series of points, which usually follow a chronological order, representing individual measurements with line segments. The data to be presented are plotted at the intersection of the (imaginary) perpendicular lines extending from the axes, and straight line segments are drawn between those intersection points. Let us consider the following example.

Sam, a student of Intermediate College is observed to be gaining weight rapidly. Suspecting hormonal problem, he is advised to maintain a weight chart as his treatment is continued. His weight chart is presented in Table 11.15.

TABLE 11.15 *Sam's Weight in Kilograms for Five Months*

Month	Weight (kg)
January	49
February	54
March	61
April	69
May	73

The data from the table has been summarized in the line graph shown in Fig. 11.23.

Interpretation: It is seen from the table that Sam's weight continuously increased from January (49 kg) to May (73 kg). The maximum weight gain was from March to April (61 to 69 = 8 kg).

Inference: From the table, it can be inferred that Sam's weight steadily increased from 49 kg to 73 kg, that is, 24 kg in four months, on average 6 kg per month. Initially, his weight increased slowly (5 kg in a month). Between the months of March and April, the rate of increase in his weight was maximum (8 kg) and the rate again declined to 4 kg from April to May. This trend of change in Sam's weight may be corresponding to the effect of his treatment.

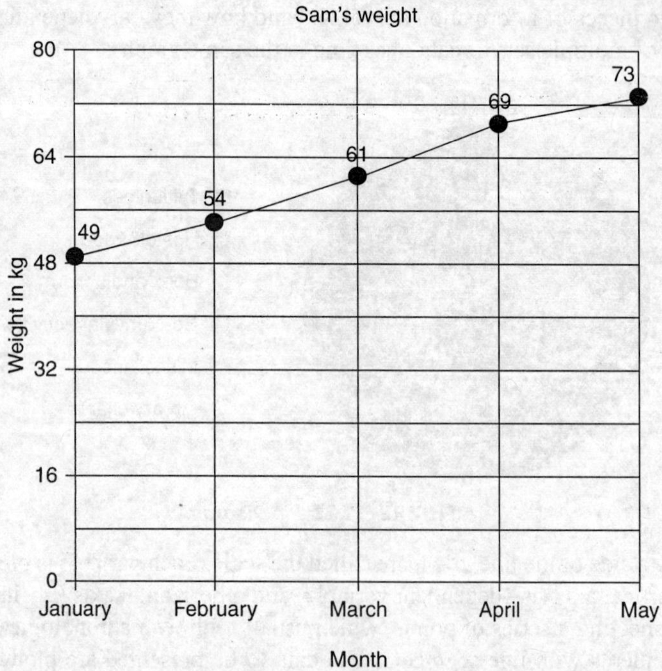

FIGURE 11.23 *Line Graph*

Data interpretation is the exact presentation of the findings, generally in numerical form. Inference is explaining the findings in depth and drawing a conclusion about the situation or issue being investigated. The diffence between these two terms are vague and they are often used synonymously.

CONCLUSION

Data analysis, especially for quantitative research studies, gives the values in numbers, frequencies, averages, percentages, and so on and also the numerical differences in values, which are easy to understand. These numerical values get further simplified by graphical presentations. However, data analysis itself is not about only numbers; it uses the numbers to understand the issues in deeper perspectives.

For example, a study of tuberculosis incidences in a selected urban area shows the number of people in different age groups and genders who are affected by the disease. Exploring into the factors leading to this health problem gives us insight into the entire life and living conditions of these people. This information cannot be that easily and perfectly presented numerically, showing differences among people of different age groups and genders, because of the qualitative aspects influencing the numbers. The quality of data also may affect the analysis outcome, making it biased.

The approach to data analysis varies depending on the study focus, objectives, hypotheses, and its theoretical and conceptual basis. Moreover, the way a researcher defines each major component of the study influences the method adopted for data analysis and interpretation. It is easy to manipulate data during analysis to obtain the desired results, but this act is unethical and against the very purpose of research. Hence, interpretation has to be very precise and has to be entirely on the basis of the research objectives, hypotheses, and the nature of data collected following appropriate methods.

KEY POINTS

- Before starting data analysis, it is important to examine the data for its suitability for the study objectives, hypotheses, and theoretical grounding.
- Sample size calculation needs to be accurate, as generalization of the findings depends on it.
- The statistical tests must be appropriate for the type and level of data.
- Careful attention must be given while using central tendency for data analysis and interpretation. The values that are very far away from the mean value can greatly affect the overall result.
- Conclusions or inferences must be true findings, whether they support or oppose the hypotheses.

QUESTIONS

I. Essay-type Questions

1. Describe the steps of data analysis
2. Explain normal distribution.
3. Illustrate the levels of measurement.
4. Explain the purposes of inferential statistics.
5. Describe the concepts of data organization and computation.

II. Short Notes

1. Differences between univariate and bivariate data
2. Generalization of research findings
3. Advanced statistical methods
4. Classification of variables
5. Types of qualitative research

III. Multiple-choice Questions

Circle the alphabet before the best answer

1. The best option to illustrate the study result of a time series trend is a
   (a) bar diagram (b) histogram
   (c) line graph (d) pie diagram
2. Multiple regression method is used to demonstrate relationship between variables, when there is/are
   1. more than one independent variable
   2. more than one dependent variable
   3. no independent variables

   (a) 1, 2, and 3 (b) 1 and 2
   (c) 1 and 3 (d) Only 1
3. A variable other than the independent variable that could cause a change in the dependent variable is known as the
   (a) extraneous variable
   (b) intervening variable
   (c) predictor variable
   (d) target variable
5. A research study measuring school children's height is collecting
   (a) categorical data
   (b) continuous data
   (c) discrete data
   (d) qualitative data

6. The level of measurement that organizes data in rank order is the
   (a) interval level (b) nominal level
   (c) ordinal level (d) ratio level

7. The storing capacity of a computer expressed as 1 kilobyte is equal to
   (a) 1000 bytes (b) 1024 bytes
   (c) 1048 bytes (d) 1072 bytes

Answer Keys

1. (c) 2. (d) 3. (a) 4. (b) 5. (c) 6. (b)

FURTHER READING

Anand. *Difference between Diagrams and Graphs*. Available at: http://www.preservearticles.com/201104125334/difference-between-diagrams-and-graphs.html.

Andersen, E. B. 1980. *Discrete Statistical Models with Social Science Applications*. Amsterdam: North Holland Publishing Company, pp. 119–121.

Babbie, Earl R. 2009. *The Practice of Social Research*. Twelfth edition. USA: Wadsworth Cengage Learning, pp. 426–433. Available at: http://books.google.co.in/books?id=QySynvetGQIC&pg=PA425&redir_esc=y#v=onepage&q&f=false.

Best, John W., Kahn, James V. 1996. *Research in Education*. Seventh edition. New Delhi: Prentice Hall India Pvt. Ltd.

Bishop, Y. M. M., Fienberg, S. E., Holland, P. W. 1975. *Discrete Multivariate Analysis: Theory and Practice*. Available at: http://en.wikipedia.org/wiki/Stephen_Fienberg.

Bivariate Analysis. 2012. Available at: http://en.wikipedia.org/wiki/Bivariate_analysis#cite_note-babbie-0.

Burns, Nancy, Grove, Susan K. 2007. *Understanding Nursing Research*. Fourth edition. Noida: Reed Elsevier India Pvt. Ltd.

Cherry, Kendra, *What is a Variable?* Available at: http://psychology.about.com/od/researchmethods/f/variable.htm.

Data Analysis. Available at: http://www.businessdictionary.com/definition/data-analysis.html#ixzz21r2kr4k0.

Data Analysis Plan. Available at: http://www.statisticssolutions.com.

Data Entry and Analysis: Evaluation Resources from Wilder Research. 2009. Available at: http://www.evaluatod.org/resources/evaluation-guides/DataEntryAnalysis_2-09.pdf.

Difference between Diagrams and Graphs. Available at: http://www.pinkmonkey.com/studyguides/subjects/stats/chap3/s0303301.asp.

Editing Line Chart. Available at: http://en.wikipedia.org/w/index.php?title=Line_chart&action=edit&section=2.

Garrett, Henry E. 1966. *Statistics in Psychology and Education*. Mumbai: Vakils, Feffer and Simons Ltd.

Hartman, Julia (ed.). 2000. *Multivariate Methods in Health Statistics*. Available at: http://bama.ua.edu/~jleeper/627/choosestat.html.

Heffner, Dr Christopher L. 2004. *Research Methods*. Available at: http://allpsych.com/researchmethods/index.html.

Leeper, James D. 2012. *Choosing Correct Statistical Test*. Available at: http://www.cengage.co.in/; http://www.ats.ucla.edu/stat/mult_pkg/whatstat/choosestat.html.

Lund, Dr Adam. 2012. *Spearman's Rank Order Correlation: A Guide*. Laerd Mathematics Site. Lund Research Ltd. Available at: https://statistics.laerd.com/statistical-guides/spearmans-rank-order-correlation-statistical-guide.php.

MathsIsFun.com. 2012. *Normal Distribution*. Available at: http://www.mathsisfun.com/data/standard-normal-distribution.html.

Merriam-Webster's Online Definition (selected, edited). 2012. *Data vs Information: Difference between Data and Information*. Available at: http://www.diffen.com/difference/Data_vs_Information.

Monotonic and Non-monotonic Relationships among Variables: Examples of Relationship. 2012. Available at: https://statistics.laerd.com/statistical-guides/spearmans-rank-order-correlation-statistical-guide.php.

Morse, J. M., Richards, L. 2002. *Read Me First for a User's Guide to Qualitative Research*. London: Sage Publications.

Munhall, Patricia L., Boyd, Carolyn Oiler. 1993. *Nursing Research: A Qualitative Perspective*. New York: National League for Nursing Press.

Negi, K. S. 2010. *Biostatistics*. Second edition. New Delhi: AITBS Publishers.

Nieswiadomy, R. M. 2008. *Foundations of Nursing Research*. Fifth edition. Delhi: Pearson Education, Inc. and Dorling Kindersley Publishing, Inc.

Polit, D. F., Beck, Cheryl T. 2010. *Essentials of Nursing Research*. Seventh edition. New Delhi: Wolters Kluwer (India) Pvt. Ltd.

Polit, D. F., Hungler, B. P. 1989. *Essentials of Nursing Research*. Second edition. Philadelphia: J. B. Lippincott Company.

Pope, C, Mays, N (eds). 2000. *Qualitative Research in Health Care*. Second edition. London: BMJ.

Rao, P. S. S. Sundar, Richard, J. 2006. *Introduction to Biostatistics and Research Methods*. Fourth edition. New Delhi: PHI Learning Pvt. Ltd.

Roberts, Dona. 1998–2012. *Univariate vs Bivariate Data*. Available at: http://www.regentsprep.org/Regents/math/ALGEBRA/AD1/unidat.htm.

Salkind, Neil J. 2007. *Statistics for People Who (Think They) Hate Statistics*. Third edition. New Delhi, London: Sage Publications.

Scatter Plot Statistics. Available at: http://mste.illinois.edu/courses/ci330ms/youtsey/intro.html and http://www.skymark.com/resources/tools/scatter_plots.asp.

Sharma, S. K. 2011. *Nursing Research and Statistics*. New Delhi: Elsevier.

Shuttleworth, Martyn. 2008. *What is Generalization?* Retrieved on 26 September 2012 from Experiment Resources: http://www.experiment-resources.com/what-is-generalization.html.

Strauss, A, Corbin, J. 1990. *Basics of Qualitative Research: Grounded Theory Procedures and Techniques.* California: Sage Publications.

Streubert, H. J., Carpenter, D. R. 1995. *Qualitative Research in Nursing: Advancing the Humanistic Imperative*. Philadelphia: Lippincott.

Trochim, William M. K. 2006. *Research Method Knowledge Base: Levels of Measurement*. Available at: http://www.socialresearchmethods.net/kb/measlevl.php.

Trochim, William M. K. 2006. *Research Method Knowledge Base: Unit of Analysis*. Available at: http://www.socialresearchmethods.net/kb/unitanal.htm.

What are Confounding Variables? Available at: http://wiki.answers.com/Q/What_are_Confounding_Variables#ixzz21uk36ZnPhttp://wiki.answers.com/Q/.

What is a Contingency Table? Available at: http://www.eumetcal.org/resources/ukmeteocal/verification/www/english/msg/ver_categ_forec/uos1/uos1_ko1.htm.

chapter 12

Critique of Nursing Research Studies

OBJECTIVES

Upon completion of this chapter the learner will be able to:

- Conceptualize critiquing nursing research
- Provide rationale for conducting research critique
- List the types of critiquing
- Explain the critiquing process
- Enumerate the factors to be considered while critiquing
- Explain the elements in a qualitative and quantitative research critique

INTRODUCTION

Nursing is a practice-based profession. The major aim of conducting nursing research is to foster optimum care to patients. When providing care, it is essential that nurses follow the evidence-informed best practices in nursing. Nurses make clinical decisions based on research evidence, their clinical expertise, and the health care preferences of their patients. To know the best practices in nursing, nurses must be able to read nursing researches, critically appraise the research report with selected criteria, and identify the best evidences for rendering the best nursing care.

All researches may not be of good quality. In order to help nurses to select good quality nursing research, this chapter aims at orienting nurses to develop the ability to appraise or critique nursing researches. A sound theoretical foundation to guide practice is enhanced by the ability to critique nursing research. This chapter provides a structured route of guidelines to question the methodology while critiquing research reports.

MEANING AND CONCEPTS OF CRITIQUE

Meaning of Critique

As a noun, critique is explained as an article or essay criticizing a literary or other work, providing a detailed evaluation or review. The following are the meanings of critique:

1. Criticism or critical comment on some problem, subject, and so on
2. The art or practice of criticism

As a verb, it means to review or analyse critically.

Concepts of Critique

1. Critique is the process of objectively and critically evaluating a research report's content to practice, theory, and education. It requires some knowledge of the subject matter and knowledge of how to critically read and use critiquing criteria.
2. Research critique is a careful appraisal of the strengths and weaknesses of a study.
3. An intellectual research critique is a careful and complete examination of a study to judge its strengths, weaknesses, logical link, meaning, and significance.
4. The ultimate aim of any critique undertaken by a nurse is to consider its applicability to practice.
5. Critique is a critical review or commentary, especially one dealing with works of art or literature, a critical discussion of a specific topic, or the art of criticism.

To conclude, a research critique is a careful appraisal of the strengths and weaknesses of a research study or report.

Purposes of Nursing Research Critique

The following are the purposes of critiquing nursing research reports or articles:

1. Nursing research critique is carried out to determine the appropriate application to practice.
2. Research critique is a mechanism to provide feedback for improvement. Written critique serves as a guide to researchers and practitioners. It also suggests possibilities for design replication. Critique helps nurses to decide how the findings from a study can be incorporated into their practice.
3. The ultimate goal of nursing research is to build up a body of nursing knowledge and determine the credibility and applicability to nursing practice.

Types of Critique

1. Nursing students learn to critique in their graduate or postgraduate programme as a part of curriculum log requirement.
2. Nursing faculty critique from the aspect of evaluation of nursing research done by postgraduates, M.Phil. students, and doctoral scholars to improve the dissertation and thesis.
3. Practising nurses analyse studies for evidences on which to base the care for their patients.
4. Nurse researchers focus on studies in one specific area of their interest.
5. The participants attending the conference critically evaluate the strengths and weaknesses of the study and clarify doubts during discussion session.
6. Critique of research report is conducted for publications in journals.
7. Peer review of research is conducted to identify the quality and credibility of the research work.
8. Funding agencies critique research proposals to provide funding assistance for a research study to be undertaken by a research scholar.

PROCESS OF CONDUCTING A RESEARCH CRITIQUE

There are four processes to be followed by nurses for conducting a research critique:

1. Comprehension
2. Comparison

3. Analysis
4. Evaluation

Comprehension

It is the first process in research critiquing. It denotes the understanding of research in terms of concepts utilized in the report and identification of the elements or steps of the research process.

Comparison

Based on the guidelines or criteria, the evaluator compares what is observed in the study with the guidelines or criteria developed. That is the objective of comparison.

Analysis

Analysis denotes critiquing the logical links connecting one study element to another. For example, the objectives and hypothesis written by the researcher should have a logical link with the problem statement.

Problem Statement

A study to evaluate a specific nursing intervention on knowledge regarding breastfeeding among primipara mothers in a selected health facility.

Objectives

1. Assess the pre- and post-interventional knowledge regarding breastfeeding among primipara mothers
2. Compare the pre- and post-interventional knowledge regarding breastfeeding among primipara mothers

Hypothesis

H1: The post-interventional knowledge score on breastfeeding is higher than that of pre-interventional knowledge score among primipara mothers at .05 level of significance.

The problem statement, objectives, and hypothesis in this example have a logical link.

Evaluation

In this process, the evaluator examines the meaning and significance of the study relevant to nursing.

Steps in Conducting Nursing Research Critique

A nurse engaged in critiquing a nursing research study needs to go through the following steps:

1. Read the entire study first. A research critique involves examining the quality of all steps of the research process. Polit and Hungler explain the process in 18 steps comprising 5 dimensions:
   (a) Substantive and theoretical dimension
   (b) Methodological dimension

   (c) Interpretive dimension
   (d) Ethical dimension
   (e) Presentational and stylistic dimensions
2. Examine whether the study has a nursing relevance.
3. Identify the strengths and weaknesses of the study.
4. Be realistic and objective in identifying the study's strengths and limitations.
5. Be balanced in the critique. Identify both the positive and negative points and give rationale for the critique.
6. Suggest modifications for future studies. Specify the feasibilities for replication of the study.
7. Examine the organization and presentation of the research report in terms of completeness, conciseness, clarity of presentation, and logical organization.
8. Examine the usefulness of the findings for nursing practice.

CRITIQUING QUANTITATIVE RESEARCH STUDIES

There are numerous guidelines available to help nursing professionals to critique research studies. The elements of critiquing research are as follows:

1. **Writing Style:** A research report should be well written, grammatically correct, concise, and well organized. The use of jargon should be avoided wherever possible. The style should be such that it attracts the reader to read on.
2. **Researcher(s) Qualification:** Examine the qualification and credentials of the researcher(s). In the past, most of the nursing studies were conducted by non-nursing personnel. Ensure the qualification and position of the researcher(s) indicates a degree of knowledge in nursing field, particularly in the area of study. However, the research study should be evaluated on its own merits and not assumed to be valid and reliable simply because of the qualification of the author(s).

   A brief biographical sketch of the author will assist the evaluator in evaluating the author's current affiliation with a university or health care institution. If the researcher has been funded by a reputable organization or agency, the report could have more confidence in the study result.

Researcher's Qualification

Title of the Study

Thesis Submitted in Partial Fulfilment for the Award of

Degree of Doctor of Philosophy

Name ________ R.N., R.M., M.Sc.(N)

Name of the University ________ State ________

Year ________

Title of the Study
Researcher's Name ______ Qualification ______ Position in Nursing ______ Email ID ______ University ______ State ______ Country ______
Funding Agency
Name ______ (Chairman of Funding Agency)
Year of Submission ______

3. **Title of the Report:** In evaluating the title of the report, clarity and conciseness are the major criteria. The focus should be visible in the title. It should contain major variable(s) and population under study. It should not have more than 10–15 words. Extraneous variables such as 'a study of', 'relationship between', or 'the effect of' should be avoided. Nouns serve as the keywords in the title. The title should be accurate and unambiguous. It should clearly identify the purpose of the study. Titles that are too long or too short can be confusing or misleading.

Title of the Study
Parental martial conflict and behavioural impact on adolescent's academic performance

4. **Abstract:** A research report published in a journal, communicating research thesis, or dissertation frequently contains an abstract at the beginning. It is a summary of the whole study written in about 100–200 words depending upon the university protocol. The abstract contains the purposes of the study, hypothesis, sample size, tools, main findings, conclusion, and recommendation. It will enable the reader to determine whether the study is of interest and whether or not to read the main study.
5. **Introduction:** An interesting and effective introduction to the research study motivates the reader to identify the background of the study, magnitude of the problem selected (globally, nationally, or locally) with the latest statistics, description of variables, and need and significance of the study specific to nursing. If any interventions are proposed in the study, the researcher may also address the traditional and current practices related to the present intervention.
6. **Purposes of the Study:** In the introduction, after providing the background and the need and significance of the current study to nursing, the research problems are presented. Some authors present it as the purpose of the study, depending on what is to be investigated. For appropriate scientific investigation, the researcher presents a broad purpose of the study and this broad purpose is made very specific in the form of objective.
7. **Problem Statement:** The research problem statement should always be written in the interrogative or declarative form. It should contain complete and grammatically correct sentences. The language should be simple and the research consumer should be able to understand and respond to it. The research problem includes the population and the variable(s) under study. The population must be delimited to the main study group of interest. For example, instead of writing the broad area 'nurses', it would be better to identify the population as 'intensive care unit nurses'. Regarding the variables, the evaluator should examine whether it is a one-variable, two-variable, or multi-variable study. The problem stated should also be empirically testable and ethically sound.

> **Research Problem Statement**
>
> A study to assess the correlation of knowledge and attitude of breastfeeding with breastfeeding practices among primipara mothers in a selected health facility

This is a co-relational study; knowledge and attitude of breastfeeding are the independent variables and breastfeeding practices is the dependent variable. Primipara mothers are the population.

8. **Logical Consistency:** The steps used to conduct a research study must follow a logical and sequential order. There should be a clear link between the statement of the problem, purpose, literature review methodology, data analysis, data interpretation, and research finding.
9. **Aims and Objectives:** The researcher should state the objectives, which should be specific, clear, concise, observable, and in measurable terms. The evaluator should examine whether the objectives are derived from the problem statement, relevant to the study, and written differently from the hypothesis. The objectives should be clearly stated and be congruent with the data presented in the literature.
10. **Literature Review:** The evaluator should examine the relevance of literature reviewed by the researcher according to the problem, objectives, and hypotheses stated. Another important factor to be noted is whether the reviews are concise, comprehensive, and recent. A good review includes classic, current, and primary sources. The writing of review should have a logical flow. A good review begins with an introduction followed by specific areas related to the study. The researcher should end the review indicating how the present study contributes to the existing body of knowledge in that subject area.
11. **Operational Definitions:** In nursing research, the researcher needs to ensure that the reader or evaluator understands the meaning of the terms and concepts used in the study. The evaluator must examine whether the key concepts in the study are operationalized. Very often, novice researchers write the conceptual definition from the dictionary or books, which is to be avoided. The outcome variable should be clearly defined along with the measuring instrument, which may be researcher-made or a standardized instrument. All the concepts used in the problem statement need to be defined.
12. **Hypothesis(es):** Studies that examine comparison, correlation, and association should have a clear and specific hypothesis. However, studies purely on descriptive nature and methodological studies usually do not contain hypothesis. The reader needs to examine whether the framing of hypothesis is of the directional or non-directional type. A good hypothesis should contain at least one independent variable and one dependent variable, population, relationship of variables, direction, and level of significance.

> **Directional Hypothesis**
>
> H1: The post-interventional level of depression score is lower than that of pre-interventional depression score among post-natal mothers at .05 level of significance.

In this study,

Independent variable: Intervention
Dependent variable: Depression
Population: Post-natal mothers

Relationship: Cause and effect (Comparison)
Direction: Lower than
Level of significance: $p < .05$

The hypothesis is empirically testable and contains one prediction.

The hypothesis should be clear, concise, stated in declarative form, and written in the present tense. Experimental and quasi-experimental studies should clearly state the hypothesis, identifying the variables to be manipulated, the population that is being studied, and the predicted outcome.

13. **Theoretical Framework:** Theoretical framework is the foundation stone for developing nursing research. After presenting the problem statement, objectives, and the review of literature, the researcher should present the theoretical framework. As nursing profession endeavours to build a body of knowledge, nursing research needs to have a strong theoretical foundation as a means to achieve the desired outcome. The reader or evaluator should be able to identify whether the study has a theoretical base that is relevant and appropriate and whether the theory is selected from the nursing discipline. All concepts in the theory should be clearly defined and the relationship between concepts should be indicated and explained thoroughly. The evaluator should examine the application of these concepts relevant to the present study.

14. **Methodology:** In this chapter, the evaluator must examine the research approach, research design, setting, population, sampling (including sample, sample size, and sampling technique), development and description of instrument, validity and reliability of the tools, intervention strategy, if any, pilot study, data collection procedure, and plan for data analysis.

    The evaluator needs to identify the *research approach*—qualitative, quantitative, or mixed method—undertaken by the researcher. The research design should be clearly identified and described in detail and the evaluator has to check its appropriateness for the present study.

    When an *intervention* is planned in the experimental study, the evaluator should examine in detail its description and appropriateness and how the treatment is administered to the group. With regard to *the setting* of the study, the researcher must give a clear picture of the setting, for example, 'maternity hospital run by the government at a particular district in South India, having 3000 deliveries conducted per year'. This may give a hint to the evaluator regarding whether the setting is appropriate for the present study.

    On critiquing *population* and *sample*, the evaluator must be able to identify the target population. With regard to sampling, the evaluator should examine who the research subjects were and how they were selected, inclusion and exclusion criteria, determination of the sample size and its adequacy, and sampling technique used by the researcher (probability or non-probability sampling).

    With regard *to data collection instruments*, the evaluator must identify the type of instruments used in the study and their description, scoring, appropriateness, and relevancy to achieve the outcome.

    The researcher needs to describe the data collection instrument and the interventions in detail. The evaluator must examine how the researcher tested the *content validity* and *reliability* of the tool and what is the content validity index and reliability score of all the instruments used in the study. He/she should also examine the *pilot study* undertaken, including the pilot study report. The researcher must ensure that the subjects used for the pilot study were excluded from the main study. It is essential that the evaluator examines the data collection procedure within the time frame.

15. **Ethical Consideration:** The researcher must get approval from Institutional Review board and ethical committee for the acceptance of the study. Furthermore, he/she should take permission from the authority of the setting to conduct research in that setting. Moreover, the researcher is required to take informed consent from the subjects for their willingness.

16. **Data Analysis and Results:** The researcher should ensure that the data collected are grouped, organized, and described under various sections. The evaluator should examine the data for their clarity and accuracy. Presentation of data in tables, graphs, and figures ensures that the researcher is confident in reporting the data in various forms of presentations.

    Usually, researchers use both descriptive and inferential statistics. Descriptive statistics include frequency, percentage, mean, and standard deviation. Inferential statistics include t test for comparison, *r* test for correlation and chi-square test or ANOVA for association or other methods according to the preference of the researchers. Inferential statistical tests are used to identify whether the relationship between variables, difference between variables, or association between variables is statistically significant. The evaluator needs to identify clearly what statistical methods were undertaken, why those methods were undertaken, and what was the statistical significance reported by the researcher. Statistical significance helps the researcher to rule out one important threat to validity, which is the possibility that the result could be due to chance rather than to real difference in the population.

    Quantitative studies usually identify the lowest level of significance as $p < .05$ (p = probability). The evaluator must determine whether the results were presented clearly, answered the research questions, and were summarized accurately and clearly through tables, figures, and graphs. The percentage of the sample who participated in the study is an important element in considering the generalizability of the results. At least 50 per cent of the sample is needed to participate if a response bias is to be avoided.
17. **Discussion:** The discussion chapter is very important; the findings should flow logically from the data and should be related back to the literature review, thus placing the study in context. The data collected are usually discussed based on the objectives and theoretical framework used in the study. While critiquing the findings, the evaluator should examine whether the hypotheses stated were accepted or rejected and, if accepted, on what level of significance they were accepted. The evaluation of testing the hypothesis is also important. For example, if the hypothesis is tested for comparison, the researcher must present the mean and standard deviation of the pre-test and post-test values of the attribute (knowledge). Then, the t value, table value, and level of significance are calculated. According to the findings, the evaluator should also examine whether the researcher had given supportive studies or, if not, the researcher's inference to support the present study findings.
18. **Conclusions:** Conclusions are derived from the in-depth examination of each step in the research process. Writing the conclusion is a tedious job. Through conclusion, the researcher attempts to communicate the worth of the research and whether there is a scope to implement the present study in nursing practice. The evaluator must examine the conclusion for its objectivity, generalizability, and clinical significance.
19. **Implications:** The evaluator needs to examine whether the researcher has explicitly identified the implications of the study findings for nursing practice, nursing education, nursing administration, and nursing research.
20. **Recommendations:** The evaluator must examine the recommendations made by the researcher for future research generated from the present study findings.
21. **Limitations:** In every study, there will be some limitations. The researcher is expected to communicate the study limitation so as to improve future studies by avoiding such shortcomings. The evaluator should examine the study limitations in terms of the problem statement, objectives, hypothesis stated, variables, study design, data collection tools, sample size, sampling techniques, and methods of data analysis and suggest possible ways to address the limitations observed.

ELEMENTS OF RESEARCH CRITIQUE

Quantitative Research	Qualitative Research
• Writing style • Author(s) • Title of the report • Abstract • Purpose or research problem • Review of literature • Logical consistency • Aims or objectives • Operational definition • Hypothesis • Theoretical framework • Methodology • Ethical consideration • Data analysis/results • Discussion, conclusion, and recommendation	• Writing style • Author(s) • Title of the report • Abstract • Statement of the phenomena of interest • Purposes or significance of the study • Literature review • Theoretical framework • Methods and philosophical underpinning • Ethical consideration • Methods of data collection • Data analysis • Rigor • Conclusion, implication, and recommendation • Reference

Guidelines for Critiquing Quantitative Research Studies in Nursing

To perform a true, objective critique of a quantitative research report, the entire study must be read and the questions provided in Table 12.1 considered.

TABLE 12.1 *Questions to be Considered in Critiquing Quantitative Nursing Research Studies*

S. No.	Criteria	Comment	Suggestions for Improvement
1.	**Title of the Report** • Does the title show clarity and conciseness in describing the nature of the study? • Does the title contain major variables? • Does the title include population? • Is the title stated within 10–15 words? • Does the title identify the purpose of the study?		
2.	**Statement of the Problem** • Is the problem statement clear? • Is the problem statement written in declarative or interrogative form? • Are the study variables and population included in the problem statement? • Does the problem statement indicate that empirical data could be collected on the topic of study? • Does the problem statement indicate that the study would be ethical? • Does the problem statement have significance to nursing?		

(Continued)

TABLE 12.1 *Questions to be Considered in Critiquing Quantitative Nursing Research Studies* (*Continued*)

S. No.	Criteria	Comment	Suggestions for Improvement
3.	**Theoretical or Conceptual Framework** • Is the framework clearly identified? • Is the conceptual framework described? • Are the concepts to be studied identified and defined? • Are the measures for each of the concepts identified and described? • Does the research problem flow naturally from the conceptual framework?		
4.	**Protection of Human Rights** • Is there evidence of an independent ethics review by a committee or an IRB? • Has the study been designed to minimize risk and maximize benefits to participants? • Is there an indication that participants gave voluntary informed consent? • Is there evidence in the study that the study participants' confidentiality and anonymity are maintained?		
5.	**Research Questions or Hypotheses** • Are research questions or hypotheses formally stated? • Are the hypotheses stated clearly? • Do the research questions and hypotheses naturally flow from the research problem and theoretical framework? • Does each research question or hypothesis contain at least two variables? • Does the hypothesis contain the population? • Are the research questions or hypotheses worded clearly and objectively?		
	• Is a prediction evident? • Is the hypothesis written in the declarative form? • Is it apparent that each hypothesis can be empirically tested?		
6.	**Review of Literature** • Is the review comprehensive, logical, and relevant to the problem? • Is the review of literature concise? • Are the sources relevant to the study topic? • Are the sources critically examined? • Are all the sources used in the study referenced?		

TABLE 12.1 *Questions to be Considered in Critiquing Quantitative Nursing Research Studies* (*Continued*)

S. No.	Criteria	Comment	Suggestions for Improvement
7.	**Research Design** • What design has been used for the study? • Is the design appropriate for the research question and purpose of research? • What are the means used to control the extraneous variables? • Has enough information been given to permit replication? • If the design was non-experimental, would an experimental design have been more appropriate?		
8.	**Sampling Procedures** • Is the target population carefully described? • Is the accessible population identified? • Are sample selection procedures clearly defined? • Does the sampling method fit the research design? • Are potential sample biases described? • Is the sample sufficiently large? How has the size been justified? • To whom can the study results be generalized? • Are subject dropouts described?		
9.	**Data Collection Methods** • What are the types of instruments used for the study? • Are the instruments relevant and appropriate? • How did the researcher develop the data collection tools? • Does the study identify content validity and reliability done by the researcher? • Is the content validity index given by the researcher? • Is it evident that the researcher took permission to use a standardized scale? • Has the researcher undertaken a pilot study? • Has the researcher given justification after the pilot study to go for the main study?		
10.	**Data Analysis and Interpretation** • Are the data grouped, organized, and described sectionwise? • What type of statistical analysis is used by the researcher to analyse the data? • Are the statistical methods appropriate? • Are tables, figures, and graphs used to present data? • Does the researcher ensure that all the data collected are analysed?		

(*Continued*)

TABLE 12.1 *Questions to be Considered in Critiquing Quantitative Nursing Research Studies* (*Continued*)

S. No.	Criteria	Comment	Suggestions for Improvement
	• Are results of data analysis clearly explained in reference to research questions, hypotheses, and theoretical framework? • Has there been appropriate generalization of significant findings beyond the study sample to the population?		
11.	**Discussion** • Are the data collected discussed based on the objectives? • Does the researcher ensure that all the hypotheses stated were tested? • Is the significance of the hypotheses identified? • Does the discussion highlight whether the hypotheses were accepted or rejected? • Does the study identify supportive studies to strengthen the present study findings? • Has the researcher brought his/her own inference where the studies were not available?		
12.	**Conclusion** • Is the conclusion made by the researcher appropriate? • Is the conclusion consistent with the present study? • Does the conclusion have a relevance and scope for nursing?		
13.	**Implications** • Does the study identify the implications of the study? • Is it relevant to nursing practice? • Is it relevant to nursing education? • Is it relevant to nursing administration? • Is it relevant to nursing research?		
14.	**Recommendations** • Are the recommendations listed clearly and consistent to the present study? • What are the recommendations for nursing practice and future? • Are these recommendations supported by the data?		
15.	**Limitations of the Study** • Does the study identify its limitations? • Does the study identify the limitations in terms of the sample size, study design, variables, study settings, statistical analysis, or any other aspect? • Does the researcher provide suggestions for overcoming the limitations?		

TABLE 12.1 *Questions to be Considered in Critiquing Quantitative Nursing Research Studies* (*Continued*)

S. No.	Criteria	Comment	Suggestions for Improvement
16.	**Presentation of Research Report** • Does the study present all aspects of research starting from introduction to limitations of the study? • Is the report well written without grammatical errors? • Is the report presented in simple language and jargon avoided? • Is the report orderly and presented in a sequential order or is it confusing? • Is the report relevant and unbiased? • Does the abstract adequately summarize the study problem, methods, and findings?		

CRITIQUING QUALITATIVE RESEARCH DESIGN

Of late, practicing nurses, nurse academicians, and nurse researchers have shown more interest towards qualitative research, which focuses on gaining an insight about individuals' perceptions of events and circumstances. There needs to be a clear-cut framework to critique qualitative research, so that the evaluator can answer questions and make critical judgment according to the questions given in the critiquing framework.

Careful evaluation of qualitative research gives the nurse practitioner a better understanding of how a group of people view or understand a particular situation. It is very difficult to evaluate qualitative research using a standard set of critiquing criteria because each qualitative method is unique in nature. Streubert and Carpenter identified five methods of qualitative research—phenomenology, grounded theory, ethnography, historical method, and action research.

In their study, Burns and Grove discussed six types of qualitative research—phenomenology, ethnography, grounded theory, philosophical enquiry, historical method, and critical social enquiry. Polit and Beck identified eleven types of qualitative research. Qualitative researches are difficult to critique because they are subjective in nature and use distinct terminology and discrete ways of reasoning. However, there are some similarities among these methods. On the basis of these similarities, the following guidelines are provided for critiquing qualitative research studies.

The guidelines for critiquing qualitative research, for the following topics are the same as those given earlier for critiquing quantitative research:

1. **Writing Style**
2. **Researcher(S) Qualification**
3. **Title of the Report**
4. **Abstract**

The guidelines for other elements of critiquing qualitative research studies are as follows:

1. **Statement of the Phenomenon of Interest:** The researcher must clearly interpret the phenomenon of interest as it should be understood by the reader. It may be written as a broad statement, indicating the general nature of the phenomenon.

2. **Purpose and Significance of the Study:** The researcher should clearly explain why the study has been undertaken and what would be the ultimate expectation from the study. The researcher must also emphasize why the study would be of significance and how it would add to the general body of information on the phenomenon under study.
3. **Literature Review:** In quantitative research, the researcher starts the framework for research with the review of literature as the first step, whereas in qualitative research, most of the researchers do not initially review the literature because they believe it will lead to bias. They do not want to know what others think or believe about the phenomenon prior to the collection of their data. However, the researcher conducting a qualitative research does a review of literature at the conclusion phase of his/her study to analyse review findings and to determine how they will fit in the present study.
4. **Research Hypothesis:** A research hypothesis is never used in qualitative research as done in qualitative research. The research question may be modified depending on the qualitative research method adopted and the researcher needs to explain and justify the modification.
5. **Theoretical Framework:** Usually, qualitative studies are theory-generating research and do not test theories, unlike quantitative studies. Therefore, the researcher does not use any existing or known theory.
6. **Research Design:** Depending on the phenomenon of interest, the researcher selects the method or design regarding the setting of the study; the researcher conducts the study in the field where the actual participants live or work. However, the researcher must take permission from the authority of the setting for ethical reasons. Compared with quantitative studies, the *sample size* is small in qualitative designs. There is no hard and fast rule about the determination of the sample size. The quality of information obtained from each sample is more important than the sample size.
7. **Ethical Consideration:** Since the researcher works very closely with research participants, people tend to share very personal or private information with him/her. Therefore, the researcher must maintain anonymity and confidentiality of the subjects and data.
8. **Methods of Data Collection:** In-depth interviews, participation observation, open-ended questionnaires, diaries, personal collection of letters and photographs, and focus group discussion are some of the instruments used by the researchers depending upon the method of the qualitative study. The researcher needs to justify why such instruments are used for data collection.
9. **Data Analysis:** Data analysis and interpretation is done as the data are collected. The researcher does the content analysis and creates categories of data. Then coding of data is done into the categories. The researcher identifies the pattern and theme from the clusters identified.
10. **Rigour:** Rigour means trustworthiness. The aim of qualitative research is to understand human experiences, which ultimately helps in theory development. The researcher should discuss the credibility, dependability, trustworthiness, and goodness of the report.
11. **Conclusion, Implication, and Recommendation:** The researcher should conclude by explaining the research findings in a context that emphasizes how the information is of interest and its implications for nursing practice. The conclusion should reflect the study findings and follow realistic recommendations.

Table 12.2 lists the questions that will help in critiquing qualitative research studies.

TABLE 12.2 *Questions to be Considered in Critiquing Qualitative Nursing Research Studies*

S. No.	Criteria	Comments	Suggestions
1.	**Title of the Report** • Is the title appropriate? • Does it suggest the key phenomenon of interest? • Does it identify the group or population under study?		
2.	**Statement of the Problem** • Is the problem stated clearly? • Is the problem easy to identify? • Does the problem statement build a rationale for the present study? • Does the problem yield significance for nursing? • Is there a good relation between the research problem and the methods used?		
3.	**Research Questions** • Are the research questions explicitly stated? • Are the questions consistent with the study's philosophical basis, underlying tradition, and conceptual framework?		
4.	**Literature Review** • Does the report adequately summarize the existing body of knowledge related to the problem or phenomenon of interest? • Does the literature review provide a solid basis for the new study?		
5.	**Conceptual Framework** • Are the key concepts adequately defined conceptually? • Is the framework appropriate? • Does the framework provide a link to the research process?		
6.	**Protection of Participants' Rights** • Are appropriate procedures used to safeguard the rights of study participants? • Is consent or permission taken from the study settings? • Is the study designed to minimize risks and maximize benefits to participants? • Are anonymity and confidentiality maintained about participants and data?		
7.	**Research Design and Research Tradition** • Is the study design identified research tradition (if any) congruent with the methods used to collect and analyse data? • Is an adequate amount of time spent in the field or with study participants? • Are there an adequate number of contacts with study participants?		

(Continued)

TABLE 12.2 *Questions to be Considered in Critiquing Qualitative Nursing Research Studies* (*Continued*)

S. No.	Criteria	Comments	Suggestions
8.	**Data Collection Procedure** • Are the methods of gathering data appropriate? • Are the data gathered through two or more methods to achieve triangulation? • Does the researcher ask the right questions or make the right observations and were they recorded in the appropriate manner? • Is sufficient amount of data gathered? • Are the data of sufficient depth and richness? • Are the data collection and recording procedures adequately described and do they appear appropriate? • Are the data collected in a manner that minimized bias or behavioural distortions?		
9.	**Data Analysis** • Are the data collection and data analysis methods sufficiently described? • Is the data analysis strategy compatible with the research tradition and with the nature and type of data gathered? • Does the analysis yield an appropriate theory or a thematic pattern? • Does the analytic procedure suggest accuracy?		
10.	**Interpretation of the Findings** • Are the findings interpreted within an appropriate frame of reference? • Are major findings interpreted and discussed within the context of prior studies?		
	• Are the interpretations consistent with the study's review of literature? • Does the report address the issue of the findings clearly?		
11.	**Findings** • Are the findings effectively summarized, with good use of excerpts and supporting arguments? • Does it appear that the research satisfactorily conceptualized the themes or patterns in the data? • Does the analysis yield an insightful and meaningful picture of the phenomenon under study?		
12.	**Theoretical Integration** • Are the themes or patterns logically connected to each other to form a convincing and integrated whole? • Are the figures, maps, or models used effectively to summarize conceptualizations?		

TABLE 12.2 *Questions to be Considered in Critiquing Qualitative Nursing Research Studies* (*Continued*)

S. No.	Criteria	Comments	Suggestions
13.	**Summary** • Do the study findings appear to be trustworthy and have confidence in the true value of the results? • Does the study contribute any meaningful evidence that can be used in nursing practice or that is useful to the nursing discipline?		
14.	**Implications and Recommendations** • Does the researcher discuss the implications of the study for clinical practice? • Are the recommendations made by the researcher based on the study findings? • Are the recommendation made appropriate and feasible for further study?		
15.	**Presentation** • Was the report well written, well organized, and sufficiently detailed for critical analysis? • Were the descriptions of the methods, findings, and interpretations sufficiently rich and vivid?		

KEY POINTS

- A research critique is not just a review or summary of a research report, but it is a careful and critical appraisal of the strengths and weaknesses of a research study.
- The critique is meant for nurse practitioners, nurse academicians, and nurse researchers who must identify to what extent the study findings could be incorporated in their professional dealings.
- A sound theoretical foundation to guide practice is enhanced by the ability of nurses to critique research reports, which they may not find in journals or published reports.
- Successful critiquing of research report requires a balanced appraisal.
- A balanced appraisal requires logic and objectivity in identifying the systematic route of enquiry that underpins the research.
- The framework or guidelines stimulate the reader or evaluator to objectively question each section of the research report.
- The framework or guidelines may differ in qualitative and quantitative researches because of their unique nature.
- All qualified nurses must develop competency in critiquing a research report to consider its applicability to practice so as to enable them to perform evidence-informed best practices.

QUESTIONS

I. Essay-type Questions

1. Discuss the rationale for conducting critique in nursing research.
2. Explain the critiquing process with examples from nursing studies.

3. Describe the elements involved in critiquing the methodological dimension of nursing research with examples.
4. Discuss the factors to be considered while critiquing qualitative research studies.
5. Prepare guidelines for critiquing quantitative research studies.

II. Short Notes

1. Concept of research critique
2. Types of research critique
3. Critiquing review of literature
4. Appraisal of hypothesis and objectives
5. Assessing interpretation of study results

III. Multiple-choice Questions

Circle the alphabet before the best answer

1. A research critique in nursing study is a careful appraisal of the
   (a) quality of a research study
   (b) strengths and weaknesses of a research study
   (c) qualification of the researcher
   (d) strength of assumption and hypothesis
2. The various dimensions of critiquing nursing research include the following except
   (a) substantive and theoretical dimension
   (b) methodological dimension
   (c) analytical dimension
   (d) evaluative dimension
3. While appraising operational definitions of the terms used in a study, the evaluator looks for
   (a) explanation of the term from its dictionary meaning
   (b) explanation of the term with regard to its concept
   (c) explanation of the term as used by previous researchers
   (d) explanation of the term meant by the researcher used in the present study, including the measuring instrument if the term is an outcome variable
4. The discussion part of the research study should be based on
   (a) objectives and hypothesis(s)
   (b) methodology and ethical aspects
   (c) data analysis
   (d) conclusion and recommendations
5. While appraising sampling procedures in a research study, the evaluator examines the following except whether
   (a) sampling technique is clearly defined
   (b) sample setting is described in detail
   (c) sample size has been justified
   (d) sample biases are described

Answer Keys

1. (b) 2. (d) 3. (d) 4. (a) 5. (b)

FURTHER READING

Boswell, Carrol, Cannon, Sharon. 2006. *Critique Process*. California: Jones and Bartlett Publishers, p. 202.

Burns, N., Grove, S. 1999. *The Practice of Nursing Research: Conduct, Critique and Utilization*. Second edition. Philadelphia: W B Saunders Company.

Burns, N., Grove, S. 2005. *The Practice of Nursing Research: Conduct, Critique and Utilization*. Fifth edition. St Louis: Elsevier Saunders.

Clegg, F. 1990. *Simple Statistics: A Course Book for the Social Sciences*. Second edition. Cambridge: Cambridge University Press.

Connel, Mechan. 1999. *Research Critique: Nursing Research and Design*. Dublin: UCD Press, pp. 57–74.

Critique. American Heritage Dictionary. www.dictionaryboss.com.

Critique.www.my-free dictionary.com.

Evaluating and Critiquing Nursing Research. Nursing planet.com/nursing_research/critiquing_nursing_research.html.

Ingham-Broomfield, Rebecca. 2008. 'A Nurse's Guide to the Critical Reading of Research', *Australian Journal of Advanced Nursing*, 26(1):102–109.

Nieswiadomy, Rose Marie. 2004. *Foundations of Nursing Research*. Fifth edition. New Delhi: Pearson Education, p. 380.

Nordquist, Richard. *Critique*. About.com. Grammar and Composition. grammar.about. com/od/c/g/critiqueterm.htm.

Parahoo, K. 2006. *Nursing Research: Principles, Process and Issues*. Second edition. Houndmills Basingstoke: Palgrave Macmillan.

Polit, D. F., Beck, C. T. 2006. *Essentials of Nursing Research; Methods, Appraisal and Utilization*. Sixth edition. Philadelphia: Lippincott Williams and Wilkins.

Russel, C. L. 2005, 'Evaluating Quantitave Research Reports.' *Nephrol Nursing journal*, 32(1):61–64.

Ryan-Wenger, N. 1992. 'Guidelines for Critique of a Research Report', *Heart Lung*, 21(4):394–401.

Streubert, H. J., Carpenter, D. R. 2002. *Qualitative Research in Nursing. Advancing the Human Imperative*. Third edition. Philadelphia: Lippincott Williams and Wilkins.

Tanner, J. 2003. 'Reading and critiquing research', *British Journal of Perioperative Nursing*, 13(4):162–164.

Valente, S. 2003. 'Research Dissemination and Utilization: Improving Care at the Bedside', *Journal of Nursing Care Quality*, 18(2):114–121.

chapter 13

Communication of Research Results: Oral and Written

OBJECTIVES

Upon completion of this chapter the learner will be able to:

Examine the strategies adopted for communicating research results

Identify the methods of oral communication of research results

Describe the methods followed for written communication of research results

INTRODUCTION

The research utilization process involves communicating study findings from investigators to practising nurses. Communication of research findings includes developing a research report and disseminating that report through presentations and publications to audiences of nurses, health care professionals, policy makers, and health care consumers. Dissemination of research findings can happen by one individual communicating to another or by one individual communicating to several others by the use of mass media such as journals, books, newspapers, and television.

STRATEGIES ADOPTED FOR COMMUNICATING RESEARCH RESULTS

Nurses communicate research results either through oral presentations or by writing them as research reports, or sometimes through both means.

Oral Presentations

The following are some of the oral presentations:

1. Nursing research conferences
2. Clinical practice conferences and meetings
3. Videotaped and audiotaped presentations from conferences and meetings
4. In-service education programs
5. Agency-based research committees and journal clubs

Written Reports

The following are some of the written reports:

1. Research publications in professional journals
2. Research publications in books

3. Monographs from research and clinical conferences and meetings
4. Theses and dissertations
5. Nursing research newsletters
6. Electronic databases (http://www...)

ORAL COMMUNICATION OF RESEARCH RESULTS

The most rapid means of disseminating one's research finding is to discuss it during formal or informal professional meetings, public lectures, or interviews with the media. A researcher typically elects to present scientific papers at research or clinical conferences. These presentations are usually for 10–30 minutes, within which an in-depth discussion of an entire project is rarely possible. However, conference participants can often ask the investigator more about the project or study. The contents of such presentation can be targeted to the audience in attendance and might focus on conceptual or methodological issues, selected research findings, or implications for practice.

Presentations at Professional Conferences

Numerous professional organizations sponsor annual meetings at which nursing studies are presented, either through the reading of a research report or through visual display in a poster session. The Nursing Research Society of India (NRSI) is an example of an organization that holds meetings at which nurses have an opportunity to share their knowledge with others interested in their topic. Presentation of research results at a conference has two distinct advantages over journal publication. First, there is usually less time elapsed between the completion of a study and its communication to others when a presentation is made at a meeting. Second, there is an opportunity for dialogue between the researchers and the audience at a conference. Listeners can request clarification on certain points or make useful suggestions. Hence, professional conferences are particularly good forums for presenting results to clinical audiences. While attending such conferences, researchers can also take advantage of meeting and talking with others working on similar problems in different parts of the world.

The mechanism for submitting a presentation to a conference is comparatively simpler than that for journal submission. The association sponsoring the conference usually publishes an announcement or 'Call for Abstracts' in its newsletter, journal, or website about 6–9 months before the meeting date. The notice indicates topics of interest, submission requirements, and deadlines for submitting a proposed paper or poster. Most universities and major health care agencies receive and post these Call for Abstracts notices.

Oral Reports

Most conferences require prospective presenters to submit an abstract of 500–1000 words rather than a complete paper. Abstracts can usually be (and in some cases must be) submitted online. Each conference has its own guidelines for abstract content and form. In some cases, abstracts are submitted to the organizer of a particular session on a given topic; in other cases, conference sessions are organized after receiving all the abstracts with related papers grouped together. Abstracts are evaluated on the basis of the quality and originality of the research and the appropriateness of the paper for the conference audience and conference theme. If abstracts are accepted, researchers are committed to appear at the conference to make a presentation.

Research reports presented at professional meetings usually follow a traditional format. The time allotted for presentation usually is about 10–15 minutes, with up to 5 minutes for questions from the audience. Therefore, only the most important aspects of the study—with special emphasis on the results—can be included. It is especially challenging to condense a qualitative report to a brief oral summary without losing the rich, in-depth character of the data. A handy rule of thumb is that a page of double-spaced text requires 2.5–3 minutes to read aloud. Although most conference presenters do prepare a written paper or a script, presentations are most effective if they are delivered informally or conversationally rather than being read verbatim. The presentation should be rehearsed to gain familiarity and comfort with the script and to ensure that time limits are not exceeded.

The question-and-answer session can be a fruitful opportunity to expand on various aspects of the research and to get early feedback about the study. It is useful to make note of audience comments because these can be helpful in turning the conference presentation into a manuscript for journal submission.

Poster Presentations

Researchers sometimes elect to present their findings in poster sessions. (Abstracts, often similar to those required for oral presentations, must be submitted to conference organizers according to specific guidelines.) In poster sessions, several researchers simultaneously present visual displays summarizing the highlights of their study, and conference attendees circulate around the exhibit area perusing the displays. In this manner, those interested in a particular topic can devote time to discussing the study with the researcher and bypass posters dealing with topics of less interest. Poster sessions are thus efficient and encourage one-on-one discussions. These sessions are typically 1–2 hours in length; researchers should stand near their posters throughout the session to ensure effective communication.

It is challenging to design an effective poster. The poster must convey essential information about the background, design, and results of a study in a format that can be perused in minutes. Bullet points, graphs, and photos are especially useful devices on a poster for communicating a lot of information quickly. Large, bold fonts are essential, because posters are often read from a distance of several feet. Another issue is that posters must be sturdily constructed for transport to the conference site. It is important to follow the conference guide-lines in determining such matters as poster size, format, and allowable display materials.

Wilson and Hutchinson recommend a three-phase process for presenting effective posters.

Pre-presentation Phase: Researchers target the audience, obtain official guidelines, write an abstract or title, and design a poster based on principles of visual literacy.

Presentation Phase: Researchers need to carry the following items to the actual poster session: Data collection instruments, bibliographic information, business cards, and pages of stick-on mailing labels so that those interested in additional information can write their names and addresses on the labels.

Post-presentation Phase: Presenters should evaluate the effectiveness of their poster. One approach is to ask viewers to complete a simple evaluation form regarding the poster. Qualitative researchers face special challenges with regard to designing a poster.

WRITTEN COMMUNICATION OF RESEARCH RESULTS

Quantitative Research Report Communication

Quantitative reports follow a conventional format referred to as the IMRAD format. This format involves organizing study material into four sections:

1. Introduction
2. Method
3. Results
4. Discussion

These sections, respectively address the following questions:

1. Why was the study done? (I)
2. How was the study done? (M)
3. What was learnt? (R)
4. What does it mean? (D)

Introduction

The introduction section deals with the research problem, its significance, and the context in which it was developed. It sets the stage for the study by describing the existing literature, the study's conceptual framework, the problem, research questions, or hypotheses, any underlying assumptions, and the rationale for doing the study. Introductions are often written in a funnel-shaped structure, beginning broadly to establish a framework for understanding the study and then narrowing to the specifics of what researchers sought to learn.

Method

To evaluate the quality of evidence a study offers, readers need to understand exactly what researchers did to address the research problem. This section ideally provides a sufficiently detailed description of the research methods such that another researcher could replicate the study. In theses or dissertations, this goal should almost always be satisfied. In journal articles and conference presentations, this section may need to be condensed.

The method section usually begins with the description of the research design and its rationale. In experimental and quasi-experimental studies, the researcher should indicate what specific design was adopted, what variables were manipulated, how subjects were assigned to groups, and whether blinding or double blinding was used.

A description of the method used to collect the data is a critical component of the method section. In an interview study, information should be provided about where the interviews were conducted, who conducted them, and how long the average interview lasted. In an observational study, the report should indicate what the role of the observer in relation to the subjects was. When questionnaires are used in the study, this section should describe how they were delivered to respondents and whether follow up procedures were used to increases responses.

Results

In a quantitative study, the results of the statistical analyses are summarized in a factual manner. If both descriptive and inferential statistics have been used, descriptive statistics come first, to provide an overview of the study variables.

Three pieces of information are normally included when reporting the results of a statistical test: value of the calculated statistic, degrees of freedom, and significance level. When results from several statistical analyses are reported, it is useful to summarize them in a table.

Discussion

A typical discussion section addresses the following questions:

1. What were the main findings?
2. What do the findings mean?

3. What evidence is there that the results and the interpretations are valid?
4. What limitations might threaten validity?
5. How do the results compare with prior knowledge on the topic?
6. What can be concluded about the findings and their use in nursing practice, in nursing theory, and in future nursing research?

Typically, the discussion section begins with a summary of the main findings. The summary should be brief. Interpretation of results is a global process, encompassing knowledge of the results, method, sample characteristics, related research findings, clinical dimensions, and theoretical issues.

Other Aspects of the Report

Title: Every research report should have a title indicating the nature of the study. The phrases *research report* and *report of a nursing research study* are inadequate. The dependent and independent variables should be named in the title. It is also desirable to indicate the study population. The title should be brief and writers must balance clarity with brevity.

Abstract: Research reports usually include an abstract or summary, with brief descriptions of the problem, methods, and findings of the study, so that readers can decide whether to read the entire report.

References: Each report concludes with a list of references cited in the text, using a referenced style required by those reviewing the manuscript or report.

Acknowledgements: People who helped with the research but whose contributions do not qualify them for authorship are sometimes acknowledged at the end of the report. This might be statistical consultants, data collectors, and reviewers of the manuscript.

Qualitative Research Reports

Introduction

Qualitative research reports also often follow the IMRAD format. They usually begin with a statement of the problem similar to quantitative reports, but the focus is more on the phenomenon under study. In qualitative studies, especially in ethnographic ones, it is critical to explain the cultural context of the study. In studies with an ideological orientation, it is also important to describe the socio-political context.

Method

The method section should provide a solid description of the research setting, so that readers can assess the transferability of the findings. Study participants and methods by which they were selected should also be described. Even when the samples are small, it may be useful to provide a table summarizing the participants' main characteristics. Qualitative reports usually cannot provide specific information about data collection, inasmuch as formal instruments are not used and questions and observations evolve in the field. Some researchers do provide sample questions and observation guidelines in the field. The description of data collection methods should include how data were collected, how long data collection sessions lasted, who collected the data, how data collectors were trained, and what methods were used to record the data.

Results

In qualitative results sections, researchers summarize their thematic analysis and, in the case of grounded theory studies, the theory that emerged. This section can be organized in a number of ways.

Discussion

The discussion section of a qualitative report is not designed to give meaning to the results, but it is to summarize them, link them to other research, and suggest their implications for theory, practice, or future research. In some cases, researchers offer explicit recommendations about how their research can be corroborated through quantitative studies.

Other Aspects of Qualitative Reports

Qualitative reports, like quantitative ones, include abstracts, key words, references, and acknowledgments. Abstracts for journals that feature qualitative reports tend to be the traditional single-paragraph type, that is, they are not structured abstracts.

TYPES OF WRITTEN RESEARCH REPORTS

There are three major kinds of research reports:

1. Theses and dissertations
2. Traditional journal articles
3. Online reports or electronic publications

Theses and Dissertations

Thesis is the product of slow, painstaking, and accurate inductive work. It involves the following steps:

1. **Logical Analysis of the Subject Matter:** Researchers are interested in developing the content either in a logical or chronological manner. The logical organization of the content is well done by sequencing the content from 'simple to complex', from 'known to unknown', or from 'general to specific'. In the manuscript, the researcher gives emphasis to the 'clarity' of the content with logical flow, whereas the chronological organization of the content is based on the 'time' that the occurrence has taken place. Usually, the researcher goes from the 'latest occurrence' to the 'past occurrence', that is, in the descending order; for example, while explaining the concept of personality development, what is being said in '2013' is first explained, then what was said in 2000, 1995, 1991, and so on are quoted. It can also be given in the ascending order.
2. **Preparation of the Final Outline:** It is the next step in writing the research report. Outline is the framework upon which work is done. It is an aid to the logical organization of the material and a reminder of the points to be stressed in the report.
3. **Preparation of the Rough Draft:** This step is of utmost importance for the researchers as it involves actually writing down what they have done in the context of their research studies. They write down the procedures adopted by them in collecting the material for their study along with various limitations, the techniques of analysis adopted by them, the broad findings and generalizations, and the various suggestions they want to offer regarding the problems encountered.
4. **Rewriting and Polishing the Rough Draft:** After writing the manuscript, it is necessary that the researcher reads through the draft to check the flow of content, language difficulties, and grammar mistakes, if any. More time and effort invested by the researcher in refining the manuscript results in the higher and the better understanding in the readers.
5. **Preparation of Final Bibliography:** Next in the order comes the task of the preparation of the final bibliography. It is a list of books, journal articles, papers presented, and so on that have contributed

or are in some way pertinent to the research currently done. The bibliography should be arranged alphabetically and may be divided into two parts; the first part may contain the names of books and journals and the second part may contain the names of magazines and newspaper articles.

6. **Writing the Final Draft:** This constitutes the last step. The final draft should be written in a concise and objective style and in simple language, avoiding vague expressions such as 'it seems' and 'there may be'. While writing the final draft, the researcher must avoid abstract terminology. It must be remembered that every report should be an attempt to solve some intellectual problem; it must contribute to the solution of a problem and must add to the knowledge of both the researcher and the reader.

Layout of a Thesis

Table 13.1 provides the layout of a thesis, indicating the purpose of each section.

TABLE 13.1 *Layout of a Thesis*

Section	Purpose
Title (Cover) page	Title of report Student name/student number Course/subject Date due
Certification of work from the guide/supervisor and principal	This is to certify that Ms/Mr X has carried out the study titled *Title of the Study*, which is the original work of the above-said person and is conducted with full honesty and compassion. Name of guide/supervisor Qualification Designation Name of principal/Head of the Department Qualification Address
Acknowledgement	It must include words of gratitude and appreciation for the people who have contributed in the compilation of the research task, including the guide, co-guide, principal or head of the department, other faculty members, ethical committee, other authorities who have facilitated the access of the data collection sources, study participants, friends, family members, and other people who have directly and indirectly facilitated the conduction of the research study.
Table of contents	It shows the various sections of the report (facilitates the reader to easily access the desired information from the research report without wasting time).
Executive summary (Abstract)	It includes the following: • Gives a summary of the whole report in one or one and a half page • Outlines the purpose, research method, findings, main conclusions, and recommendations Mainly past tense is used for writing abstracts.

TABLE 13.1 *Layout of a Thesis* (*Continued*)

Section	Purpose
Chapter I: Introduction	It outlines the following: • Context, background, and purpose • Significance or need of the study • Research problem or questions • Objectives • Hypothesis or assumptions • Scope and delimitation • Operational definitions • Conceptual framework
Chapter II: Literature review	It shows what previous researchers have explored and discovered about the phenomenon under study. Literature review should cite similar areas of study or studies that led to the current research.
Chapter III: Methodology (Materials and methods)	Provides the following • Design of the research study • Research setting • Target population • Sampling technique and sample size • Development and description of research instrumentation (include copy in appendix) • Validity and reliability of research tool(s) • Procedure and time frame of data collection (may present as an algorithm) • Pilot study • Feasibility of the study • Ethical considerations • Analysis plan (state critical alpha level and type of statistical tests expected to be used)
Chapter IV: Analysis and interpretation of data (Results or Findings)	It presents the following: • Findings of the research • Description of study sample • Analysis and interpretation of the data through descriptive and inferential statistics It uses graphic form to present data (e.g., tables and graphs).
Chapter V: Discussion	• Provides explanation of findings • Analyses results—draws together different aspects of the findings and findings of other studies and refers to literature • Presents the verdict on whether the findings support existing theories
Chapter VI: Conclusion (may be combined recommendations) ↓	It provides a brief statement of what was found.
Recommendations	It suggests suitable changes or solutions.

(*Continued*)

TABLE 13.1 *Layout of a Thesis* (*Continued*)

Section	Purpose
References	• Lists all references used • May be written in American Psychological Association (APA) or Vancouver style
Bibliography	It provides a list of all the materials that have been consulted while conducting a research study or writing an academic article, a paper, or a book based on research. References, on the other hand, are those that have been directly referred to and referenced in a research report, article, or book.
Appendix	It refers to attachments of additional information (e.g., surveys, questionnaires, and glossary).

Referencing

Referencing is a standardized way of acknowledging the sources of information and ideas that one has used in his/her assignments and allows the sources to be identified. It is important to be consistent when one is referencing.

The following are the types of referencing for various types of publications:

1. **Books: Print**

   Author/Editor (if it is an editor/editors, always insert (ed./eds) after the name)
   Title (should be in italics)
   Series title and number (if part of a series)
   Edition (if not the first edition)
   Place of publication (if there is more than one place listed, use the first named)
   Publisher
   Year of publication

   Lalitha, K., *Mental Health and Psychiatric Nursing: An Indian Perspective*, Bangalore: VMG Publications, 2011.
2. **Journal Articles: Print**

   Author
   Title of journal article
   Title of journal (should be in italics)
   Year of publication
   Volume number
   (Issue number)
   Page numbers of the article

   Usha, V. K., Lalitha, K., Social Problems of Senior Citizens, *Nightingale Nursing Times*, 2011, 7(5), 12–5, 64.
3. **Theses**

   (Final written work by PhD and postgraduate students or dissertations, project reports, discourses, and essays by any student)

Author
Title (should be in italics)
Type of thesis
Academic institution
Year of publication
Sreepriya, M., *Self Instructional Module on Care of Elderly*, M.Sc. nursing thesis, Bangalore: NIMHANS, 2009.

Vancouver Style of Reference: The Vancouver style, or uniform requirement style, is based on an American National Standards Institute (ANSI) standard adapted by the National Library of Medicine (NLM) for database such as Medline. It was developed in Vancouver in 1978 by the editors of medical journals who now meet annually as the International Committee of Medical Journal Editors (ICMJE). Over 500 medical journals, including prestigious journals such as British Medical Journal (BMJ), Canadian Medical Association Journal (CMAJ), and Journal of American Medical Association (JAMA), use this style.

Traditional Journal Articles

Before writing begins, there should be a clear idea of the journal to which a manuscript will be submitted. Journals differ in their goals, types of manuscript sought, and readership; these factors need to be matched against personal interests and preferences. All journals issue goal statements as well as guidelines for preparing and submitting a manuscript. This information is published in the journals and on their websites.

Types of Papers Sent for Journal Publication

There are different types of scientific papers. Most standard journals distribute the articles under different heads, such as Continuing Medical Education (CME)/tutorial, invited paper, review article, original article, research column, case reports, and communications. The order and nomenclature vary from journal to journal.

1. **Case Report:** The simplest type of paper of any author is a case report. When one encounters an unusual case, whether in presentation, diagnostic difficulty, or histopathology, the full details should be noted down and all relevant details should be documented. The paper should contain a couple of relevant photographs such as clinical picture, operative picture, and histopathology slide authentication. A literature survey should be done to see how frequently such cases have been reported. The report of the case with a short discussion on the importance of the case will make the paper complete. A few relevant references should be incorporated.
2. **Original Article:** Original article is based on at least four or more cases. A scientific study case can be a case control or case series (retrospective) study or a cohort (prospective) study. The article is usually written under the following headings:
   (a) Introduction—why the paper is presented on the particular subject and what are the lacunae in the existing knowledge
   (b) Materials and methods used, including the details of methodology utilized
   (c) Observations—depicted in texts, graphs, or figure tables
   (d) Discussion
   (e) Conclusion
   (f) Bibliography

3. **Review Article/Meta-analysis:** Even if one finds that there is nothing to publish in original, there is still a chance for publishing. It is possible to publish papers such as a review article or meta-analysis. In a review article, one reviews the data presented by different authors. If one scans around twenty articles on a particular subject and organizes all the observations of the different authors, discusses the issue at length, and explains the various opinions expressed in the articles reviewed, it forms a review article. In meta-analysis, one makes statistical comparison of data presented by different authors and comes to his/her own conclusions.
4. **Research Article:** There is not much difference between an original article and a research article in the case of clinical study. However, a research article can also be a purely experimental work, and hence is called an analytical study. After identifying a suitable topic, the work is performed and then a paper is written. A scientific paper should ideally consider statistical aspects, namely randomization of cases, matching controls, and blinding.
5. **Tutorial/CME:** These papers are usually written by experts in the concerned subject. Even though it is ideal to write such articles in the prescribed format of original articles, it may be acceptable to have a pattern of unformatted material as in a descriptive study, which is superficial, giving expert opinion about a particular problem based on the author's experience.

Writing the Manuscript for Journal Publication

Prior to writing the manuscript, query letters must be sent to several journals at the same time to gauge the appropriateness of one's matter for the journal. The preparation of an article for a journal is a service to the profession as well as a means of obtaining recognition for the author or authors.

Writing manuscript requires *willingness* to share the research findings. Oral and written communication skills are also necessary. The researcher has to get trained in writing a research report to the journals for publication. Repeatedly venturing to write makes the researcher to gain skill and confidence. It is very rewarding to a researcher to see his/her write-up getting published in the scientific journals. The happiness that the researcher gets becomes the motivating factor for further writing.

To write a manuscript, some people prefer creative writing whereas others prefer mind mapping. Mind mapping technique may be productive, but while creating a document, structured creative writing methods may be used. The momentum of writing can be started by imagining oneself writing a letter or an email to a friend. The researcher should think of what he/she would say to a friend about the activity and describe the problem that is being encountered.

Narrating the story to someone is often easier than writing the manuscript; so, the researcher should start by writing what he/she would tell his friend and start working from there. It is possible to develop one's writing skills by following a few steps:

1. Thinking aloud about the content that is to be sent for publication
2. Speaking out the content as if describing the content to a group of students in the classroom
3. Putting it in writing as the flow of thought continues
4. Reading the draft and checking for language clarity, content adequacy, and sentence construction
5. Repeating the readings until the writer is confident of having communicated clearly what he/she wanted to say

The Beginning Exercise: Every budding author should decide when and where to start writing a paper. The earlier the process is started, the better. One must have something worthwhile to say in the paper and it must be said well. Before commencing on writing the paper, one must have a work done to write about. The topic should be in a scientific area of interest and relevant in the modern context.

1. **Subject of the Paper:** There are two ways of writing a paper. One is to write on a subject in which original work has been done. The postgraduate thesis is an example of this situation, where the work is done and the findings have to be presented in the form of a paper. The second is to write a paper for a journal on invitation or after investigation. This may end up as a review article or a retrospective study based on already available data.

   The purpose of writing a paper is either to present to the scientific world something new an author has identified in his/her work or experience or to convey to the community modifications in existing knowledge, which has risen out of the experience of the author.

   There is, however, nothing called total originality in any work. The term *research* clearly conveys that it is re-searching. This means one is redoing something that someone else has already done. In the process, one comes across new findings not reported earlier. A thesis is 20 per cent originality and 80 per cent chaff, which is reproducing knowledge already existing in literature.
2. **Organization of Work:** Whatever the type of work, a research paper should be written in the actual format incorporating basic headings. Journal guidelines may vary but the usual pattern would include the abstract, key words, introduction (why did you start?), methods (what did you do?), research terminologies such as aims and objectives, research question, null hypothesis, alternate hypothesis, study design, results or observations, discussion, and conclusion. The paper should be planned before starting to write. A mental outline should be ready on what is going to be presented. The abstract highlights the key points and is presented separately.
3. **Presentation of the Paper:** Presentation of the paper includes giving an appropriate title, proper headings and subheadings, and presentation of the data under the different subheads.
   (a) **Title:** The title of the paper can be given in different ways from being very short to very elaborate and descriptive, depending on personal preferences. Ideally, the title should be as short as possible, preferably less than ten words, but exhibiting the full nature of the subject presented. It should be able to attract the attention of the reader. The title should express the subject of the paper but never the conclusion.

   (b) **First Draft:** The first draft is the most difficult step in the entire writing process. It should be written freely as the thought flows, continuously and unhurriedly in a quiet atmosphere, without bothering about the order of the subheadings. The initial writing should not concentrate on language, grammar, or spellings. Language and grammar should not be barriers to writing a paper. The primary author should transform any idea that comes to his/her mind to words and jot down every point on paper. It is always better to write down these points in a book rather than on sheets of paper to ensure the safety of the matter. The written matter may be unorganized, which can be organized later.

   (c) **Subsequent Versions:** Revising and polishing are undertaken in the subsequent versions. Many revisions, sometimes up to eight times, may be needed. The sentences undergo reorganization and reorientation. Language and grammar creep into the writing. In scientific writing, the sentences should be short and crisp. Simple common words should be used in short simple sentences, avoiding repetition. It is also essential to keep the writing interesting. Lengthy sentences will confuse the reader. In each revision, the sentences should be improved to make the text simple and understandable. Monotonous duplications such as 'It was observed that' should be avoided. Continuity of the message will make the paper readable.

   Each paragraph should correspond to one message. The first sentence should be the topic sentence. This is followed by the details of that topic alone and not any other topic. Too long paragraphs are not very palatable to the reader. The concluding sentence of the paragraph should bring out the final idea clearly.

The style of writing improves with practice. The paper should be concise, clear, direct, and unambiguous. Support of language experts could be obtained before submission of the manuscript. When one is writing fast, doubts may arise. All doubts should be marked immediately and could be clarified later. The important point is to keep up the flow and momentum of one's thoughts. The numerous corrections will take care of refining the text and adding details.

(d) **Order of Presentation:** Every paper should follow a simple pattern of introduction, materials and methods, observations, discussion, conclusion, and references.

Introduction should clearly state the objectives, project the importance of the work, and suggest what is new in the paper.

Materials and methods should detail the research methodology clearly in full and the statistical methods used to validate the results. Sufficient details should be given for any reader to duplicate the work on a scientific basis. It should state the trial design, for example, randomized controlled trial, case series, and blinding, and describe the study population and sample.

Results should be presented to show how the hypotheses have been proved. The findings should be detailed in text and expressed in graphs and tables with appropriate legend. All methods should be mentioned in the methods section and all should have been statistically analysed.

Discussion should answer the objectives stated in the introduction and explain the results. It should describe how the findings of the present study differ from the works of other authors in the past. It should explain any limitations in the methods and highlight unexpected results.

Conclusion should briefly state the final opinion of the authors based on the study.

Abstract should be written last. It should state the purpose of the research, methods used, important results, and conclusions. The abstract should be written in the IMRAD format.

References must be in appropriate format specific for the journal.

(e) **Subheadings:** The subheadings are to be given in a set pattern. Readability is the crux of the issue. From the reader's point of view, there are two types of approaches. One is to scan a journal to find out if there is anything interesting to procure new knowledge. The other is for the person interested to go into the complete details of the paper since he/she is making a similar study. To suit both types of readers, the presentation of the paper must be made in such a way that the main idea is easily absorbed by the casual reader as well as those who are keen on details. This is achieved by giving appropriate headings and subheadings.

There are definite rules for the order of subheadings. All subheadings must be kept in boldface. There are six types of subheadings.

First-order subheading is the primary heading. It should be given in all capital letters, left aligned, with two spaces above and one space below. The usual presentation is made under the following first-order headings: Introduction, methods and materials, observations, discussion, and conclusion.

The second-order subheading is for topics that come under the particular first-order heading. This will be in capital and small letters, the first letter in capital and the rest in small. This will be left aligned and bold, having one space above and below. For example, 'Observations' is the first-order subheading, under which the second-order subheadings could be clinical features, investigations, and treatment.

Third-order subheading is the further detailing of the second-order subheading. The text continues on the same line using capital and small letters giving one space above. For example, if 'Clinical features' is the second-order subheading, symptoms and signs can be the third-order subheadings.

Fourth-order subheading may be added with left indent. Fifth-order subheading may be added with left and right indents. Sixth-order subheading is similar to fifth order but set in *italics.*

(f) **Presentation of the Data:** Data can be represented in the form of tables and graphs. Tables show frequency distribution. The graphs commonly used are of the following types:

(i) Frequency polygon
(ii) Dot plots
(iii) Line diagram
(iv) Bar diagram
(v) Pie diagram
(vi) Histogram
(vii) Relative frequency polygon
(viii) Scatter diagram
(ix) Regression line

(g) **Statistics:** Basic inferential statistics should ideally be included in any scientific paper. The services of a statistician can be availed of. Simple statistical tests such as t-test, Z-test, and chi-square tests can be used.

(h) **Conclusion:** All articles should end with a short conclusion, which the author has arrived at after performing the study.

(i) **Writing References:** The references quoted in the text should be listed and those not quoted need not be given in the list of references. Reference can be quoted by either giving the author's name and the year in brackets or giving the number in superscript. If there are two authors, the names of both authors (in the same order as in the original publication) should be mentioned; if there are more than two authors, et al. should be mentioned after the first author's name. Listing references should follow editorial policies.

References may be written in Vancouver, Campbell, or APA style. There are software programs to facilitate the preparation of reference lists.

(j) **Revisions:** The first draft always changes contour in the final version. The sentences should be repeatedly read and improved. The manuscript should be read by a colleague, as authors tend to overlook their own mistakes.

(k) **Finalization:** As the manuscript reaches the final stages, the following points should be verified:

(i) **Content:** Whether the matter deviates from the title of the paper
(ii) **Order:** Whether there is overlapping of matter under the different subheadings
(iii) **Clarity:** Whether the message is clearly pronounced for the reader to understand
(iv) **Paragraph:** Whether each idea represents a single collective message
(v) **Observation:** Whether all the findings are properly described in tables or in graphic form
(vi) **Discussion:** Whether the literature survey is complete and discussed in relation to the findings of the present study
(vii) **References:** Whether they are complete, names are not misspelled, abbreviations are put according to accepted norms, and patterns are followed according to the guidelines of the journal

If the author uses an abbreviation in the paper, the expansion should be given in the first instance and then the abbreviation can be used throughout. The final paper should give only one interpretation to the reader, which should be absorbed in the first reading itself. The final paper must be flawless and attractive, following the style of the journal to which it is sent. The first page should have the title, names of authors, affiliations, corresponding authors, addresses and email ids, abstract in about 200 words, and about 10 key words. This is followed by the main paper, acknowledgements, and disclaimers. The author should refer the journal's 'instruction to the authors' before sending the paper.

General Information for Writing a Paper

1. Write clearly. Articles must be written at a level that is appropriate for the audience. Active voice must be used, as it is clearer and more concise than the passive voice. The article should be written using the first person.
2. Write succinctly. While writing, the use of verbs instead of abstract nouns should be encouraged. Strong verbs should be used instead of 'to be'. Short sentences with concise terms should be used.
3. A sentence of more than 40 words should be written as two sentences.
4. Grammar, spelling, and punctuation should be carefully checked. The spellchecker should be used cautiously.
5. Unnecessary commas should be avoided.
6. Proof reading must be done carefully to see if any words are left out.
7. Arial or Times New Roman is the font currently in preference.
8. The size of the font should be maintained at 11 or 12 points with spacing of 1.5 in between the lines.
9. The number of lines per page should be restricted to 25–30 per page consisting of 400–450 words.
10. Good quality paper such as executive bond or copier paper is the expected material to be used.
11. The margins for the page should be of the following dimensions: Left 1.5", right 1", top 1", and bottom 1".
12. Continuous pagination should be maintained.

Rejection of a Paper

Rejection of a paper may lead to disastrous depression. One should not get disheartened with a single rejection. The paper should be rewritten, taking into consideration the critiques mentioned by the reviewer for rejection. A time frame should be made and must be kept to. There could be several reasons for rejection, which are enumerated as follows:

1. Poorly written article
2. Incomprehensive content
3. Inaccurate content
4. Inappropriate content for the particular journal
5. Publication of a similar article in the recent past
6. Poorly developed idea
7. Written in term paper style
8. Problems in the applied methodology
9. Unimportant content

10. Clinically not applicable
11. Problems in statistical application
12. Data interpretation problems

The editor makes specific suggestions to modify and resubmit or to submit to another journal.

Misconduct in Research Communication

In the process of communicating research, an investigator may get involved in practices such as fabrication, falsification, or plagiarisms, which needs to be avoided. Table 13.2 lists the various types of scientific misconduct along with their description.

TABLE 13.2 *Misconduct in Research Communication*

Types of Scientific Misconduct	Description
1. Fabrication	Making up data or results
2. Falsification	Manipulating research by changing or omitting data
3. Plagiarism	Stealing intellectual property or taking credit for another individual's work
3.1. Plagiarism of ideas	Using another person's ideas without giving appropriate credit
3.2. Plagiarism of text	Using another person's words without giving appropriate credit
3.2.1. Without citing the source—verbatim copying	Using the text or any materials of another person without acknowledging the source
3.2.2. Paraplagiarism	Using the text of others with a few changes or mixing the texts without acknowledging the sources
3.2.3. With citing the source—verbatim copying	Using the text of others with citing the origin without using quotation marks
3.2.4. Inappropriate paraphrasing	Using the text of others with paraphrasing but with only minor changes in the words or structure
4. Copyright infringement	Using a large part of others words (in quotation marks) that violates copyright
5. Self-plagiarism	
5.1. Duplication publication	Publication of paper or results in more than one journal
5.2. Salami publication	Publication of each part of the results of one study in several papers
5.3. Practice of text recycling	Using one's own text in several different papers as the copyright is reserved

Although writing an article appears to be highly taxing, it is definitely worth the efforts. Placing too many restrictions and insisting perfectionism in the style of writing may make the neophytes to keep themselves away from writing journal article. Repeatedly reading journal articles and making many attempts to write articles mat help to improve the skill in writing. Writing articles for journals is a skill, which needs to be mastered with sheer practice and determination.

Electronic Publication

Computers and the Internet have changed forever the way information of all types is retrieved and disseminated. Many nurse researchers are exploring opportunities to share their research findings through electronic publication. Most journals that publish in hard copy format (e.g., Nursing Research) now also have online capabilities. Such mechanisms, which serve as a document delivery system, expand a journal's circulation and make research findings accessible worldwide. There are few implications for authors, however; such electronic publication is just a method of distributing reports already available in hard copy and are subject to the journal's standard page limitations, peer review process, and so on.

There are, however, many other ways to disseminate research findings on the Internet. For example, some researchers or research teams develop their own web page with information about their studies. When there are hyperlinks embedded in the websites, consumers can navigate between files and websites to retrieve relevant information on a topic of interest. At the other extreme are peer-reviewed electronic journals (e-journals) that are exclusively in online format. Electronic publication offers numerous advantages. Dissemination can occur much more rapidly, cutting down dramatically on publication lag time. Electronic research reports are accessible to a broad, worldwide audience of potential consumers. Typically, there are no page limitations, enabling researchers to describe and discuss complex studies more fully. Qualitative researchers are able to use more extensive quotes from their raw data, for example. Research reports on the Internet can incorporate a wide variety of graphic material, including audio and video supplements not possible in hard copy journals. Raw data can also be appended to reports on the Internet for secondary analysis by other researchers. Still, there are some potential drawbacks, including technological requirements. One issue concerns peer review. Although many online journals perform peer reviews, there are many opportunities to 'publish' results on the Internet without a peer-review process. There are also non–peer-reviewed traditional journals. However, non-reviewed journal articles are not as accessible to a worldwide market as non-reviewed information on the Internet. There is a much greater risk of there being a glut of low-quality research available for consumption as a result of the Internet than there was previously. Responsible researchers who want their evidence to have an impact on nursing practice should seek publication in outlets that subject manuscripts to a review process.

Communication of research findings is the last formal step in the research process, but it is the most important phase of research—the utilization of research findings.

Several problems may be encountered by a beginner. Some of the challenges faced by a novice writer may be hesitation to start and lack of technical assistance. The suggested solutions to these problems are to keep the mind fresh before commencing on the task, to keep distractions and disturbances at bay, and to initiate the scientific thought process.

KEY POINTS

- Research results can be communicated either through oral presentation or by writing them as research reports, or sometimes through both means.
- Oral presentations are made in conferences, clinical meetings, research classes and committees, and in journal clubs.
- Written reports are published in professional journals, textbooks, monographs, theses and dissertations, newsletters, and electronic media.
- While preparing oral presentations and written reports, follow the guidelines or instructions given by the agency through whom you are trying to communicate research results.

- Use Vancouver style of writing references or follow uniform requirement style as prescribed by the agency.
- Be aware that there are different types of papers sent for journal publication, such as case report, original article, review article or meta-analysis, research articles, and tutorial or CME materials.
- Follow the steps of writing manuscript for journal publication and include specified contents.
- Do not get disheartened with a rejection of a paper to get it published in the journal. Instead rewrite the articles taking into consideration the critique mentioned by the reviewer for rejection.
- Avoid all types of scientific misconduct in research communication.
- Remember communication of research findings is the most important phase in the utilization of research findings.

QUESTIONS

I. Essay-type Questions

1. Discuss the various strategies adopted for communicating research results.
2. Explain in detail the conventional format followed in communicating the study material.
3. Describe the steps in writing a research report.
4. Illustrate the layout of a research report with suitable examples.
5. How do you write the manuscript of a research work for publication in a scientific journal?

II. Short Notes

1. Kinds of research report
2. Referencing style in research report
3. Types of papers sent for journal publication
4. General principles for writing a scientific paper
5. Reasons for rejecting publication in a paper

III. Multiple-choice Questions

Circle the alphabet before the best answer

1. The most convenient method of reporting research report is through
   (a) electronic data base
   (b) research publication in books
   (c) journal articles
   (d) oral presentation in a conference
2. A quantitative research report usually includes
   (a) research problem, objective, literature, and data analysis
   (b) introduction, method, results, and discussion
   (c) research problem, objective, conceptual model, and methodology
   (d) research plan, data plan, and analysis
3. APA format of typing (referencing) refers to
   (a) American Psychological Association
   (b) as per alphabetical order
   (c) as per administration
   (d) as per advise

4. Misconduct in research communication includes the following, except
   (a) fabrication
   (b) plagiarism
   (c) falsification
   (d) unimportant content

5. One of the requirements for the presentation of research report in a professional conference is
   (a) reference sources
   (b) photograph of the presenter
   (c) abstract of the research work
   (d) contract agreement

Answer Keys

1. (c) 2. (b) 3. (a) 4. (d) 5. (c)

FURTHER READING

Brender, A. E. 1997. 'How to Write a Scientific Paper', *The Journal for the Royal Society for the Promotion of Social Health*, 117(1): 17–19.

Crisp, J., Chick, N., Roders, J., et al. 1996. 'Publishing Workshops. Number 2. Preparing a Manuscript Reporting Quantitative Research Findings', *Nursing Praxis*, 11(2): 31–35.

Habermann, B., Broome, M., Pryor, E. R. 2010. 'Research Coordinators' Experiences with Scientific Misconduct and Research Integrity', *Nursing Research*, 59(1): 51–57.

Huth, E. J. 1990. *How to Write and Publish Papers in the Medical Sciences*. Second edition. Baltimore: Williams and Wilkins.

King, C. R. 2001. 'Ethical Issues in Writing and Publishing', *Clinical Journal of Oncology Nursing*, 5(3): 19–23.

Polit, Dense, F., Hungler, Bernadette, P. 2008. *Nursing Research, Principles and Methods*. Sixth edition, Philadelphia: Lippincott Williams and Wilkins.

Reumann, M. *Survival skills for scientific writing in the academic and professional environments*. Q & A from IEEE Webinars. Taken from www.ieee.org/documents/51764_postscripts.pdf.

Rudy, Ellen B. 2000. 'Auditing Research Studies', *Nursing Research*, 49(2): 117–120.

Sharma, Suresh K. 2011. *Nursing Research and Statistics*. New Delhi: Elsevier Publication.

Sidhu, Kulbir Singh. 1990. *Methodology of Research in Education*. First edition. New Delhi Sterling Publishers' Pvt. Ltd.

Wilson, H. S., Hutchinson S. A. 1997. 'Presenting Qualitative Research Up close: Visual Literacy in Poster Sessions'. In J. M. Morse (ed.), *Completing a Qualitative Project*. Thousand Oaks, California: Sage, pp. 63–85.

chapter 14

Research Utilization and Evidence-based Nursing Practice

OBJECTIVES

Upon completion of this chapter the learner will be able to:

- Discuss the concept of research utilization and evidence-based practice
- List the elements of research utilization
- Explain about research utilization continuum
- Describe Rogers' diffusion of innovation theory
- Discuss research utilization in nursing practice
- Explain about evidence-based practice movement
- List the types of evidence and their hierarchies
- Explain the levels of evidence hierarchy
- Enumerate the barriers to research utilization
- Discuss the process of using research in nursing practice
- Explain different phases of research utilization to facilitate evidence-based practice

INTRODUCTION

Research utilization (RU) refers to the use scientifically produced knowledge and investigation and the application of the findings to clinical practice unrelated to original research, whereas *evidence-based practice* (EBP) represents a broader concept. When clinicians use the EBP approach, they go beyond the expertise of clinicians and researchers and consider the patient's preferences and values to guide patient care.

Research utilization is a process of communicating and using research-generated knowledge to make an impact on or a change in the existing practices in health care system.

ELEMENTS OF RESEARCH UTILIZATION (RU)

The main elements of the RU process are as follows:

1. Summarizing knowledge generated through research (new idea, practice, or procedure)
2. Communicating the research knowledge to nurses, other health care professionals, policy makers, and consumers of health care
3. Achieving desired outcomes for patients, nurses, and health care agencies

Summarizing Research Knowledge

Empirical knowledge is generated by conducting quality studies, and several studies on a topic are conducted. Cognitive clustering is accomplished through integrative reviews and meta-analyses of nursing research. Integrative reviews of research are conducted to identify, analyse, and synthesize the results from independent studies to determine the current knowledge of a particular topic. These reviews are published in a variety of research and clinical journals and in the annual review of nursing research.

Using meta-analysis, we can determine the following:

1. Overall significance of pooled data from several studies
2. Average effect size, indicating the degree to which the null hypothesis is false or the degree to which the phenomenon is present in the population
3. Relationship among variables studied

Meta-analysis provides an objective rather than a subjective approach in evaluating research accuracy and the usefulness of findings for practice as well as assists in summarizing the research findings. The new intervention must be communicated in a clear and concise manner, which will promote its use by practising nurses.

Communicating Research Knowledge

The RU process involves communicating the study findings from investigators to practising nurses. Communication of research findings includes developing a research report and disseminating that report through presentations and publications to audiences of nurses, health care professionals, policy makers, and health care consumers. Dissemination of research findings can happen from one person to another or from one person to a group of persons by the use of mass media such as journals, books, newspapers, and television.

Achieving Desired Outcomes in Health Care System

The desired outcomes of RU are improving nursing care, promoting positive patient and family outcomes, and providing cost-effective services in health care systems. RU is one of the unique problems in nursing. It is difficult to promote changes based on research. RU occurs within a specific social system. A social system is a set of inter-related individuals or units who are engaged in joint problem-solving to accomplish a common goal.

Rogers studied the process for using research findings in society and formulated a theory for communicating innovations and new ideas developed through research.

RESEARCH UTILIZATION AND EVIDENCE-BASED PRACTICE (EBP)

The terms RU and EBP are sometimes used synonymously. Although there is an overlap between the two concepts, in fact they are different.

Research utilization is the use of study findings in a practical application unrelated to the original research. The research conducted by nurses can potentially play a pivotal role in improving the quality of nursing care, the efficiency with which it is delivered, and the process by which the care is delivered. In contrast, *EBP* involves making clinical decisions on the basis of the best possible evidence (research) and uses information from clinical experiences, patient preference, and other sources.

RESEARCH UTILIZATION CONTINUUM

It is from the starting point of research on the emergence of new knowledge, ideas and utilization of research. The utilization of research finding in the continuum should be discrete and clearly attempts to specific action and put at one end of continuum.

In the 1960s and 1970s, a series of studies demonstrated the optional placement time of a glass thermometer for accurate oral temperature determination to be nine minutes. The specific alteration of behaviour by nurses from shorter placement time to the research-based recommendation of nine minutes is an example of RU at this end of continuum. This type of RU is known as *instrumental utilization*.

However, the research findings can be used in a more diffuse manner, in a way that promotes cumulative awareness, understanding, or enlightenment. This end of the utilization continuum is referred to as *conceptual utilization*. It refers to situations in which the users are influenced in their thinking about an issue based on their knowledge of studies but do not put this knowledge to any specific documentable use.

The *middle ground* of this continuum involves the partial impact of research findings on nursing activities. This is frequently the result of a slow evolutionary process that does not reflect a conscious decision to use an innovative procedure but rather reflects knowledge creep and decision accretion, in which the momentum for a decision builds over time based on accumulated information gained through readings, informal discussions, meetings, and so on. However, nurses are making conscious decisions to use research in their clinical practice, and the EBP movement has contributed to this change.

TYPES OF RESEARCH UTILIZATION

Estabrooks studied RU by collecting survey data from 600 nurses in Canada and found evidence to support three types of RU:

1. *Indirect research utilization*, involving changes in nurses' thinking and, therefore, analogous to conceptual utilization
2. *Direct research utilization*, involving the direct use of findings in giving patient care and, therefore, analogous to instrumental utilization
3. *Persuasive research utilization*, involving the use of findings to persuade others (decisions-makers) to make changes in policies or practices relevant to nursing care

RESEARCH UTILIZATION IN QUALITATIVE RESEARCH

Estabrooks argues that the process of implementing research findings into practice is essentially the same for both quantitative and qualitative research. However, the difference is that qualitative findings are presented in narrative form and hence this type of research may have a privileged position in RU. Clinicians do not need a strong background in statistics to understand qualitative research. It is not necessary to translate the results into everyday language before the findings can be used conceptually.

Several theorists have developed models on how knowledge can be disseminated and used.

Rogers' Diffusion of Innovations Theory Model

According to Roger, knowledge diffusion is an evolutionary process by which an innovation or new idea is communicated over time to members of a social system. The key elements of the process that influence the adoption of innovation are as follows:

1. *Innovation* is the new idea, practice, or procedure that, if adopted, will result in a change, which affects decisions and adoption.
2. *Communication channels* are the media through which information about the innovation is transmitted, for example, journals, mass media, the Internet, and face to face.
3. *Time* is an important component of the process. Knowledge diffusion occurs over a period of time from the creation of knowledge to dissemination.
4. *Social system* is the set of inter-related units that solve problems to accomplish a common goal. The diffusion occurs within a social system and it depends on the norms and receptivity to innovations.

Stages in the Innovation Adoption Process

There are five stages in the innovation adoption process:

1. **Knowledge Stage:** Individuals or groups become aware of innovation.
2. **Persuasion Stage:** They form a positive attitude towards the innovation.
3. **Decision Stage:** A choice is made about whether to adopt or reject the innovation.
4. **Implementation Stage:** The innovation is actually put into use.
5. **Confirmation Stage:** The effectiveness of the innovation is evaluated and decisions are made about the continuation or discontinuation of the innovation.

Some of the stages can be skipped sometimes, but in general, the model has been a useful way of thinking about the RU process in nursing.

Research Utilization in Nursing Practice

Based on some studies conducted in the 1980s and 1990s, it was found that nurses were not always aware of research results, and therefore, they did not incorporate research findings in their practice. It was felt that nurses failed to use research findings as a basis for making decisions and for developing nursing interventions.

Coyle and Sokop investigated practising nurses' adoption of 14 nursing innovations that had been reported in nursing literature, replicating a study by Brett. The 14 studies were selected based on scientific merits of the studies, the significance of practice, and the suitability for practice. A sample of 113 nurses practising in 10 hospitals was taken (randomly in North Carolina) and the nurses' awareness and use of study findings were measured. The results indicated that awareness ranged from 34 per cent to 94 per cent.

Based on Roger's theory, awareness and persuasion occasionally used in practice and regularly used in practice were assessed. Out of the fourteen studies, only one study was at regular use of adoption, whereas six studies were in the persuasion stage, that is, the nurses knew the innovation and thought it should be practised but were not able to take decisions on it.

This shows that there is a need to reduce the gap between nursing practice and RU.

Steps in Research Utilization

The following are the steps in the RU process:

1. Identification and synthesis of multiple studies on a selected topic
2. Organization of research knowledge into a solution or clinical practice
3. Transformation of clinical practice into specific nursing actions (innovations) that are used for patients
4. Clinical evaluation of the new practice to determine whether it has produced the desired outcome

It has been observed that RU by practising nurses is feasible, but only if the research is relevant to practice and the results are broadly disseminated. Projects can be taken up at the institutional level to implement a change in nursing practice on the basis of research findings.

During the 1990s, RU began to be superseded by EBP.

EVIDENCE-BASED PRACTICE

It begins with a search for information on how best to solve a practice problem. EBP tries to provide solutions to sustain high health care quality in a cost-constrained environment. The EBP movement has shifted to a broader concept of using the best evidence for health care education and practice.

In EBP, the findings from rigorous research are considered the best possible sources of information. One of the basic features of EBP is that it de-emphasizes decision-making based on customs, authority, opinion, or ritual and integrates it with clinical expertise, patient input, and existing resources rather than the best available research evidence alone.

The EBP movement has given rise to debates on caution and balanced approach to health care quality in the current cost-constrained environment. A rational approach is needed to provide the best possible care to most people with cost-effective use of resources.

Overview of Evidence-based Practice Movement

Cochrane Collaboration

The EBP movement was founded in the United Kingdom based on the work of the British epidemiologist Archie Cochrane. Cochrane published an influential book in the early 1970s that drew attention to the dearth of solid evidence about the effects of health care. He called for efforts to make research summaries of the results of clinical trials available to health care decision-makers. This eventually led to the development of the Cochrane Center in Oxford in 1992, and an international collaboration called the Cochrane Collaboration, with centres now established in 15 locations throughout the world. The aim of the collaboration is to help people make good decisions about health care by preparing, maintaining, and disseminating systematic reviews of the effects of health care interventions.

At the same time, a group from McMaster Medical School in Canada developed a clinical learning strategy called *evidence-based medicine*. Dr David Sackett, the pioneer of evidence-based medicine at McMaster, who later moved to Oxford in England to promote EBP, defined evidence-based medicine as the conscientious, explicit, and judicious use of current best evidence in making decisions about the care of individual patients. The practice of evidence-based medicine means integrating individual clinical expertise with the best available external evidence from systematic research.

The evidence-based medicine movement was shifted over time to a broader conception of using best evidence by all health care practitioners and not just physicians in a multi-disciplinary team. EBP has been considered as a major paradigm shift for health care education and practice.

Critics say that the advantages of EBP are exaggerated, and individual clinical judgments and patient inputs are being devalued. However, EBP path is the one that health care professions will follow in the twenty-first century (Fig. 14.1).

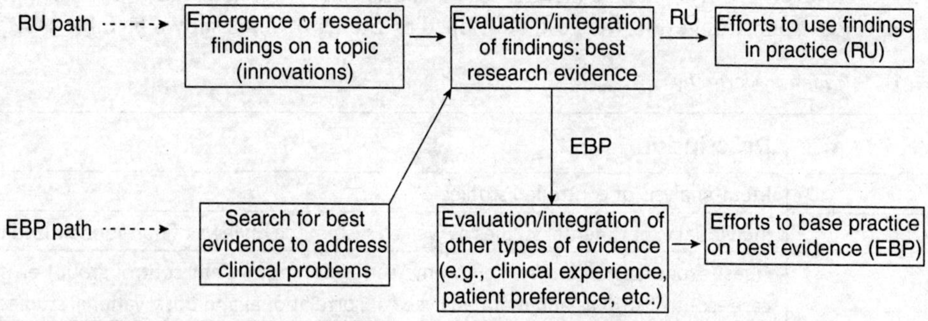

FIGURE 14.1 *Research Utilization and Evidence-based Practice (Research Results)*

Types of Evidence and Evidence Hierarchies

There is general agreement that the evidence for EBP is the findings from rigorous studies. In the initial phase of the EBP movement, there was a definite bias towards reliance on information from a randomized clinical trial (RCT). For example, the focus of Cochrane Collaboration was on evidence about interventions rather than about other aspects of the health care practices. This led to some resistance to EBP by nurses who felt that the evidence from qualitative and non-RCT studies not be ignored. Therefore the useful evidence has loosen its strength, but there have been efforts to develop an evidence hierarchy that ranks studies according to the strength of the evidence they provide (Fig. 14.2).

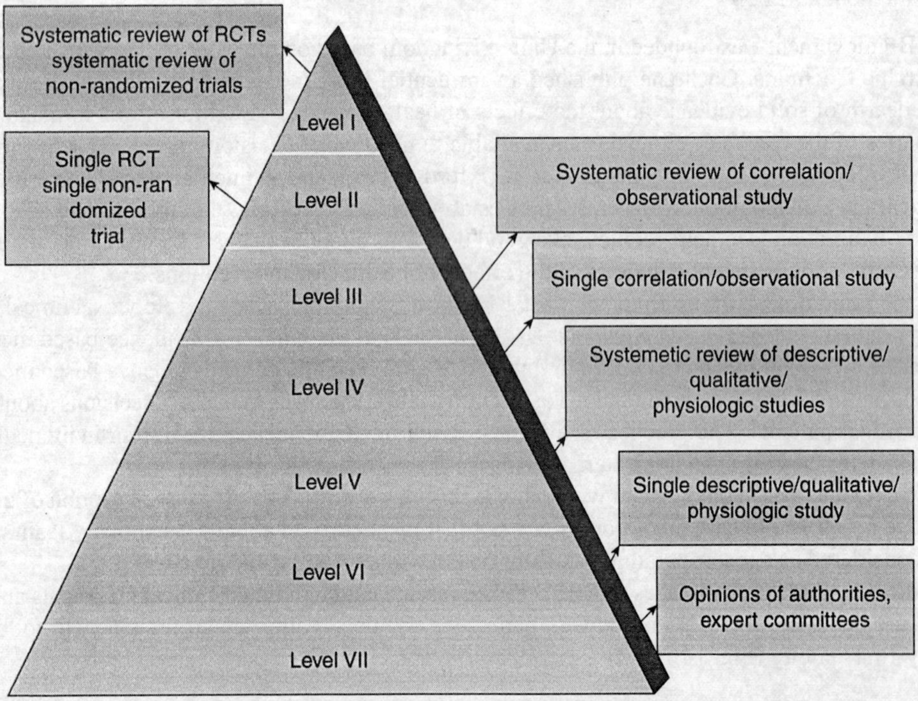

FIGURE 14.2 *Hierarchy of Evidence-based Practice*

A seven-level (levels I–VII) evidence hierarchy that also assigns grades on study quality within each of the seven levels from strongest to weakest, developed by Stetler et al., is shown in Table 14.1:

TABLE 14.1 *Evidence Hierarchy*

Level	Description
I.	Meta-analysis of controlled studies
II.	Individual experimental studies as well as systematic reviews of non-randomized trials
III.	Quasi-experimental studies (e.g., time-series non-equivalent control group) or matched case–control studies and meta-analyses of correlational and observational studies

(*Continued*)

TABLE 14.1 (*Continued*)

Level	Description
IV.	Single correlational or observational study
V.	Systemic reviews of descriptive qualitative or physiological studies, program evaluations, RU studies, quality improvement projects, and case reports
VI.	Single descriptive qualitative study
VII.	Opinions of respected authorities and expert committees

Till date, there have been relatively few published studies of RCTs (levels I and II) in nursing and even fewer published meta-analyses of RCT nursing studies. Moreover, the evidence hierarchies are applied only certain types of questions such as questions about effectiveness of interventions.

There are many important clinical questions that can best be answered by descriptive and qualitative data from level IV and V studies. Moreover, there are very few research data available on clinical practice questions. In such situations, EBP will have to draw from other sources. Thereby, Goode gives us another EBP model developed at the University of Colorado Hospital, which includes nine non-research sources of evidence that can be used as a supplement of the core. They are as follows:

1. Bench marking
2. Cost-effectiveness analysis
3. Patho-physiological data
4. Retrospective or concurrent chart review
5. Quality improvement
6. Risk data—national and international
7. Local standards
8. Institutional data collected for infection-control purposes
9. Patient preference and clinical expertise

Thus, although EBP comprises RU of both research and non-research sources of information, nurses should be able to locate, evaluate, and integrate evidence with clinical judgment and patient preference to find out the most effective solutions to health problems. An important feature of EBP is that it may not necessarily imply practice changes. The best evidence may confirm that the existing practices are effective and also cost effective.

BARRIERS TO RESEARCH UTILIZATION

The knowledge of barriers to RU and EBP in nursing is useful to plan and implement the efforts to integrate nursing research in practice.

Research-related Barriers

1. Many nursing problems do not have a solved base of valid and trustworthy study results. Most of the studies have flaws. We need to have a perfect study, basing clinical decisions on research findings.
2. Replication of research methods is limited. Repeated efforts to a research question in different settings giving similar results lead to greater confidence in the findings.
3. Research reports are sometimes inaccessible to practising nurses.

Tips to Deal with Research-related Barriers

1. **Collaborate with Clinicians:** If research questions are more clinical based, practising nurses will be able to use them efficiently.
2. **Do High-quality Research:** The quality of nursing studies has improved dramatically in the last two decades; however, we still need to ensure valid research findings.
3. **Replicate:** The research studies should be replicated repeatedly and the results should be published, so that there is a justified base to use the research results.
4. **Communicate Clearly:** Research reports should be written in a user-friendly manner.
5. **Present Findings Amenable to Meta-analysis:** An integrative review of research findings is essential for EBP.
6. **Suggest Clinical Implications:** If the suggestions for clinical practice become a standard feature of research reports, then the burden of using research evidence would be lighter for nurse clinicians.
7. **Disseminate Aggressively:** If the researchers fail to communicate the results of a study to other nurses, it is obvious that the results will never be used by practising nurses.
8. **Disseminate Broadly:** It is important from the utilization point for researchers to report their results in journals such as Journal of NRSI, NJI, IJNS, and other such journals that are read by practising nurses. Moreover, efforts should be taken to disseminate the study findings at conferences and workshops attended by nurse practitioners.
9. **Prepare Integrative Research Reviews:** There is an urgent need for high-quality integrative reviews of research. Such reviews are of help to practising nurses who do not have time to review literature or may find it difficult to evaluate individual studies. Integrative reviews are a core feature of the EBP process.

Nurse-related Barriers

1. The nurses' educational preparation and their research skills are not enough for them to judge the merits of a research study.
2. Nurses' negative attitude towards research and their poor motivation to engage in EBP are also potential barriers. Studies have found that the more positive the attitude of the nurses, the more likely they are to use the research in practice.
3. Another characteristic, which is common to most humans, is that people often are resistant to change, because change requires efforts in retraining and restructuring of work habits.
4. Change may be perceived as affecting job security, and hence, there may be opposition to a new practice.

However, in a survey of more than 1200 nurses, it was found that nurses value nursing research and they want to be involved in research-related activities.

Tips or Strategies for Nurses to Use Research Evidence

1. **Read Widely and Critically:** Professionally accountable nurses should keep themselves abreast with important developments and should read journals and research reports relating to their specialty.
2. **Attend Professional Conferences:** Many nursing conferences have presentations of research studies of clinical relevance. Moreover, nurses can meet research scholars and can explore practice implications.

3. **Learn to Expect Evidence that a Procedure is Effective:** Every time nurses are told about a standard nursing procedure based on sound rationales, they should first confirm and understand the importance of the suggested new technique and then adopt it.
4. **Become Involved in a Journal Club:** Many organizations that employ nurses sponsor journals with research articles that have potential relevance to practice.
5. **Pursue and Participate in RU or EBP Projects:** Such projects by staff nurses will help them to develop more positive attitudes towards research and better research skills.

Organizational Barriers

1. Some organizations also resist change, when there is a strong organizational perception, for example, to maintain a status quo.
2. Research review and use are often considered appropriate only when time is available but time is usually limited.
3. One of the greatest barriers to RU was found to be insufficient time on job to implement new ideas.
4. Organizations are also reluctant to expand resources for RU and EBP activities or to change organizational policy.
5. EBP can become part of organizational norms only if there is a commitment on the part of managers and administrators. Strong leadership in health care organizations is essential to make EBP a part of the organization.

Strategies for Administrators to Promote the Use of Research Evidence

1. **Foster a Climate of Intellectual Curiosity:** The administration should communicate with staff nurses that their experiences and problems are important and the administration is willing to consider innovative solutions.
2. **Offer Emotional and Moral Support:** Administrators should support their staff by forming RU and EBP committees and by serving as role models for staff nurses.
3. **Offer Financial or Resource Support for Utilization:** RU and EBP projects need resources.
4. **Reward Effort for Nursing Research:** The administration can use various criteria to evaluate nursing performance. Research can also be included as one such criterion in evaluation, which will influence the behaviour of the nurses.
5. **Seek Opportunities for Institutional RU or EBP Projects:** organizational efforts and commitments are essential for the RU and EBP projects.

Barriers Related to the Nursing Profession

It has been observed there is a big gap between research and practice. It is difficult to make practitioners or clinicians and researchers to interact and collaborate. They are in different settings and have different professional concerns and different philosophical systems.

Phillips also noted some other barriers between the research and practice:

1. One barrier is the shortage of appropriate role models (nurses) who can be appointed for their success in using or promoting the use of research in clinical practice.

2. The other barrier is the historical *baggage* that defines nursing such that practising nurses may not typically perceive themselves as independent professionals capable of recommending changes based on research results. Since nurses wait for directions from medical community, there is no power for self-direction. They, therefore, find it difficult to initiate innovations based on research findings.

In surveys, the barrier perceived by a large number of nurses was that nurses feel they do not have *enough authority* to change patient-care procedures. Yet, much progress has been made in the profession in the two barriers mentioned here. The valuing of nursing research on which practice is based must be conveyed to all categories of nurses.

General Tips to Promote the Use of Research Evidences

1. **Incorporate Research Findings into the Curriculum:** When possible, the efficacy of specific procedures should be documented by referring to relevant studies to support.
2. **Encourage Research and Research Use:** This can be done by discussing research studies done and demonstrating positive attitudes towards research and its use in nursing practice.
3. **Place Demands on Researchers:** There should be a demand for the researcher to demonstrate the potential of the research studies for clinical use and to provide a specific plan for dissemination or utilization.

THE PROCESS OF USING RESEARCH IN NURSING PRACTICE

This section describes how to use research as a basis for clinical decisions. Here, we give an overview of the RU/EBP models developed by nurses.

Models for Evidence-based Nursing Practice

During the 1980s and 1990s, a number of different models of RU were developed, which include the following:

1. Diffusion of innovations theory
2. Stetler model
3. Iowa model

The Stetler and Iowa models have been updated to incorporate EBP processes as well rather than RU processes alone.

Stetler Model

The Stetler model of RU was designed with an assumption that RU can be undertaken not only by organizations but by clinicians and managers as well. The updated and refined model provides 'an enhanced approach to overall application of research in the service setting'.

The model involves five sequential phases, which are as follows:

1. **Preparation Phase:** In this phase, nurses define the underlying purpose and outcomes of the research project, select sources of research evidence, and consider external factors and internal factors that influence their objectivity.

2. **Validation Phase:** This phase involves the utilization of evidences for potential application in practice otherwise rejected.
3. **Comparative Evaluation and Decision-making Phase:** This involves a synthesis of findings and the application of the criteria taken to determine the desirability and feasibility of the findings to nursing practice.

   The considered criteria are as follows:

   (a) Fit of setting
   (b) Feasibility
   (c) Current practice
   (d) Substantiating evidence

   These are used for comparative evaluation to make a decision about using the findings in practice or rejecting them.
4. **Translation or Application Phase:** This involves the following activities:

   (a) Confirm how the finds will be used (formally or informally).
   (b) Spell out the operational details of the application and implement them. It may be desirable to develop procedures and plan of action for organizational change.
5. **Evaluation Phase:** In this last phase, the application is evaluated.

   Initially, the Stetler model was designed as a tool for individual practitioners. However, it has become a basis of formal RU and EBP projects by groups of nurses (Fig. 14.3).

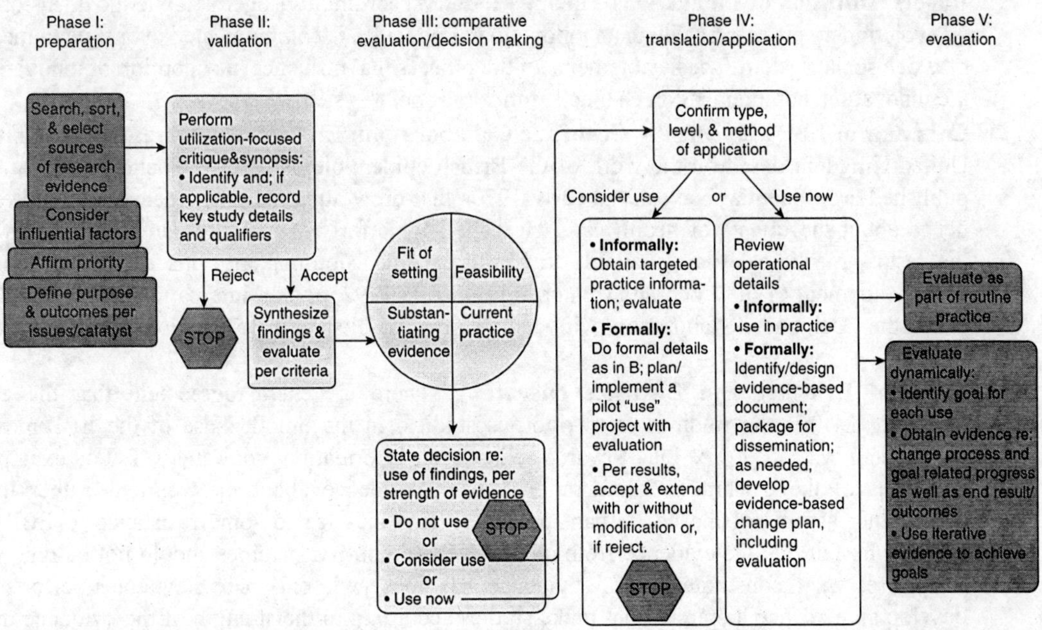

FIGURE 14.3 *Stetler Model of Research Utilization to Facilitate Evidence-based Practice*

As mentioned already, EBP de-emphasizes clinical decision based on customs and rituals and integrates the best available research evidence with other sources of data such as clinical expertise and patient preferences. In nursing EBP and RU, often face a variety of barriers. In EBP resistance to change, due to lack of organizational support, resources constraints and limited communication, and collaboration between practitioners and researchers.

KEY POINTS

- Research utilization is a process of communicating and using research-generated knowledge to make an impact on or a change in the existing practices in health care system.
- Evidence-based practice involves making clinical decisions on the basis of the best possible evidence (research) and uses information from clinical experiences, patient preference, and other sources.
- Empirical knowledge is generated by conducting quality studies, and several studies on a topic are conducted. Cognitive clustering is accomplished through integrative reviews and meta-analyses of nursing research. Integrative reviews of research are conducted to identify, analyse, and synthesize the results from independent studies to determine the current knowledge of a particular topic. These reviews are published in a variety of research and clinical journals and in the annual review of nursing research.
- **Research Utilization in Qualitative Research:** The qualitative findings are presented in narrative form and this type of research may have a privileged position in RU. Clinicians do not need a strong background in statistics to understand qualitative research. It is not necessary to translate the results into everyday language before the findings can be used conceptually.
- **Rogers' Diffusion of Innovations Theory Model:** According to Roger, knowledge diffusion is an evolutionary process by which an innovation or new idea is communicated over time to members of a social system. The key elements of the process that influence the adoption of innovation are innovation, communication channels, time, and social system.
- **Overview of EBP Movement—Cochrane Collaboration:** EBP movement was founded in the United Kingdom based on the work of the British epidemiologist Archie Cochrane. Cochrane published an influential book in the early 1970s that drew attention to the dearth of solid evidence about the effects of health care. He called for efforts to make research summaries of the results of clinical trials available to health care decision-makers. This eventually led to the development of the Cochrane Center in Oxford in 1992, and an international collaboration called the Cochrane Collaboration, with centres now established in 15 locations throughout the world.
- **Types of Evidence and Evidence Hierarchy:** There is general agreement that the evidence for EBP is the findings from rigorous studies. In the initial phase of the EBP movement, there was a definite bias towards reliance on information from an RCT. For example, the focus of the Cochrane Collaboration was on evidence about interventions rather than about other aspects of the health care practices. This bias led to some resistance to EBP by nurses who felt that the evidence from qualitative and non-RCT studies should not be ignored. Therefore, what constitutes useful evidence has loosened, but there have been efforts to develop an evidence hierarchy that ranks studies according to the strength of the evidence they provide.

- **Barriers to Research Utilization:** The knowledge of the barriers to RU and EBP in nursing is useful to plan and implement the efforts to integrate nursing research in practice. Barriers are at the nurses' level, at the institutions' level, and at professional level, and the strategies to break these barriers also need to be addressed at all these various levels.
- **Models for Evidence-based Nursing Practice:** During the 1980s and 1990s, a number of different models of RU were developed, which include the diffusion of innovations theory, Stetler model, and Iowa model.

QUESTIONS

I. Essay-type Questions

1. What is RU and how can this be achieved by practising nurses?
2. What is EBP? Discuss its levels as defined by Stetler.
3. What are the barriers to RU and EBP at professional level in nursing? Discuss.
4. How can you overcome the barriers to RU and EBP in nursing practice? Discuss.
5. Discuss the stages of Roger's *innovation adoption* process for EBP.

II. Short Notes

1. Differences between RU and EBP
2. Elements of RU process
3. Organization-related barriers to EBP
4. General tips to promote EBP in nursing practice

III. Multiple-choice Questions

Circle the alphabet before the best answer

1. Following are the models of EBP in nursing, except
   (a) Stetler model
   (b) Iowa model
   (c) diffusion of innovations theory
   (d) Maslow's model
2. The number of sequential phases involved in the Stetler model, which is 'an enhancement to overall approach of research in nursing', is
   (a) one (b) three
   (c) five (d) four
3. The strategies for enhancing the use of RU by nurses include the following except
   (a) reading widely and critically
   (b) learning by trial and error
   (c) becoming involved in a journal club
   (d) attending professional conferences
4. A research-related barrier to RU is
   (a) shortage of nurses
   (b) unqualified nurses in hospital settings
   (c) research reports inaccessible to practising nurses
   (d) dearth of qualitative research
5. The number of levels of hierarchy in EBP as given by Stetler is
   (a) one (b) three
   (c) five (d) seven

Answer Keys

1. (d) 2. (c) 3. (b) 4. (c) 5. (d)

FURTHER READING

Burns, N., Grove, Susan K. 1999. *Understanding Nursing Research*. Saunders.

Caplan, N., Rich, R. F. 1975. *The Use of Social Science Knowledge at the National Level*. N Arbor, MI: Institute for Social Research, University of Michigan.

Kothari, C. R. 1985. *Research Methodology Methods and Techniques*. New Delhi: New Age International Publisher.

Polit, Denise F., Hungler, Berandette P. 1999. *Nursing Research: Principles and Methods*. Lippincott.

Rogers, E. M. 1995. *Diffusion of Innovations*. Fourth edition. New York: Free Press.

Stetler, C. B. 1994. 'Refinement of the Stetler/Marram Model for Application of Research Findings into Practice'. *Nursing Outlook*, 42: 15–25.

chapter 15

Fundamentals of Statistics

OBJECTIVES

Upon completion of this chapter the learner will be able to:

- Define the basic terms used in statistics
- Understand the basic concepts related to statistics
- Describe the scope of statistics in health and nursing
- Present the bulky data in a meaningful manner
- Describe the uses and application of descriptive statistics
- Describe and apply inferential statistics
- Interpret and predict the statistical significance of the results
- Understand the application of various parametric and non-parametric tests (chi-square test, *Z*-test, *t*-test, ANOVA, and so on)
- Design the experiment and apply the statistical tests in nursing research
- Define statistical package
- Enlist different available statistical packages
- Enlist the uses of statistical package
- Describe in brief various statistical packages such as SPSS, Minitab, SAS, and Epiinfo
- Enumerate the steps for using SPSS
- Know the importance of statistical packages in the analysis of data

INTRODUCTION

In the present chapter, the two main branches of statistics, namely descriptive and inferential statistics, are discussed in detail. The first part of the chapter deals with the basic concepts of statistics, organization of data, diagrammatic representation of data, frequency distribution, and various descriptive statistics such as mean, median, mode, and standard deviation. The second part of the chapter deals with the inferential statistics and its applications. Here, we discuss the basics of testing of hypothesis, *t*-test, ANOVA, MANOVA, ANCOVA, chi-square test, sign test, and so on.

BASIC CONCEPTS AND DESCRIPTIVE STATISTICS

The word *statistics* comes from the Italian word *statista*, meaning 'statesman', which means a political state. In the early days, statistical data were only collected for framing important policies by the government for public welfare. The study of statistics involves methods of refining numerical and non-numerical information (data) into more useful forms. The word *statistics* today refers to either quantitative information or a method of dealing with quantitative or qualitative information. Science with statistics bears good fruits; statistics without scientific application has no roots.

Statistics has a double meaning. It is defined both in singular and plural senses. When it is defined in the sense of a group of data, it is meant for a particular purpose, called plural sense of statistics. For example, the data of height, weight, number of births, number of deaths, and so on are the collection of figures called the statistics in plural sense. Data expressed in terms of table, chart, graph, diagrams, and so on are also termed as statistics in plural sense. In daily life, we come across such statistics in newspapers, journals, and magazines. The term *statistics* is used in singular sense to refer to a specific field of study, that is, a discipline concerned with the treatment of data derived from groups of individuals. So statistics in this sense provides various methods for data collection, analysing data, and presentation of data in order to take relevant decisions. We can say that statistics is a body of various statistical methods. The various methods employed in the analysis and interpretation of statistical data are known as statistical methods.

Biostatistics is the branch of statistics applied to biological or medical sciences. Biostatistics is also called biometry and may be defined as a science of figure and variation. It is to be noted that statistics is a science as well as an art and it can neither prove nor disprove anything. It is just a tool. Statistics is widely used in various fields such as medical sciences and physical sciences. Various fields make use of statistics to solve their problems; in medical sciences, it is used to solve the biological problems. Biostatistics covers applications and contributions not only from health, medicine, and nutrition but also from the fields such as agriculture, genetics, biology, biochemistry, demography, epidemiology, anthropology, and many others.

All the tools and techniques of statistics are applied over data to draw valid conclusions relating to the characteristics under the study of the group of individuals. Data may be defined as any group of measurements that is of our interest. Data are broadly classified into two categories as quantitative data and qualitative data. Quantitative data is a numeric data having a strong level of measurement, and qualitative data non-numeric having a weak level of measurement.

The finite and infinite sets of individual under study are called population or universe. Thus, in statistics, population is an aggregate of objects, animate or inanimate under study. Any characteristic or numerical summary measure of population is called parameter. A parameter is always a constant quantity. For example, the mean *body mass index* (BMI) of the nursing students of University College of Nursing, Faridkot, is a parameter. Any characteristic of a sample is called a statistic. For example, instead of calculating the BMI for all nursing students as discussed in the previous example, we draw a sample of students and calculate the mean BMI only for the sampled students. Now, this sample mean BMI is called statistic. A statistic is a variable.

Depending upon the method used to collect the data, there are two types of data that are analysed in statistics. These are primary data and secondary data. The data that are collected first hand by someone specifically for the purpose of facilitating the study are known as primary data, and any data that have been gathered earlier for some other purpose are secondary data in the hand of an individual who is using them. Thus, primary data collected by one person may become the secondary data for another.

When we collect data, there is not one or two observations but a large number of them. It becomes necessary to organize the mass of data so that they are reduced to meaningful proportion. This brings to us a tabular representation. For example, we may present the figures of population as given in Table 15.1.

TABLE 15.1 *Population of India from 1941 to 1991*

Year	Population (in Crores)	Year	Population (in Crores)
1941	31.87	1971	54.82
1951	36.11	1981	68.33
1961	43.92	1991	84.63

Suppose there is a group of 30 patients having knee pain. An appropriate therapy is given to this group to reduce the pain level. The following are the measurements of pain on 0–5 scale after the therapy:

3, 2, 0, 4, 1, 2, 3, 2, 5, 3, 3, 1, 1, 3, 5, 4, 2, 2, 3, 1, 0, 4, 3, 2, 2, 4, 2, 3, 3, and 1

It is seen that even with only 30 observations, the data need some better display. One way of doing this is to show the data in a certain order as follows:

0, 0, 1, 1, 1, 1, 1, 2, 2, 2, 2, 2, 2, 2, 2, 3, 3, 3, 3, 3, 3, 3, 3, 3, 4, 4, 4, 4, 5, and 5

The same data can be shown differently. We can condense these data by pairing each of that value with its frequency. This is shown in Table 15.2

TABLE 15.2 *Frequency Distribution of Pain Levels of 30 Patients*

Observation (X)	Frequency (Y)
0	2
1	5
2	8
3	9
4	4
5	2

The arrangement and display of data in this form where the observed value is paired with its frequency are called frequency distribution. Since X is taking non-fractional values, it may also be called a discrete frequency distribution.

In order to draw the grouped frequency distribution, the following steps are applied:

1. Deciding the appropriate number of class groupings
2. Choosing a suitable size or width of a class interval
3. Establishing the boundaries of each class interval
4. Classifying the data into appropriate classes
5. Counting the number of items in each class

For example the following data pertain to the weights (in kg) of 33 students of a class.
42, 74, 40, 60, 82, 115, 41, 61, 75, 83, 63, 53, 110, 76, 84, 50, 67, 65, 78, 77, 56, 95, 68, 69, 104, 80, 79, 79, 54, 73, 59, 81, and 110.

Prepare a suitable frequency table.

Solution:

Class Interval	Tally Marks	Frequency
40–50	111	3
50–60	~~1111~~	5
60–70	~~1111~~ 11	7

(Continued)

Class Interval	Tally Marks	Frequency
70–80	~~1111~~ 111	8
80–90	~~1111~~	5
90–100	1	1
100–110	1	1
110–120	111	3
Total		**33**

The comprehension of the different essential features of a distribution becomes quite easy even for a laymen if the data are presented graphically. Graphs are interesting, attractive, and impressive where no knowledge of mathematics is required. This is the simplest method of presenting the data.

Histogram is one of the important graphical techniques to present the data. A histogram is a graphical representation of a frequency distribution of a continuous series. It represents the class frequencies in a frequency distribution by vertical rectangle, meeting each other from left to right. For each class interval, a rectangle is constructed to the frequency density of the class so that the area of the rectangle above each class is proportional to the frequency of that class. The total area covered under a histogram is proportional to the total frequency. In histograms, the key factor is the area of the rectangles erected on each class interval and not the height of the rectangle. Bars touch each other but never overlap.

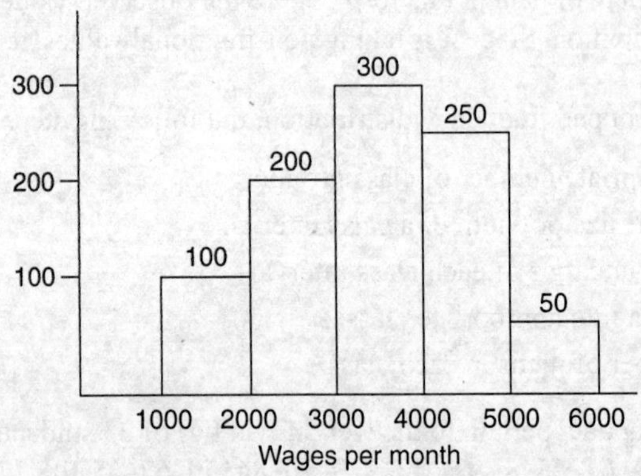

FIGURE 15.1 *Histogram Showing Frequency Distribution of Wages Received by Employees*

Measures of Central Tendency

Every datum has the tendency to cluster around a single value called measure of central tendency or average, which is considered to be the representative of the group. We will discuss three averages in this chapter: mean, median, and mode. Before discussing the various averages, a question arises. Why should we use such averages? There are two main objectives of using averages:

1. First, to get a single value that indicates the characteristics of the entire data.
2. Second, to facilitate comparisons. For example, the mean height of Bengali boys is less than that of Punjabi boys. Such comparisons are made.

Arithmetic Mean

This is the most familiar measure. The arithmetic mean is obtained by adding all the observations and dividing the sum by the number of observations.

(i.e.,)

$$\bar{X} = \frac{\sum_{i=1}^{N} X_i}{N}$$

For example the gain in weights of five albino rats over a period of five days is 5, 6, 4, 8, and 7. The mean is

$$\bar{X} = \frac{5+6+4+8+7}{5} = \frac{30}{5} = 6$$

When the frequency distribution of the variable is given, the mean is obtained as

$$\bar{X} = \frac{\sum_{i=1}^{n} f_i X_i}{\sum_{i=1}^{n} f_i}$$

For example the following table gives the marks of 58 students in statistics. Calculate the mean marks.

Marks	No. of Students
0–10	4
10–20	8
20–30	11
30–40	15
40–50	12
50–60	6
60–70	2
Total	**58**

Solution:

Marks	Mid-point (*X*)	*F*	*fX*
0–10	5	4	20
10–20	15	8	120
20–30	25	11	275
30–40	35	15	525
40–50	45	12	540
50–60	55	6	330
60–70	65	2	130
Total		**58**	**1940**

$$\bar{X} = \frac{\sum_{i=1}^{7} f_i X_i}{\sum_{i=1}^{7} f_i} = \frac{1940}{58} = 33.45 \simeq 33 \text{ marks}$$

Median

Median is the value of the variable which divides the total distribution (data) into two equal parts. It is a positional average.

In the example of albino rats, the gains in weight are arranged in ascending order.

4, 5, 6, 7, and 8

No. of observations (N) = 5 (odd)

Therefore,
$$\text{median} = \left(\frac{N+1}{2}\right)^{\text{th}} \text{item}$$
$$= \text{third item} = 6$$

If the number of observations is even, say, 4, 5, 6, 7, 8, and 9,

then,
$$\text{median} = \frac{\left(\frac{N}{2}\right)^{\text{th}} \text{item} + \left(\frac{N}{2}+1\right)^{\text{th}} \text{item}}{2}$$
$$= \frac{\text{Third item} + \text{Fourth item}}{2}$$
$$= \frac{6+7}{2} = 6.5$$

The calculation of the median is done after arranging the given series in a particular order. When grouped frequency is given, then median is calculated as

$$\text{Median} = l + \frac{\left(\frac{N}{2} - c\right)}{f_m} \cdot h$$

where

l = the lower limit of the median class

f = the frequency of the median class

h = the class interval

c = the cumulative frequency of the class preceding the median class

Let us calculate the median weight (kg) of 30 adults for the following data:

Class Interval	Mid-point (x)	Frequency (f)	Cumulative Frequency (cf)
45–50	47.5	2	2
50–55	52.5	3	5
55–60	57.5	6	11

Class Interval	Mid-point (x)	Frequency (f)	Cumulative Frequency (cf)
60–65	62.5	4	15
65–70	67.5	6	21
70–75	72.5	4	25
75–80	77.5	5	30
	Total	**30**	

$$\text{median} = 60 + \frac{(15-11)5}{4} = 60 + 5 = 65$$

Mode

The most frequency-occurring value of the variable is mode.

For example the gains in weight of ten rats are 4, 8, 6, 7, 3, 9, 2, 6, 5, and 0. As 6 occurs more frequently, the mode is 6.

Median is considered to be the robust average as it is not effected by the extreme values.

Measures of Variability (Dispersion)

The word *dispersion* literally means scatterings, deviation, or spread of group of observations from their average value. It refers to the deviation of the various observations of a series from their central value or the difference between only two extreme values of the series. The phrase 'measures of dispersion' means the various possible methods of measuring the dispersions.

Decisions are taken based on the average value for the improvement of the situation. But average value may not be reliable. In order to verify the reliability of the average and stability of the series, dispersion is calculated.

The various types of dispersions that are mostly in use may be outlined as under:

1. Range
2. Quartile deviation
3. Average deviation
4. Standard deviation

The above measures of dispersion are discussed in the following paragraph.

Range

It is the difference between the largest and smallest items of the sample of observations. If samples of observations are 5, 6, 7, 8, and 10, the range is 10 – 5 = 5.

Quartile Deviation

Quartile deviation or semi-interquartile range is given by the following formula:

$$Q_D = \frac{Q_3 - Q_1}{2}$$

where Q_1 and Q_3 are the first and third quartiles, respectively.

For example from the following series, determine the interquartile range and quartile deviation.

Roll No.	1001	1002	1003	1004	1005	1006	1007	1008
Marks	94	95	96	93	87	79	73	69

Solution:
Arrange the given series in ascending order:

69 73 79 87 93 94 95 96

Now,

$$Q_1 = \left(\frac{N+1}{4}\right)^{\text{th}} \text{ item}$$
$$= \left(\frac{8+1}{4}\right)^{\text{th}} \text{ item}$$
$$= 2.25^{\text{th}} \text{ item}$$
$$= \text{Value of second item} + \frac{1}{4} \text{ (value of third} - \text{value of second item)}$$
$$= 73 + 1.50 = 74.50$$

And

$$Q_3 = 3\left(\frac{N+1}{4}\right)^{\text{th}} \text{ item}$$
$$= 6.75^{\text{th}} \text{ item}$$
$$= 94 + \frac{3}{4}(95 - 94)$$
$$= 94 + 0.75 = 94.75$$

Thus,

$$IQR = Q_3 - Q_1 = 94.75 - 74.50$$
$$= 20.25$$
$$QD = \frac{Q_3 - Q_1}{2} = \frac{20.25}{2} = 10.125$$

Average Deviation (Mean Deviation)

Average deviation may be defined as the arithmetic average of the deviations of the items of a series taken from its average value, ignoring the plus and minus signs. Average may be taken as either mean, median, or mode.

For example from the following data relating to the marks obtained by 11 students, determine the (a) mean deviation about mean and (b) mean deviation about median.

Roll No.	1	2	3	4	5	6	7	8	9	10	11
Marks	21	54	63	49	67	33	35	59	66	32	38

Solution:

(a) **Mean Deviation about Mean**

Roll No.	Marks X	$\lvert X-\bar{X}\rvert$
1	21	26
2	54	7
3	63	16
4	49	2
5	67	20
6	33	14
7	35	12
8	59	12
9	66	19
10	32	15
11	38	9
Total	**517**	**152**

where $$\bar{X} = \frac{\Sigma X}{N} = \frac{517}{11} = 47$$

$$\text{MD(Mean)} = \frac{\Sigma\left|(X-\bar{X})\right|}{N} = \frac{152}{11} = 13.82 \text{ (approx.)}$$

(b) **Mean Deviation about Median**

Values in Ascending Order X	$\lvert X-M\rvert$
21	28
32	17
33	16
35	14
38	11
49	0
54	5
59	10
63	14
66	17
67	18
Total	**150**

where median $$(M) = \left(\frac{N+1}{2}\right)^{\text{th}} \text{ item}$$

$$= \left(\frac{11+1}{2}\right)^{\text{th}} \text{ item} = 6^{\text{th}} \text{ item} = 49$$

$$\text{MD(Median)} = \frac{\Sigma|X - M|}{N} = \frac{150}{11} = 13.64\text{(approx.)}$$

Standard Deviation

This is the most commonly used measure of dispersion. It takes into account all the values of the series for its calculation. It is defined as the square root of the arithmetic mean of the squared deviations of the individual values from their arithmetic mean. It is also known as the root mean square deviation from mean. The formula to calculate standard deviation is

$$SD(\sigma) = \sqrt{\frac{1}{N}\sum_{i=1}^{N}(X_i - \bar{X})^2}$$

$$= \sqrt{\frac{1}{N}\left[\sum_{i=1}^{N} X_i^2 - \frac{\left(\sum_{i=1}^{N} X_i\right)^2}{N}\right]}$$

For example calculate the standard deviation for the following data:

X	5	10	15	20	25	30

Solution:

	X	*X*²
	5	25
	10	100
	15	225
	20	400
	25	625
	30	900
Total	**105**	**2275**

$$\sigma^2 = \frac{1}{N}\left[\sum X^2 - \frac{(\Sigma X)^2}{N}\right]$$

$$= \frac{1}{6}\left[2275 - \frac{(105)^2}{6}\right]$$

$$= 72.92$$

$$\sigma = \sqrt{72.92} = 8.54 \text{ approx.}$$

Coefficient of Variation: It is the relative measure of standard deviation. Here standard deviation is expressed as percentage of mean.

(i.e.,) $$CV = \frac{\sigma}{\overline{X}} \cdot 100$$

It is used to compare the dispersion of two series.

Properties of Standard Deviation:

1. It is independent of the change in the origin.
2. It is dependent of the change in scale
3. It determines the number of items that face within a specific range of a symmetrical distribution with following relationship.

$$\overline{X} \pm 1\sigma = 68.27\%$$
$$\overline{X} \pm 2\sigma = 95.45\%$$
$$\overline{X} \pm 3\sigma = 99.73\%$$
$$\overline{X} \pm 1.96\sigma = 95\%$$

That is, it is used to calculate the standard error.

Normal Distribution

It is a theoretical continuous distribution. The theory of normal distribution was developed by a famous English mathematician Abraham Dr. Moivre in 1733. Many statistical problems are solved by using normal distribution.

Properties of Normal Distribution

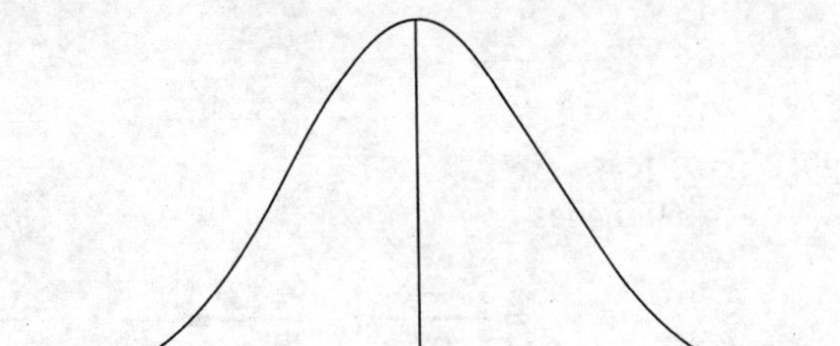

FIGURE 15.2 *Properties of Normal Distribution*

1. It is a famous bell-shaped symmetric curve.
2. Mean, median, and mode coincide for this distribution.
3. The area under the curve represents the probability; hence, total area is 1 (unity).
4. The line X = mean divides the total area into two equal parts.
5. The maxima of the curve occurs at X = mean, and the curve starts declining if we move either side of the point X = mean.
6. The tails of the curve never touches the x axis.
7. Normal distribution has two parameters, mean and standard deviation.

Standard Normal Curve

A normal curve in which the x scale is converted into z scale on which the mean (μ) is taken at 0, and the standard deviation (σ) taken at a unit (1) is called standard normal curve.

This kind of conversion of normal curve into a standard normal curve is called z– transformation.

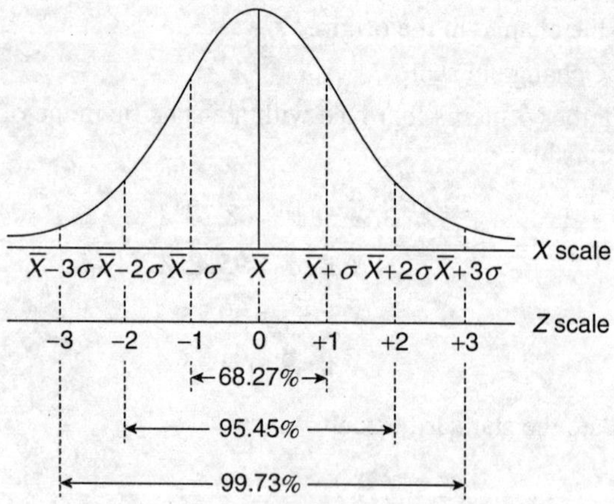

FIGURE 15.3 *A Standard Normal Curve*

For example the mean height of the students of a certain college is 66 inches with a standard deviation of 3 inches. How many of the said college consisting of 2000 students would you expect to be over 5 feet height? Give your answer through a normal curve.

Solution:

Mean (μ) = 66 inches

SD (σ) = 3 inches

Value of the desired height (X) = 5 feet

= 60 inches

$$Z = \frac{X-\mu}{\sigma} = \frac{60-66}{3} = -2$$

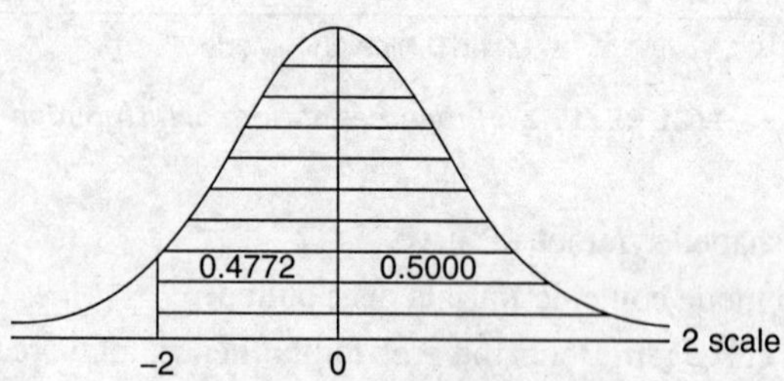

FIGURE 15.4 *Example of Standard Normal Curve*

For example in a normal curve, the area between 2 at 0 and at −2 = 0.4772. The area to the right of 2 at 0 = 0.5000. So the total area to the right of 2 at −2 would be 0.4772 + 0.5000 = 0.9772. This is shown through the shaded portion of the normal curve.

The proportion of the area in normal curve for the students having the height above 5 feet is = 0.9772.

The total number of students (N) = 2000. Hence, the number of students expected to have height above 5 feet would be $0.9772 \times 2000 = 1954.4 \simeq 1954$

Measures of Relationship

For assessing the linear relationship between the variables, correlation analysis and regression analysis are generally employed. Such analyses are called bivertical analyses. Correlation analysis and regression analysis are discussed below.

Correlation Analysis

It is the study of linear relationship between two or more than two variables. When the relationship between any two variables is studied, then the correlation analysis is said to be the simple correlation analysis.

If both the variables move in the same direction, then the correlation is said to be the positive correlation, and if in the opposite direction, then negative correlation.

One can have an idea about the type and degree of correlation by drawing scatter plot. A scatter plot as given in Figure 15.5 is an arrangement of dots obtained after plotting a pair as a dot in the graph.

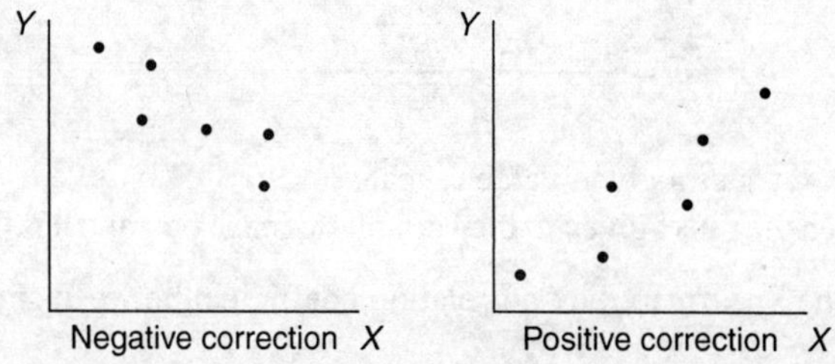

FIGURE 15.5 *Scatter Plot Showing Correlation Analysis*

More spread of points from the straight line indicates the low degree of correlation and vice versa. If all the points (dots) fall on an exact straight line, then we have perfect correlation (negative or positive).

These are the methods to calculate the numeric value of the coefficient of correlation.

1. Karl Pearson's coefficient of correlation or product moment correlation
2. Spearman rank correlation coefficient

Karl Pearson's Coefficient of Correlation: The following formula is used to calculate the correlation coefficient:

$$r_{XY} = \frac{N\Sigma XY - \Sigma X \Sigma Y}{\sqrt{N\Sigma X^2 - (\Sigma X)^2}\sqrt{N\Sigma Y^2 - (\Sigma Y)^2}}$$

For example calculate the correlation coefficient between the variables – gains in height and weight in 10 children by using the following information.

Gain in weight (kg) – X
Gain in Height (cm) – Y
$\Sigma X = 32.5$ $\quad \Sigma Y = 28.4$ $\quad \Sigma XY = 101.69$
$\Sigma X^2 = 113.31$ $\quad \Sigma Y^2 = 93.06$

Solution:

$$r_{XY} = \frac{N\Sigma XY - \Sigma X\Sigma Y}{\sqrt{N\Sigma X^2 - (\Sigma X)^2}\sqrt{N\Sigma Y^2 - (\Sigma Y)^2}}$$

$$r_{XY} = \frac{10\times 101.69 - 32.5\times 28.4}{\sqrt{10\times 113.31 - (32.5)^2}\sqrt{10\times 93.06 - (28.4)^2}}$$
$$= 0.9620 \simeq +0.96$$

The result indicates that there is a very high degree of positive correlation between the gain in weight and the gain in height of the 10 children under study.

Spearman Rank Correlation Coefficient: This method uses the ranks of the observations for the calculation of correlation coefficient instead of actual magnitude. The formula to calculate the rank correlation is

$$r = 1 - \frac{6\Sigma d^2}{n(n^2-1)}; \quad \text{when there is no tie}$$

$$r = 1 - \frac{[6\Sigma d^2 + AF]}{n(n^2-1)}; \quad \text{when there is a tie}$$

where,
$$AF = \frac{m_1^3 - m_1}{12} + \frac{m_2^3 - m_2}{12} \ldots$$

m's denotes the number of times a given value repeats.
d is the difference between the ranks given to the variables of each pair and *n* is the number of pairs studied.

For example calculate the Spearman rank correlation coefficient between smoking and lung cancer for the following data:

S. No.	**1**	**2**	**3**	**4**	**5**	**6**	**7**	**8**	**9**	**10**
Grates of Smoking	1	2	3	4	5	6	7	8	9	10
Severity of Cancer	2	1	4	3	6	7	5	9	8	10

Solution:

Rank (*X*) R_X	**Rank (*Y*) R_Y**	***D***	***d*²**
1	2	−1	1
2	1	1	1
3	4	−1	1
4	3	1	1
5	6	−1	1
6	7	−1	1
7	5	2	4
8	9	−1	1

Rank (X) R_X	Rank (Y) R_Y	D	d^2
9	8	1	1
10	10	0	0
Total			**12**

$$r = 1 - \frac{6\Sigma d^2}{n(n^2-1)} = 1 - \frac{6 \times 12}{10(10^2-1)}$$
$$= 1 - 0.073$$
$$= 0.927$$

For example for the following data relating to the marks obtained in paediatric (X) and anatomy (Y) of eight students, calculate the rank correlation coefficient.

Paediatric Marks (X)	60	80	90	60	91	100	95	93
Anatomy Marks (Y)	30	40	50	40	60	70	40	75

Solution:

X	Y	R_X	R_Y	d	d^2
60	30	7.5	8	–0.5	0.25
80	40	6	6	0	0
90	50	5	4	1	1
60	40	7.5	6	1.5	2.25
91	60	4	3	1	1
100	70	1	2	–1	1
95	40	2	6	–4	16
93	75	3	1	2	4
Total					**25.50**

$$m_1 = 2, m_2 = 3$$
$$AF = \frac{m_1^3 - m_1}{12} + \frac{m_2^3 - m_2}{12}$$
$$= \frac{2^3-2}{12} + \frac{3^3-3}{12} = \frac{1}{2} + 2 = 2.5$$
$$r = 1 - \frac{6[\sum d^2 + AF]}{n(n^2-1)}$$
$$= 1 - \frac{6[25.50 + 2.5]}{8(8^2-1)} = 1 - \frac{6 \times 28}{504}$$
$$= 1 - 0.33 = 0.67 \text{ approx.}$$

We find that there is a positive correlation between the marks in paediatric and anatomy.

Properties of the Correlation Coefficient: The following are the main properties of the correlation coefficient:

1. Correlation coefficient is symmetric in nature; that is, $r_{xy} = r_{yx}$
2. There is no cause-and-effect relationship.
3. It can take values range from −1 to +1, that is, $-1 \le r \le +1$.
4. It is independent of change in origin and scale.
5. It is a relative measure of covariance; hence a pure number is free from the system of units.

Regression Analysis

In the last topic, we have discussed the concept of the correlation analysis. If correlation is detected between two variables, then we can go for regression analysis for the prediction purpose.

Regression analysis is an attempt to represent a linear average relationship between two or more than two variables.

If there are only two variables under study, then regression analysis is called simple regression analysis. This analysis is applicable if there is a cause-and-effect relationship between the variables. It involves dependent and independent variables in its mathematical model. The variable which is to be predicted is called dependent variable and the other variable is called independent variable. The following is the mathematical form of simple regression model:

$$Y = a + bX$$

where, Y is the dependent variable, X is the independent variable, a is the Y intercept, b is the regression coefficient, and a and b are also called the parameters of the regression line and are given by

$$a = \overline{Y} - b\overline{X}$$

$$b = \frac{N\Sigma XY - \Sigma X \Sigma Y}{N\Sigma X^2 - (\Sigma X)^2}$$

For example fit a regression line for the following data to predict diastolic blood pressure as a function of time periods.

Time Periods (*X*)	0	5	10	15	20
Diastolic Blood Pressure (*Y*)	72	66	70	64	66

Solution:

	X	***Y***	***X*²**	***XY***
	0	72	0	0
	5	66	25	330
	10	70	100	700
	15	64	225	960
	20	66	400	1320
Total	**50**	**338**	**750**	**3310**

$$\bar{X} = \frac{\sum X}{N} = \frac{50}{5} = 10$$

$$\bar{Y} = \frac{\sum Y}{N} = \frac{338}{5} = 67.6$$

The required regression equation is

$$Y = a + bX \tag{15.1}$$

$$b = \frac{N\Sigma XY - \Sigma X \Sigma Y}{N\Sigma X^2 - (\Sigma X)^2}$$

$$= \frac{5 \times 3310 - 50 \times 338}{5 \times 750 - (50)^2}$$

$$= -0.280$$

$$a = \bar{Y} - b\bar{X}$$

$$= 67.6 - (-0.28) \times 10$$

$$= 67.6 + 2.8 = 70.4$$

Hence, the required regression line is

$$Y = 70.4 - 0.28\,X$$

The above regression equation is obtained after substituting the values of *a* and *b* in the Eq. 15.1.

For example for the following data on height, find out the regression equation of height of an adult son (*Y*) on the height of the father (*X*).

Adult Son(*Y*)	68	66	68	65	69	66	68	65	71	67	68	70
Father (*X*)	65	63	67	64	68	62	70	66	68	67	69	71

$$n = 12 \qquad \Sigma X = 800 \qquad \Sigma X^2 = 53418 \qquad \Sigma Y = 811$$

$$\Sigma Y^2 = 54849 \qquad \Sigma XY = 54107 \qquad \bar{X} = 66.667 \qquad \bar{Y} = 67.583$$

Solution: The required equation is

$$Y = a + bX \tag{15.2}$$

$$b = \frac{N\Sigma XY - \Sigma X \Sigma Y}{N\Sigma X^2 - (\Sigma X)^2}$$

$$= \frac{12 \times 54107 - 800 \times 811}{12 \times 53418 - (800)^2}$$

$$= \frac{40.33}{84.67} = 0.4764$$

$$a = \bar{Y} - b\bar{X}$$

$$= 67.583 - 0.4764 \times 66.667$$

$$= 67.583 - 31.759 = 35.824$$

Substituting the value of r and b in the Eq. 15.2, we get the required regression equation as

$$Y = 35.824 + 0.4764\,X$$

Now, using the above regression equation, one can predict the value of the height of the adult son for a given value of the height of the father. For example, what would be the height of the adult son if the height of the father is 75? Put $X = 75$ in the above regression model, we get

$$\begin{aligned} Y &= 35.824 + 0.4764 \times 75 \\ &= 35.824 + 35.73 \\ &= 71.554 \end{aligned}$$

Hence, we conclude that the height of the adult son would be 71.554 if his father is 75.

Regression coefficient may be defined as the rate of change in the value of the dependent variable (Y) with a unit change in the value of the independent variable (X). So we can interpret the value of the regression coefficient for the above example as $b = 0.4764$, which means a change in height of the father by one unit will produce a change of 0.4764 unit in the height of the adult son.

Remark: A regression equation X on Y is given by

$$X = a' + b'y$$

where

$$a' = \overline{X} - b'\overline{Y}$$

$$b' = \frac{N\Sigma XY - \Sigma X \Sigma Y}{N\Sigma Y^2 - (\Sigma Y)^2}$$

These expressions can be obtained by interchanging X and Y in the expressions of the regression equation Y on X.

Properties of Regression Coefficients: The following are the important properties of the regression coefficients:

1. Regression coefficient is not symmetric; that is, $b_{YX} \neq b_{XY} (b \neq b')$
2. Regression coefficient is independent of the change in the origin but not of scale.
3. The sign of the regression coefficient is same as that of the correlation coefficient and vice versa.
4. If the magnitude value of one of the regression coefficient is greater than one, then another must be less than one; that is, if $b_{YX} |>|$ then $(b_{XY}) < 1$.
5. Both the regression coefficients have the same sign; that is, both are either positive or negative.
6. Correlation coefficient is the geometric mean of the regression coefficients

$$r = \pm\sqrt{b_{XY} b_{YX}}$$

INFERENTIAL STATISTICS AND ITS APPLICATIONS IN NURSING RESEARCH

As we know statistics is broadly classified into two categories: descriptive statistics and inferential statistics. In the last section, we have discussed about the descriptive statistics where the sole purpose is to describe the data. In the present section, we will discuss about the inferential statistics.

Inferential statistics is a branch of statistics that deals with drawing the inferences about the population characteristics under study based on the random sample drawn from the population of interest. This branch of statistics heavily depends upon the assumption that the population from which the sample has been drawn follows normal distribution. Generally, two types of statistical problems are dealt with in statistical inference: theory of estimation and testing of hypothesis.

Theory of estimation deals with the *point* estimation and *interval* estimation. *Point estimation* is a procedure to calculate the unknown population parameter based on the sample. It is called point estimation because we get single value of the parameter in their procedure. The formula used to estimate the unknown parameter involving the sample observations is called 'estimator' and the numeric value obtained after calculation is called an estimate.

Interval estimation is a procedure to set up a range with lower limit and upper limit using the sample observations, where unknown parameter is expected to lie within this range with some confidence. That is why, it is also known as confidence limit.

Testing of hypothesis is a procedure to test the statistical hypothesis for its truthfulness based on the sample observations. There are basically two types of testing procedures in statistics: parametric and non-parametric statistical tests. Before discussing the statistical procedure in detail, we discuss some basic terms involved in the testing procedure below:

Hypothesis is a tentative statistical statement which is to be verified for its truthfulness by using the sample information.

For example, 'prevalence of cancer in Faridkot district is 132/100000' is a hypothesis regarding the cancer cases in Faridkot district.

Null hypothesis is a hypothesis of no difference. It indicates that the result is insignificant and denoted by H_0. The above-mentioned statement regarding cancer can be put in null hypothesis as

H_0: The prevalence of cancer in Faridkot district is 132/100000

or

$$H_0 : P = 132/100000$$

where P denotes the prevalence of cancer.

Alternate hypothesis is a tentative statistical statement, contrary to null hypothesis. It is denoted by H_1. For example,

$$H_1 : P \neq 132/100000$$

This type of alternative hypothesis is called two-tailed or two-sided hypothesis. An alternate hypothesis is said to be the right-tailed (sided) hypothesis if it is of greater than left-tailed type. For example, $H_1 : P > 132/100000$. An alternate hypothesis is said to be the left tailed if it is of less than right-tailed type. For example, $H_1 : P < 132/100000$.

From here, it is clear that there are three types of alternate hypothesis. One hypothesis is considered at a time in a problem. Every testing problem has two hypothesis; one is null hypothesis and other alternative hypothesis, and one is refuted based on the testing procedure.

Error in Testing

Two types of errors may creep out in testing of hypothesis procedure:

1. **Type-I Error:** It is the probability of rejection of null hypothesis when actually it is true. It is denoted by α. For example, suppose we know that the *oral contraceptive pills* (OCP) are not responsible for weight gain among the females. If one testing procedure rejects this hypothesis, this implies that we are committing type I error. If an X-ray machine reports a fracture in a bone but actually there is no fracture, then the testing procedure is committing type-I error.
2. **Type-II Error:** It is the probability of acceptance of null hypothesis when actually it is false. It is denoted by β. Considering the above example of X-ray machine, if fracture is there, but as per the testing procedure, it is claimed that there is no fracture. This is a case of type-II error.

Level of Significance: It is the amount of error that is acceptable to the researcher. It is denoted by α. Level of significance is same as that of the type-I error. And the quantity $(1 - \alpha)$ is known as confidence. Generally, α value is considered either 1% or 5%. This implies a confidence of 99% or 95%, respectively.

Now, first of all, we will discuss the parametric tests and then non-parametric tests.

Parametric Tests

Parametric statistical methods are based on a stringent assumption that the population from which the random sample has been drawn follows normal distribution with mean *m* and variance σ^2. Also, the parametric testing procedures are applicable primarily to the data which are measured in interval or ratio scale. The various parametric tests are *Z*-test, *t*-test, and *F*-test. *Z*-test is a large sample test, and *t*-test a small sample test. A sample is said to be a large sample if its size is more than thirty; that is, $n > 30$. Otherwise it is said to be a small sample. Small sample testing procedure can be used in place of large sample testing procedure, but the large sample testing procedure can't be used in place of the small sample testing procedure. This implies that the small sample testing procedures are valid in all the situations. Therefore, we will discuss *t*-test and *F*-test only. *F*-test will be in analysis of variance (ANOVA), multivariate analysis of variance (MANOVA) and analysis of covariance (ANCOVA). *t*-test and *F*-test are discussed in this section.

t-test for Testing the Single Mean

Suppose the hypothesis to be tested are

$$H_0 : \mu = \mu_0$$
$$H_1 : \mu = \mu_0$$

where μ_0 is the specified value of the mean of the population characteristic. In order to test this hypothesis, the following *t*-test statistic is used:

$$t = \frac{\bar{X} - \mu_0}{S/\sqrt{n}} \text{ with } (n - 1)\ d.f.$$

where $\bar{X}$ is the sample mean, *d.f.* stands for degrees of freedom, and *S* is the sample standard deviation which is given by,

$$S = \sqrt{\frac{1}{n-1}\left[\sum X^2 - \frac{(\sum X)^2}{n}\right]}$$

or $$S = \sqrt{\frac{1}{n-1}\left[\sum d^2 - \frac{(\sum d)^2}{n}\right]};\ d = X - A, A \text{ is assumed mean}$$

After calculating the above-mentioned t-test statistic (t_{cal}), a theoretical value of t-statistic at $\alpha/2$ level of significance is drawn from t-table denoted by $t_{\alpha/2}$. If $|t_{cal}| > t_{\alpha/2}$, then the null hypothesis is rejected; otherwise, accepted. For one-tailed test, if $t_{cal} > t_\alpha$ or $-t_{cal} < -t_\alpha$, then the null hypothesis is rejected; otherwise, accepted. This procedure of rejection or acceptance of null hypothesis will be same for F-test also.

For example a random sample of 10 boys had the following IQs: 70, 120, 110, 101, 88, 83, 95, 98, 107, and 100. Do these data support the assumption of a population mean IQ of 100? Find the reasonable range in which most of the mean IQ values of the samples of 10 boys lie.

Solution: Let us first set up the hypothesis of the given problem as follows:

$$H_0 : \mu = 100$$

$$H_1 : \mu \neq 100$$

The test statistic used to test this hypothesis is

$$t = \frac{\bar{X} - \mu_0}{S/\sqrt{n}} \text{ with } (n-1)\ d.f \tag{15.3}$$

where $\bar{X}$ and S are to be calculated from the sample values of IQs as follows:

X	d = X − 90	d²
70	−20	400
120	30	900
110	20	400
101	11	121
88	−2	4
83	−7	49
95	5	25
98	8	64
107	17	289
100	10	100
Total	**72**	**2352**

Here, $$\bar{X} = A + \frac{\sum d}{n} = 90 + \frac{72}{10} = 97.2$$

$$S^2 = \frac{1}{n-1}\left[\sum d^2 - \frac{(\sum d)^2}{n}\right]$$

$$= \frac{1}{9}\left[2352 - \frac{(72)^2}{10}\right]$$

$$= 203.73$$

or $$S = \sqrt{203.73} = 14.27$$

Substituting the values of $\bar{X}$ and S in (15.3), we get

$$t = \frac{97.2 - 100}{14.27/\sqrt{10}} = \frac{-2.8}{4.52} = -0.62$$

and $$|t| = 0.62 \quad \text{with } 9\ d.f.$$

$$t_{0.05/2}(9) = 2.262$$

Since $|t| < 2.262$, the null hypothesis is accepted at 5% level of significance. Hence, we conclude that the data are consistent with the assumption of mean IQ of 100 in the population.

For example the mean haemoglobin level of 25 preschool children was observed to be 10.50 gm/dl with standard deviation of 1.16 gm/dl. Is it significantly different from the mean of 11 gm/dl?

Solution:

$$H_0 : \mu = 11$$
$$H_1 : \mu \neq 11$$
$$\bar{X} = 10.5 \qquad SD = 1.16 \qquad n = 25$$

Now,

$$t = \frac{\bar{X} - \mu_0}{SD/\sqrt{n}}$$
$$= \frac{10.5 - 11}{1.16/\sqrt{25}} = -2.16$$

$$|t| = 2.16 \quad \text{and} \quad t_{0.05/2}(24) = 2.06$$

Since $|t| > 2.06$, the null hypothesis is rejected. Hence, we conclude that the mean haemoglobin level of 25 preschool children is significantly different from 11.

For example the mean serum vitamin A level of 10 students has 23 μg/dl with a variance of 40 μg/dl. Does this mean value differ from a mean value of 25 μg/dl observed in another study?

Solution:

$$H_0 : \mu = 25$$
$$H_1 : \mu \neq 25$$
$$\bar{X} = 23 \qquad S^2 = 40 \qquad n = 10$$

Now, $$t = \frac{\bar{X} - \mu_0}{S/\sqrt{n}} = \frac{23 - 25}{6.32/\sqrt{10}}$$

$$= \frac{-2}{2} = -1$$

and $$|t| = 1$$

$$t_{0.05/2}(9) = 2.262$$

Since $|t| < 2.262$, the null hypothesis is accepted. Hence, the difference in the mean values is not significant.

t-test for Testing the Difference of Mean of Two Independent Sample

This is also called an unpaired *t*-test. In this case, the hypotheses are

$$H_0 : \mu_1 = \mu_2$$
$$H_1 : \mu_1 \neq \mu_2$$

The test statistic to be applied to test the significant difference is

$$t = \frac{(\bar{X}_1 - \bar{X}_2)}{\sqrt{S^2\left(\frac{1}{n_1} + \frac{1}{n_2}\right)}} \quad \text{with } (n_1 + n_2 - 2) \ d.f.$$

where $\bar{X}_1, \bar{X}_2, n_1, n_2$, and S^2 are the mean of the first sample, mean of the second sample, size of the first sample, size of the second sample, and combined variance of both the samples, respectively, and S^2 is calculated as follows:

$$S^2 = \frac{(n_1 - 1)S_1^2 + (n_2 - 1)S_2^2}{n_1 + n_2 - 2}$$
$$= \frac{\Sigma(X_1 - \bar{X}_1)^2 + \Sigma(X_2 - \bar{X}_2)^2}{n_1 + n_2 - 2}$$

The formula of *t*-statistic is given above by assuming the equal variance of both the samples.

For example the mean values of birth weight with standard deviations and sample sizes are given below by socioeconomic status. Is the mean different in the birth weight significant between socioeconomic groups?

Detail	High Socioeconomic Group	Low Socioeconomic Group
Sample size	15	10
Man birth weight (kg)	2.91	2.26
Standard deviation	0.27	0.22

Solution: In this case, the hypotheses are

$$H_0 : \mu_1 = \mu_2$$
$$H_1 : \mu_1 \neq \mu_2$$
$$n_1 = 15 \quad \bar{X}_1 = 2.91 \quad S_1 = 0.27$$
$$n_2 = 10 \quad \bar{X}_2 = 2.26 \quad S_2 = 0.22$$

Test statistic *t* is given by,

$$t = \frac{(\bar{X}_1 - \bar{X}_2)}{\sqrt{S^2\left(\frac{1}{n_1} + \frac{1}{n_2}\right)}} \tag{15.4}$$

$$S^2 = \frac{(n_1 - 1)S_1^2 + (n_2 - 1)S_2^2}{n_1 + n_2 - 2}$$

$$S^2 = \frac{14 \times (0.27)^2 + 9 \times (0.22)^2}{15 + 10 - 2}$$

$$= \frac{1.02 + 0.44}{23} = 0.06$$

$$\frac{1}{n_1} + \frac{1}{n_2} = \frac{1}{15} + \frac{1}{10} = 0.17$$

Substituting the results of S^2 and $\left(\frac{1}{n_1} + \frac{1}{n_2}\right)$ in (15.4), we get

$$t = \frac{2.91 - 2.26}{\sqrt{0.06 \times 0.17}} = \frac{0.65}{0.10} = 6.5$$

$$d.f. = n_1 + n_2 - 2 = 23$$

$$t_{0.05/2}(23) = 2.398$$

Since $|t_{cal}| > 2.398$, the null hypothesis is rejected. Hence, we conclude that the mean difference in birth weight is significant between socioeconomic groups.

For example twenty-four experimental animals with vitamin D deficiency are divided equally into two groups. Groups I receives treatment with vitamin D and group II without vitamin D. At the end of the experimented period, serum calcium determination was made, and the results are provided below:

Details	Serum Calcium (Mean ± SD)	Sample Size
Group I	11.1 ± 0.50	12
Group II	7.8 ± 0.75	12

Can we conclude that the mean serum levels are not different between the two groups?

Solution:

$$H_0 : \mu_1 = \mu_2$$

$$H_1 : \mu_1 \neq \mu_2$$

$$n_1 = 12 \quad \bar{X}_1 = 11.1 \quad S_1 = 0.50$$

$$n_2 = 12 \quad \bar{X}_2 = 7.8 \quad S_2 = 0.75$$

$$t = \frac{(\bar{X}_1 - \bar{X}_2)}{\sqrt{S^2\left(\frac{1}{n_1} + \frac{1}{n_2}\right)}} \tag{15.5}$$

$$S^2 = \frac{(n_1 - 1)S_1^2 + (n_2 - 1)S_2^2}{n_1 + n_2 - 2}$$

$$= \frac{11\times(0.50)^2 + 11\times(0.75)^2}{12+12-2}$$

$$= \frac{11(0.25+0.56)}{22}$$

$$= \frac{8.91}{22} = 0.405$$

$$\frac{1}{n_1} + \frac{1}{n_2} = \frac{1}{12} + \frac{1}{12} = \frac{1}{6} = 0.17$$

Using the value of S^2 and $\frac{1}{n_1} + \frac{1}{n_2}$ in (15.5), we get

$$t = \frac{11.1-7.8}{\sqrt{0.405\times 0.17}} = \frac{3.3}{0.26}$$

$$= 12.69$$

$$d.f. = n_1 + n_2 - 2 = 22$$

$$t^{(22)}_{0.05/2} = 2.406$$

Since $|t_{cal}| > 2.406$, the null hypothesis is rejected. Hence, we calculate that the mean serum calcium levels are significantly different between the two groups.

Dependent Samples t-test or Paired t-test

Such a situation arises when any two samples are drawn in paired observations such that the second sample is dependent upon the first one. The purpose of this test is to test the significance of the intervention (treatment) given to a group. Such experiments result in two observations per individual: one before giving the treatment and other after treatment. For example, effects of a drug on a disease or on certain development are studied using paired *t*-test.

The test statistic is given by

$$t = \frac{\bar{d}}{s/\sqrt{n}} \quad \text{with } (n-1)\ d.f.$$

where, *d* is the change in the value of the variables; that is, $d = X_1 - X_2$ or $X_2 - X_1$

$$\bar{d} = \frac{\Sigma d}{n} \quad \text{and} \quad S = \sqrt{\frac{1}{n-1}\left[\Sigma d^2 - \frac{(\Sigma d)^2}{n}\right]}$$

For example the fat fold at triceps (mm) were recorded on 12 children before the commencement of the feeding programme and also at the end of the programme. Is there any change in the fat fold at triceps indicating the effect of the feeding programme?

	Fat Fold at Triceps	
Child No.	**At the Beginning (X_1)**	**At the End (X_2)**
1	6	8
2	8	8

(Continued)

Child No.	Fat Fold at Triceps	
	At the Beginning (X_1)	At the End (X_2)
3	8	10
4	6	7
5	5	6
6	9	10
7	6	9
8	7	8
9	6	5
10	6	7
11	4	4
12	8	6

Solution:

H_0: Feeding programme is not effective
H_1: Feeding programme is effective

X_1	X_2	$d = X_2 - X_1$	d^2
6	8	2	4
8	8	0	0
8	10	2	4
6	7	1	1
5	6	1	1
9	10	1	1
6	9	3	9
7	8	1	1
6	5	–1	1
6	7	1	1
4	4	0	0
8	6	–2	4
Total		**9**	**27**

$$\bar{d} = \frac{\Sigma d}{n} = \frac{9}{12} = 0.75,\ \Sigma d^2 = 27$$

$$S^2 = \frac{1}{n-1}\left[\Sigma d^2 - \frac{(\Sigma d)^2}{n}\right]$$

$$= \frac{1}{11}\left[27 - \frac{(9)^2}{12}\right] = \frac{1}{11}[27 - 6.75] = 1.84$$

$$S = 1.36$$

t-test statistic is given by

$$t = \frac{\bar{d}}{s/\sqrt{n}} = \frac{0.75}{1.36/\sqrt{12}}$$
$$= \frac{0.75}{0.39} = 1.92$$

$$d.f. = n - 1 = 11$$

$$t_{0.05}(11) = 2.20$$

Since $|t_{cal}| < 2.20$, the null hypothesis is accepted. Hence, we conclude that there is no change in fat fold at triceps, which means the feeding programme is not effective.

Analysis of Variance (ANOVA)

The analysis of variance is a powerful statistical tool for tests of significance. t-test is an adequate procedure only for testing the significance of the difference between two sample means. In order to test the significance of the difference among three or more than three sample means, ANOVA technique is applied.

For example, responses to four different treatments of anaemia, energy intake of individuals engaged in different activity levels, and so on. According to Prof. R. A. Fisher, ANOVA is the 'separation of variance ascribable to one group of causes from the variance ascribable to other group.' It is an application of F-test.

For example suppose four different treatments are given to four groups of patients, and we wish to test whether these treatments have had an effect on the percentage Hb level in blood. Random samples of 7 were taken from the groups, and the blood levels of Hb percentage were observed after one month. Can we say that the average Hb levels in four groups are significantly different?

	Treatments			
Patients	**A**	**B**	**C**	**D**
1	10.2	11.7	10.8	12.1
2	11	10.1	11.3	11.8
3	9.8	9.7	12.1	11.2
4	12.4	11.4	11.6	12.7
5	11.6	10.6	12.2	13.2
6	13.1	10.3	10.9	14.1
7	10.5	11.9	12.5	13.4

Solution:

H_0: $\mu_1 = \mu_2 = \mu_3 = \mu_4$
H_1: At least one pair is different

	A	B	C	D	Total (G)
	10.2	11.7	10.8	12.1	
	11	10.1	11.3	11.8	
	9.8	9.7	12.1	11.2	
	12.4	11.4	11.6	12.7	
	11.6	10.6	12.2	13.2	
	13.1	10.3	10.9	14.1	
	10.5	11.9	12.5	13.4	
Total	**78.6**	**75.7**	**81.4**	**88.5**	**324.2**

We calculate the various terms one by one as follows:

1. Raw sum of square (RSS) $= (10.2)^2 + (11.0)^2 + \ldots + (13.4)^2$
   $= 3788.46$

2. Correlation factor (CF) $= \dfrac{G^2}{N} = \dfrac{(324.2)^2}{28}$
   $= 3753.7728$

3. Total sum of square (TSS) $=$ RSS $-$ CF
   $= 3788.46 - 3753.7728$
   $= 34.6872$

4. Sum of square due to treatment (SST) $= \frac{1}{7}\left[(78.6)^2 + (75.7)^2 + \ldots + (88.5)^2\right] - \text{CF}$
   $= 3766.6657 - 3753.7728$
   $= 12.8929$

5. Error sum of square $=$ TSS $-$ SST
   $= 21.7943$

Now, we construct the ANOVA table to perform the rest of the calculations as given in the following table:

Source of Variation	Degrees of Freedom (*d.f.*)	Sum of Squares (SS)	Mean Sum of Squares (MSS)	*F*-ratio
Treatment	3	12.8929	$\dfrac{12.8929}{3} = 4.2976$ 21.7943/24 = 0.9081	4.2976/0.9088 = 4.7325
Error	24	21.7943		
Total	**27**			

Therefore
$$F_{\text{cal}} = 4.7325$$
$$F_{0.05}(3, 24) = 3.49 \quad \text{and} \quad F_{0.01}(3, 24) = 5.95$$

At 5% level of significance, $F_{cal} > 3.49$; therefore, the null hypothesis is rejected. Hence, we conclude that at least one pair is significantly different.

At H level of significance, $F_{cal} < 5.95$; therefore, the null hypothesis is accepted. Hence, we conclude that there is no significant difference among the average of four groups.

Multivariate Analysis of Variance (MANOVA)

MANOVA technique is multivariate ANOVA. This is used when we have more than one study variable along with the categorical variables. When we apply ANOVA on the multivariate data, it is called MANOVA. Detail of this topic is beyond the scope of this book.

Analysis of Covariance (ANCOVA)

ANCOVA technique is used when the initial value of the variable influences the final value, for example, studying the differences in average systolic BP values of two groups of heart patients after giving two different drugs, taking into consideration the information on BP values before and after giving the drugs. Hence it is known that BP values after giving the drugs are influenced by values before giving the drugs. If this fact is not taken into consideration, the conclusion arrived at only from the final values would be misleading. The most appropriate design used in such situations is ANCOVA, which takes care of such influences. It is again an application of F-test.

Design of Experiment

Experience has shown that proper consideration of the statistical analysis before the experiment is calculated forces the experiments to plan more carefully the design of the experiment. The design of the experiment may be defined as 'the logical construction of the experiment in which the degree of uncertainty with which the inference is drawn may be well defined'.

Randomized Block Design (RBD)

This design is generally applied when the experimental material is not homogeneous. To achieve the homogeneity, total heterogeneous materials are divided into relatively more homogeneous groups called blocks. Each block contains equal number of cases, and a block is considered to be the homogeneous group. For example, in some circumstances, littermates may be more alike in response than the members of different litters. If, say, five treatments are to be compared, one could take litters of five animals and allocate treatments at random to the individual animals in each litter so that each treatment occurs once in each litter. RBD controls the variation in one direction. In this case, either rows are blocks or columns are blocks. The number of treatments is equal to the size of the block.

Latin Square Design (LSD)

LSD controls the variations in two directions. Here, rows as well as columns are considered as blocks. LSDs are the more efficient designs as compared to the RBD as the former controls more variations than the later. In this design, the number of treatments is equal to the number of replications.

Non-parametric Tests

The hypothesis tests t-tests, F-test, and so on are called the parametric tests. These testing procedures depend upon the assumption of normal distribution that population from which the sample has been drawn follows normal distribution. But the assumption of normality can't be met all the time. So, in such situations, non-parametric tests are applied. Non-parametric testing procedures do not require any assumption regarding population distribution. Therefore, sometimes non-parametric tests are called distribution-free tests. Some important non-parametric tests are discussed below:

Chi-square (χ^2) Test for Association

Here, the procedure for conducting the χ^2 test for testing the association between two attributes is best explained by an example.

For example the distribution of 100 individuals by their hair colour and eye colour is given below. Is there any association between these two attributes?

	Hair Colour			
Eye Colour	**Black**	**Fair**	**Brown**	**Total**
Blue	25	12	8	45
Green	20	5	5	30
Brown	15	5	5	25
Total	**60**	**22**	**18**	**100**

Solution:
H_0: There is no association between hair colour and eye colour.
First, we have to estimate various expected frequencies as

$$E(25) = \frac{45 \times 60}{100} = 27$$

$$E(12) = \frac{45 \times 22}{100} = 12$$

Similarly,

$$E(8) = 8$$
$$E(20) = 18$$
$$E(5) = 7$$
$$E(5) = 5$$
$$E(5) = 15$$
$$E(5) = 5$$
$$E(5) = 5$$

Calculations are performed in the following table:

O	*E*	*O* – *E*	$(O-E)^2$	$(O-E)^2/E$
25	27	–2	4	0.1481
12	10	2	4	0.4000
8	8	0	0	0

O	*E*	*O*−*E*	$(O-E)^2$	$(O-E)^2/E$
20	18	2	4	0.2222
5	7	−2	4	0.5714
5	5	0	0	0
15	15	0	0	0
5	5	0	0	0
5	5	0	0	0
				$\chi^2 = 1.3417$

$$d.f. = (\text{rows} - 1)\,(\text{columns} - 1)$$
$$= (r-1)\,(c-1) = (3-1)\,(3-1)$$
$$= 4$$
$$\chi^2_{0.05}(4) = 9.49$$

Since $\chi^2_{\text{cal}} < 9.49$, the null hypothesis is accepted. We conclude that there is no association between the two attributes.

Sign Test

Sign test is the simplest test of all the non-parametric tests. This test is based on the direction of a sample of observations (i.e., + or – signs). Under this test, we examine the null hypothesis that + and – signs are values of a random variable having the binomial distribution with $p = \frac{1}{2}$. In this test, the null hypothesis is

$$H_0\colon p = \frac{1}{2} \quad \text{or} \quad \mu = \mu_0$$

For example from the following mark percentages of 16 students selected at random from a coaching institute, test the claim of the institute through sign test that all its students get 80% marks on an average in the competitive tests.

Roll No.	1	5	9	13	17	21	26	31	36	41	46	51	61	71	81	91
Marks	82	75	95	90	80	83	77	79	81	92	76	74	72	97	98	74

Solution:

$$H_0\colon \mu = 80$$
$$H_1\colon \mu \neq 80$$

Marks	82	75	95	90	80	83	77	79	81	92	76	74	72	97	98	78
Signs	+	–	+	+	0	+	–	–	+	+	–	–	–	+	+	–

Total number of signs (n) = 15 (ignoring one zero)
Total number of fewer sign (S) = 7 (–)

The critical value of the fewer sign (–) at 5 + level of significance is given by

$$K = \frac{n-1}{2} - 0.92\sqrt{n}$$

$$= \frac{15-1}{2} - 0.92\sqrt{15}$$

$$= 7 - 3.8 = 3.2$$

Thus, $S > K$; therefore, the null hypothesis is accepted.

Mann–Whitney Test

This non-parametric test was devised by the joint efforts of Mann and Whitney. This test is an improvement over the sign test, which ignores the actual magnitude of the observations. This test is applied to test whether two independent samples have come from the same population or not. This test is also known as U-test and utilizes the results to estimate the test statistic. Mann–Whitney U-test is an alternative to the independent t-test. The test statistic U is defined in terms of T as

$$U = n_1 n_2 + \frac{n_2(n_2+1)}{2} - R_2$$

or

$$U = n_1 n_2 + \frac{n_1(n_1+1)}{2} - R_1$$

where n_1 and n_2 are the sample sizes and R_1 and R_2 are the rank totals of group one and two, respectively.

STATISTICAL PACKAGES AND ITS APPLICATIONS IN NURSING AND ALLIED HEALTH SCIENCES

A statistical package is a suite of computer programmes that are specialized for statistical analysis. It enables people to obtain the results of standard statistical procedures and statistical significance tests, without requiring low-level numerical programming. Most statistical packages also provide facilities for the data management.

Statistical analysis is a vital component in every aspect of research. Nursing and allied sciences research are based on the social surveys, laboratory experiments, clinical trials, and so on. All these require statistical treatment of the data before arriving to the valid research findings and conclusions. Today's researchers require the use of statistical techniques and packages to reduce the time consumption for the analysis of bulky data. The findings of any research are required to be justified in the light of statistical logic, but manually, it is very difficult for a researcher to do even simple statistics such as averages, percentages, and standard deviation for a large number of data.

With the availability of standard computer packages, it is now an easy job to compute all the statistical parameters, by even having some basic knowledge of computer and Microsoft Window's applications. The researcher has only to decide which tool to be used for a particular analysis, and the rest of the job will be done by the computer and software package. Graphical aids of software package would also help in the proper interpretation of the results.

Due to the arrival of computers and software for data analysis, the task of data analysis is considerably reduced. The researcher has to decide on appropriate technique and understand how to interpret the result of the analysis. The actual analysis part is performed by the computers. There are many versatile software packages available. The most widely known and used software package is statistical package for social sciences (SPSS) package.

SPSS was released in its first version in 1968 after being developed by Norman H. Nie and C. Hadlai Hull. Norman Nie was then a political science postgraduate at Stanford University and now a research professor in the Department of Political Science at Stanford, and Professor Emeritus was in the Department of Political Science at the University of Chicago. Several computer packages are available to be used for the statistical analysis; among them, the commonly used packages are Microsoft Excel, SPSS, SAS, Minitab, Stata, Systat, NCSS, and so on.

Microsoft Excel

Microsoft Excel is a very popular and useful spreadsheet programme that can be used for data entry. It has the capacity to generate random numbers, and it can be used for the computation of many standard statistical applications such as computation of mean, range, standard deviation, and so on. It can also be used for relatively sophisticated work such as computing regression and ANOVA.

SPSS

SPSS was developed in 1960 at Stanford University to help solve problems in the social sciences. SPSS now stands for statistical product and services solutions and is among the most comprehensive and popular statistical packages. In addition to its provisioning for the standard procedures needed in descriptive statistics, it can also provide for regression analysis and analysis of variance (ANOVA). It is also capable of multivariate analysis involving sophisticated techniques namely, cluster analysis, time series analysis, and so on. The product is also capable of determining the sample size and estimating the power of a statistical procedure. To know more about SPSS, visit the web site www.spss.com.

The SPSS, now known as PASW (predictive analytics software), is a widely used statistical package worldwide for the analysis of data. The release history of software is as follows:

1. SPSS 15.0.1—November 2006
2. SPSS 16.0.2—April 2008
3. SPSS statistics 17.0.1—December 2008
4. PASW statistics 17.0.3—September 2009
5. PASW statistics 18.0—August 2009
6. PASW statistics 18.0.1—December 2009

SAS

The statistical analysis system (SAS) is very comprehensive software developed by North Carolina State University. This software is divided into many modules, and its licensing is flexible, based upon the need for functions. This system contains a very large variety of statistical methods and is the software of choice of many major businesses, including the entire pharmaceutical industry. SAS has also developed a PC SAS, which is compatible with personal computer and has a user-friendly Windows interface. The more useful components of SAS are Base SAS, SAS/STST, SAS/GRAPH, and so on. An advantage of SAS is its capability to transport data files in various formats and convert them to SAS data set without much efforts. To learn more, visit their web site www.sas.com.

Minitab

This is another statistical package designed to facilitate the teaching of statistical methods by using computer. The Minitab is also a very user-friendly product with well-designed documentation facilities that are being used widely in educational institutions. To learn more about Minitab, visit their web site www.minitab.com.

THE SPSS ENVIRONMENT

There are excellent tests that give introduction to the general environment within which SPSS operates. The best ones include Kinnear and Gray (1997) and Foster (1998). Once SPSS has been activated, the programme will automatically load two Windows: *the data editor* and the *output Window.*

1. **Data Editor:** This is where you input your data and carry out statistical functions.
2. **Output Window:** This is where the results of any statistical functions.

There are a number of additional Windows that can be activated. Another Window that is useful is the syntax Window, which allows to enter SPSS commands manually.

Data Editor

The main SPSS Window includes a data editor for entering data. This Window is where most of the actions happen. At the top of this screen is a menu bar similar to the ones you might have seen in other programmes such as Microsoft Word. There are several menus at the top of the screen that can be activated by using the computer mouse to move the on-screen arrow onto the desired menu and then pressing the left menu button once. When you have clicked on the menu, a menu box will appear that displays a list of options that can be activated by moving the on-screen arrow so that it is pointing at the desired option and then clicking with the mouse. Often, selecting an option from a menu makes a Window appear; these Windows are referred to as dialogue boxes.

Within these menus, you will notice that some letters are underlined; these underlined letters represent the keyboard shortcut for accessing that function. It is possible to select many functions without using the mouse, and the experienced keyboard user may find these shortcuts faster than maneuvring the mouse arrow to the appropriate place on the screen.

Coding

The data can be categorized into two types. The first one is qualitative data, which signify an attribute such as affection, gender, level of satisfaction, colour, and taste, which cannot be expressed on an interval scale or in some measured units. The second one is quantitative data, which signify a measurement on an interval scale such as body mass index, blood cholesterol level, plant height, distance, and income of a person.

For the analysis of data through statistical package, the collected data are required to be coded in numeric form. The coded data have to be later decoded for the purpose of interpretation. Example of qualitative data is a questionnaire or tool when there is an option such as 'Yes' and 'No' or 'Male' and 'Female'. The option can be coded as '1' for 'Yes' and '0' for 'No'; similarly, '1' for 'Male' and '0' for 'Female'. In the same way, if there are more than one option, they require a multilevel code. For instance, the level of agreement over an issue may be coded giving '2' for 'Strongly Agree', '1' for 'Agree', and '0' for 'Disagree'. In the case of quantitative data, one may use the code '1' for the monthly income of a responded less than 10,000, code '2' if it is between 10,001 and 20,000, code '3' if it is between 20,001 and 30,000, and so on. Other example of quantitative data coding is, age group 'less than 20' may be coded as '1', age group with '20–30' may be coded as '2' and the age group 'more than 30' may be coded as '3', and so on.

Menu

File: This menu allows you to do general things such as saving data, graphs, or output. You can previously save files and print graphs, data, or output.

Edit: This menu contains the edit functions for the data editor. In SPSS for Windows, it is possible to cut and paste blocks of numbers from one part of the data editor to another.

Data: This menu allows you to make changes to the data editor. The important features are insert variable, which is used to insert a new variable into the data editor, and insert case, which is used to add a new role of data between two existing rows of data.

Transform: You should use this menu if you want to manipulate one of your variables in some way. The computer function is also useful for transforming data. This function allows you to carry out any number of calculations on your variables.

Analyse: This menu is called statistics in version 8 and earlier. The fun begins here because the statistical procedure lurks in this menu. Brief guide to the options in the statistics menu is as follows:

1. Descriptive statistics
2. Compare means
3. General linear model
4. Correlate
5. Regression
6. Data reduction
7. Nonparametric
8. Graphs

Inputting Data

When you first load SPSS, it will provide a blank data editor with the title 'New Data'. When inputting a new set of data, you must input your data in a logical way. The SPSS data editor is arranged in such a way that each row represents the data from one subject, while each column represents a variable: both types should be placed in a separate column. The key point is that each row represents one participant's data. Therefore, any information about that case should be entered across the data editor.

The Output Viewer

Alongside the main SPSS Window, there is a second Window known as the output viewer (or output navigator in version 7 and 7.5). In the earlier versions of SPSS, this is simply called the output Window, and its functions is, in essence, the same. However, the output Window of the previous version displayed only statistical result; the new, improved and generally amazing output viewer will happily display graphs, tables, and statistical result and all in a much nicer front. On the right-hand side, there is a large space, in which the output is displayed. SPSS displays both graphs and the result of the statistical analyses in this part of the viewer. It is also possible to edit graphs, and to do this, you simply double-click on the graph you wish to edit (this creates a new Window in which the graph can be edited). There are a number of icons in the output viewer Window that help you to do things quickly without using the drop-down menus. Some of these icons are the same as those described for the data editor Window.

However, you can save data in different formats such as Microsoft Excel files and tab-delimited text.

Steps to be Followed for Data Analysis Using the SPSS

The following are the steps to be followed for data analysis using the SPSS:

1. Coding of questionnaire/data or transferring of data directly into the spreadsheet of software
2. Preparation of manual spreadsheet (MSS)
3. Entering of data into package's spread sheet
4. Calculation of results or tests

Coding of Questionnaire

The whole questionnaire or data collection tool should be numerically coded for the purposes of data analysis because coding technique is a time-saving device. An example of questionnaire after assignment of numeric codes is given in Fig. 15.6:

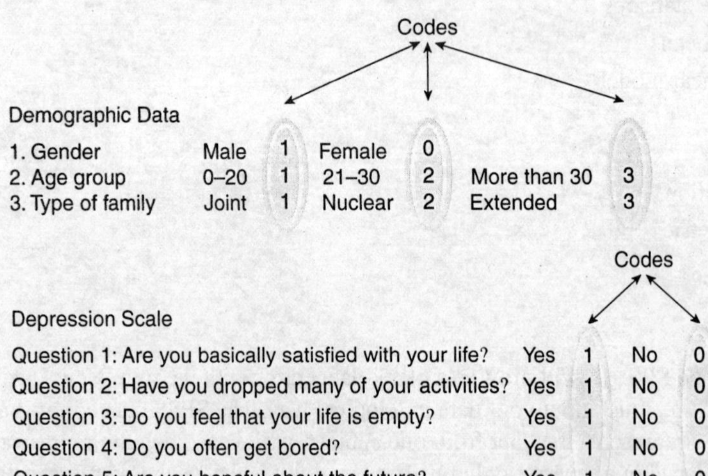

FIGURE 15.6 *Sample of Coded Questionnaire or Tool*

The same coding procedure is to be followed for other questions as well.

Preparation of MSS

MSS may be prepared for all the coded data. An example of MSS is given in Fig. 15.7.

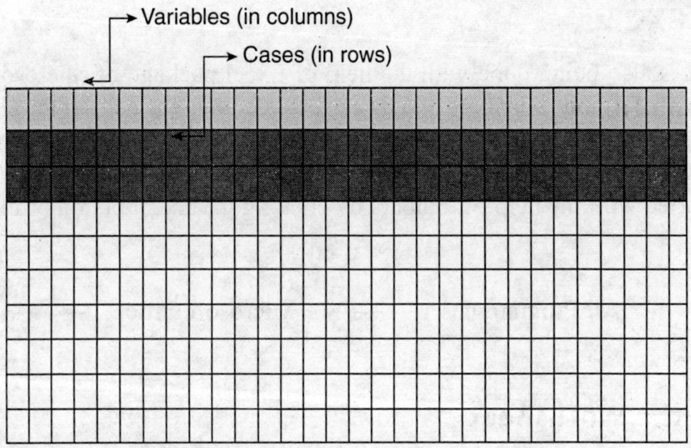

FIGURE 15.7 *Preparation of Master Data Sheet*

Note: It can be prepared according to the number of variables in the questionnaire. But 30 columns and 30 rows sheet can be a sufficient data sheet for data analysis. More sheets can be pasted on the right-hand side of the sheet, if variables are more than 30, and more sheets can be used, if cases are more than 30.

Entering Data in the Spreadsheet of SPSS

Opening a new spreadsheet:

1. Click on start menu.
2. Choose the SPSS icon from programme files or click the shortcut of SPSS package on the desktop.

The window shown in Fig. 15.8 will be opened:

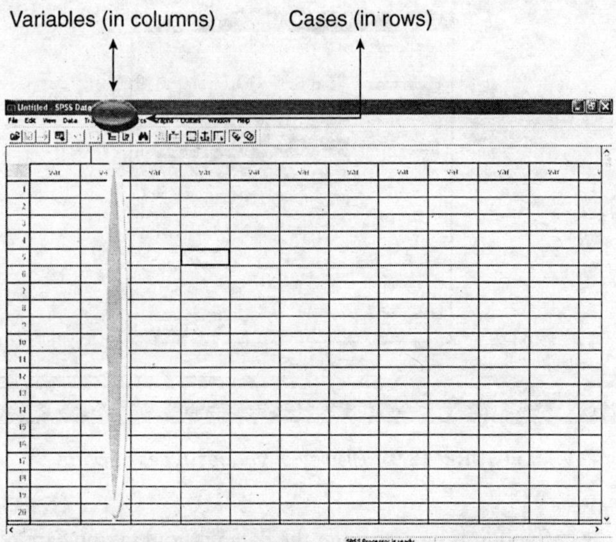

FIGURE 15.8 *Opening of SSPS System*

Results can be calculated as per the need and options available in the package.

MICROSOFT EXCEL

Data analysis work is also being done with the help of Excel package of Microsoft Office. It is a big worksheet in the form of a table. Any type of data can be entered in the cells of the table, but calculations can be done for numeric data only. It is helpful to perform several statistical calculations without writing any kind of programmes and also helpful to draw high-quality graphs to represent data.

Excel can be started with the help of toolbars by clicking the Excel button or through using the following steps:

Start ⟶ All Programmes ⟶ Microsoft Office ⟶ MS Excel

Data Entry on the Worksheet

In the worksheet, both the numeric and the character data can be entered in any cell. There are several types of data formats available, which can be viewed by clicking

Format ⟶ Cells

The screen shown in Fig. 15.9 will be displayed, in which various types of defining the data are given:

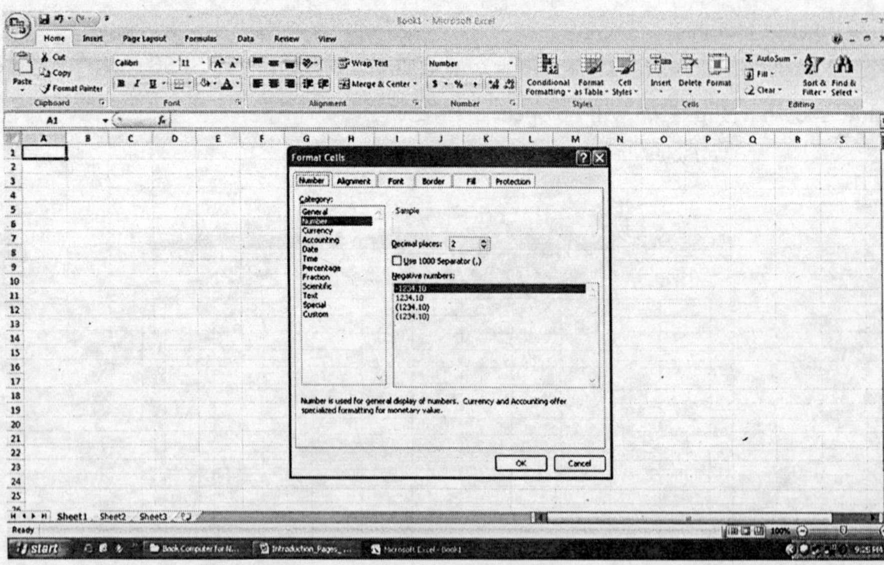

FIGURE 15.9 *Display of Various Types of Data*

Once the type of cells is defined, it is easy to enter the data without taking care of the format. The default setting will be general, in which one can enter both numeric and non-numeric data. For example, if data related to date, month, and year are required to be entered, then field 'date' can be chosen. Similarly, other fields can be opted on the basis of need and data.

Calculations on the Worksheet

Excel can be used to do the routine calculations such as sum, difference, average, standard deviation, and percentage. For example, in Fig. 15.10 the average of the data shown is calculated.

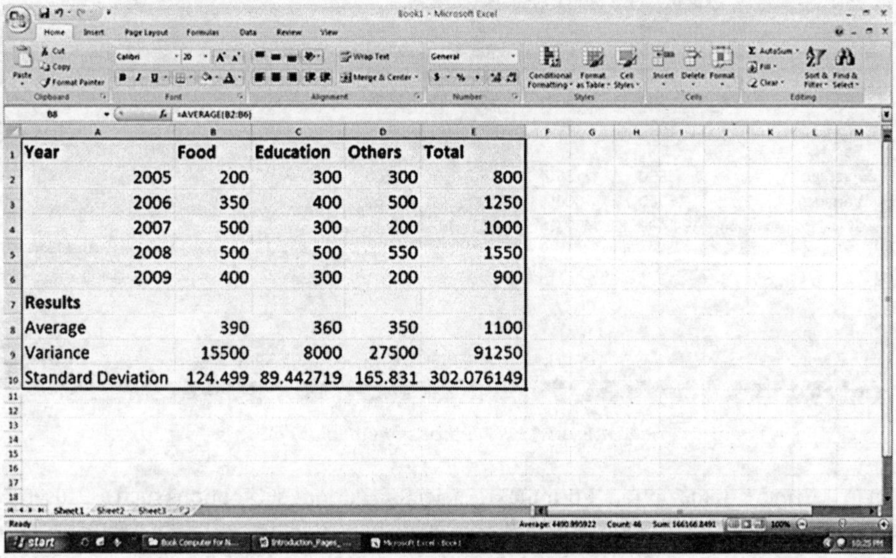

FIGURE 15.10 *Calculation Methods in EXCEL Work Sheet*

To do this, leave one row as a gap between the data and the results. The following steps are required to follow to calculate the results:

1. Keep the cursor at cell B8.
2. In this cell, type the command @AVERAGE(B2:B6) and press the Enter button. This will display the average values of data from B2 to B6.
3. Now put the cursor at B9 and type @VAR(B2:B6) and press the Enter button. The variance values will be displayed for the data from B2 to B6.
4. To calculate the standard deviation of the above-mentioned data, type @STDEV(B2:B6) and press the Enter key.
5. To get the results of other two columns, the facility of Copy and Paste can be used.

Built-in Functions for Quick Use

Excel has many built-in functions to perform special calculations without typing any formula. To calculate the desired results, selection of that particular function is required along with the selection of the range of values on which it should be applied. In order to see the function, click on the icon *fx* or just select the buttons on the menu bar (Fig. 15.11).

Insert ⟶ Function (In case of MS Excel 2003)

Formulas (In case of MS Excel 2007)

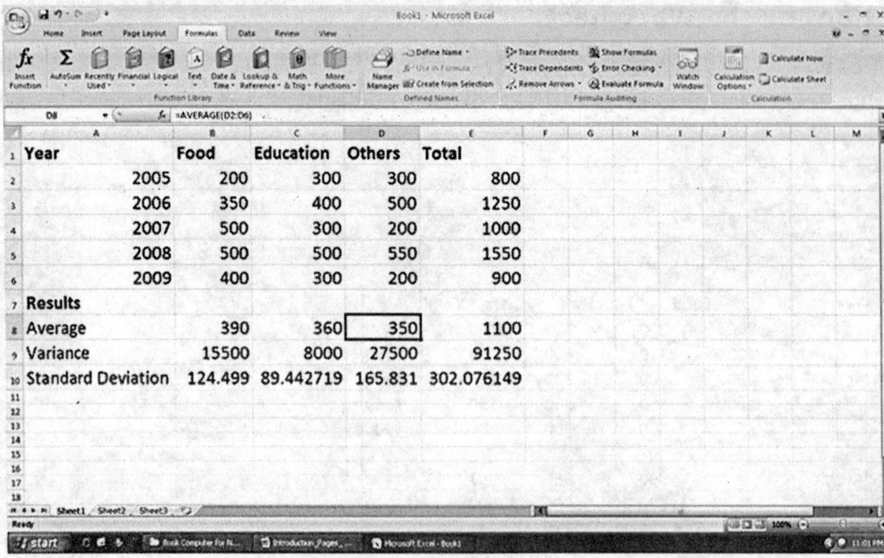

FIGURE 15.11 *Methods of Calculating Sums*

As shown in the figure, if the option 'Formulas' is selected, various sub-options such as 'Insert Function', 'Auto Sum', 'Recently Used', and so on will also be displayed. After selecting the category, the list of available functions will be displayed in the down pane. For instance, if we choose the category 'Auto Sum', we will get a list of functions in the down pane. If we click on 'Sum', we will get a screen asking for various input parameters such as the cells to be included in the calculation of Sum. The results of SUM function will be displayed in the cell where the cursor is placed.

Thus, Excel can be a very useful package for any kind of statistical calculations.

KEY POINTS

- **Statistics:** The word *statistics* refers to either quantitative information or a method of dealing with quantitative or qualitative information.
- **Biostatistics** is the branch of statistics applied to biological or medical sciences. Biostatistics is also called biometry and may be defined as a science of figure and variation.
- **Data** may be defined as any group of measurements that is of our interest. Data are broadly classified into two categories as quantitative data and qualitative data.
- **Central Tendency or Average** is considered to be the representative of the group.
- **Dispersion:** The word literally means scatterings, deviation, or spread of group of observations from their average value.
- **Measures of Dispersion:** Means the various possible methods of measuring the dispersions.
- **Normal Distribution:** It is a theoretical continuous distribution. The theory of normal distribution was developed by a famous English mathematician Abraham Dr. Moivre in 1733. Many statistical problems are solved by using normal distribution.
- **Measures of Relationship:** For assessing the linear relationship between the variables, correlation analysis and regression analysis are generally employed.

- **Inferential Statistics** is a branch of statistics that deals with drawing the inferences about the population characteristics under study based on the random sample drawn from the population of interest.
- **Parametric Tests:** Parametric statistical methods are based on a stringent assumption that the population from which the random sample has been drawn follows normal distribution with mean *m* and variance *s* 2. Also, the parametric testing procedures are applicable primarily to the data which are measured in interval or ratio scale.
- **Non-parametric** testing procedures do not require any assumption regarding population distribution. Therefore, sometimes non-parametric tests are called distribution-free tests. Some important non-parametric tests are chi square, *Mann–Whitney Test, etc.*
- **Statistical Package:** A statistical package is a suite of computer programmes that are specialized for statistical analysis.
- **Statistical Package for Social Sciences:** The SPSS, now known as PASW (predictive analytics software), is a widely used statistical package worldwide for the analysis of data.
- **SAS:** The statistical analysis system (SAS) is very comprehensive software developed by North Carolina State University.
- **Minitab:** This is another statistical package designed to facilitate the teaching of statistical methods by using computer.

QUESTIONS

I. Essay-type Questions

1. Describe frequency distribution and graphical presentation of data.
2. (a) What do you mean by confidence interval?
   (b) Why median is used when there are extreme scores in a distribution?
   (c) Calculate median for the following series:
   48, 35, 36, 40, 42, 54, 58, 60, 64, 66, and 25
3. Define Statistical package?
4. Enumerate various statistical packages available in market?
5. Describe about SPSS package in detail?

II. Short Notes

1. Mann–Whitney test
2. Correlation and its types
3. Descriptive and inferential statistics
4. Normal distribution
5. Measures of variability
6. Write briefly about SAS?
7. Enlist the steps for using SPSS?

III. Multiple-choice Questions

Circle the alphabet before the best answer

1. The class interval of the continuous grouped data

   10–19
   20–29
   30–39
   40–49
   50–59

   is:

   (a) 9 (b) 10
   (c) 14.5 (d) 4.5

2. With the help of histogram, we can prepare
   (a) frequency polygon
   (b) frequency curve
   (c) frequency distribution
   (d) all the above

3. In a bar diagram, the baseline is
   (a) horizontal (b) vertical
   (c) false baseline (d) all of the above

4. Which of the following is a measure of the central value?
   (a) Standard deviation
   (b) Median
   (c) Mean deviation
   (d) Range

5. If two observations are 20 and –20, the arithmetic mean is
   (a) 10 (b) 20
   (c) 0 (d) 40

6. Which of the following is a unitless measure of dispersion?
   (a) Standard deviation
   (b) Mean deviation
   (c) Coefficient of variation
   (d) Range

7. Variance of the following distribution

Classes	Frequency
2–4	2
4–6	5
6–8	4
8–10	1

   is approximately equal to
   (a) 2.5 (b) 2.9
   (c) 5 (d) 3.9

8. Whether a test is one sided or two sided depends on
   (a) alternative hypothesis
   (b) level of significance
   (c) null hypothesis
   (d) all of the above

9. Paired *t*-test is applicable when the observations in two samples are
   (a) paired
   (b) correlated
   (c) equal in number
   (d) all of the above

10. Degrees of freedom for statistic chi-square in case of contingency table of order (2×2) is
    (a) 3 (b) 4
    (c) 2 (d) 1

11. SPSS stands for
    (a) Statistical Package for Social Sciences
    (b) Statistical Process of Social sciences
    (c) Social Package for Statistical Sciences
    (d) None of the above

12. Once SPSS has been activated, the programme will automatically load two Windows:
    (a) Crosstab and the descriptive statistics
    (b) the data editor and output Window.
    (c) File and MS Excel
    (d) All of the above

13. Statistical package for Social Sciences, SPSS was developed in
    (a) 1950 (b) 1954
    (c) 1960 (d) 1964

Answer Keys

1. (b)	2. (d)	3. (b)	4. (b)	5. (c)	6. (c)	7. (b)	8. (a)
9. (d)	10. (b)	11. (a)	12. (b)	13. (c)			

FURTHER READING

Bhaskara Raj D. Elakkuvana, 2010. *Nursing Research and Biostatistics*. Bangalore: Emmess Medical Publishers. pp. 465–468.

Sarma, K. V. S. *Statistics Made Simple: Do It Yourself on PC.* New Delhi: PHI. pp.1–99.

www.minitab.com.

www.sas.com.

www.spss.com.

www.wikipedia.com.

Appendix: Statistical Tables

TABLE A1 *Random Digits*

49487	52802	28667	62058	87822	14704	18519	17889	45869	14454
29480	91539	46317	84803	86056	62812	33584	70391	77749	64906
25252	97738	23901	11106	86864	55808	22557	23214	15021	54268
02431	42193	96960	19620	29188	05863	92900	06836	13433	21709
69414	89353	70724	67893	23218	72452	03095	68333	13751	37260
77285	35179	92042	67581	67673	68374	71115	98166	43352	06414
52852	11444	71863	34534	69124	02760	06406	95234	87995	79560
98740	98054	30195	09891	18453	79464	01156	95522	06884	55073
85022	58736	12138	35146	62085	36170	25433	80787	96496	40579
17778	03840	21636	56269	08149	19001	67367	13138	02400	89515
81833	93449	57781	94621	90998	37561	59688	93299	27726	82167
63789	54958	33167	10909	40343	81023	61590	44474	39810	10305
61640	81740	60986	12498	71546	42249	13812	59902	27864	21809
42243	10153	20891	90883	15782	98167	86837	99166	92143	82441
45236	09129	53031	12260	01278	14404	40969	33419	14188	69557
40338	42477	78804	36272	72053	07958	67158	60979	79891	92409
54040	71253	88789	98203	54999	96564	00789	68879	47134	83941
49158	20908	44859	29089	76130	51442	34453	98590	37353	61137
80958	03808	83655	18415	96563	43582	82207	53322	30419	64435
07636	04876	61063	57571	69434	14965	20911	73162	33576	52839
37227	80750	08261	97048	60438	75053	05939	34414	16685	32103
99460	45915	45637	41353	35335	69087	57536	68414	10247	93253
60248	75845	37296	33783	42393	28185	31880	00241	31642	37526
95076	79089	87380	28982	97750	82221	35584	27444	85793	69755
20944	97852	26586	32796	51513	47475	48621	20067	88975	39506
30458	49207	62358	41532	30057	53017	10375	97204	98675	77634
38905	91282	79309	49022	17405	18830	09186	07629	01785	78317
96545	15638	90114	93730	13741	70177	49175	42113	21600	69625
21944	28328	00692	89164	96025	01383	50252	67044	70596	58266
36910	71928	63327	00980	32154	46006	62289	28079	03076	15619
48745	47626	28856	28382	60639	51370	70091	58261	70135	88259
32519	91993	59374	83994	59873	51217	62806	20028	26545	16820

(*Continued*)

TABLE A1 *Random Digits (Continued)*

75757	12965	29285	11481	31744	41754	24428	81819	02354	37895
07911	97756	89561	27464	25133	50026	16436	75846	83718	08533
89887	03328	76911	93168	56236	39056	67905	94933	05456	52347
30543	99488	75363	94187	32885	23887	10872	22793	26232	87356
68442	55201	33946	42495	28384	89889	50278	91985	58185	19124
22403	56698	88524	13692	55012	25343	76391	48029	72278	58586
70701	36907	51242	52083	43126	90379	60380	98513	85596	16528
69804	96122	42342	28467	79037	13218	63510	09071	52438	25840
65806	22398	19470	63653	27055	02606	43347	65384	02613	81668
43902	53070	54319	19347	59506	75440	90826	53652	92382	67623
49145	71587	14273	62440	15770	03281	58124	09533	43722	03856
47363	36295	62126	42358	20322	82000	52830	93540	13284	96496
26244	87033	90247	79131	38773	67687	45541	54976	17508	18367
72875	39496	06385	48458	30545	74383	22814	36752	10707	48774
09065	16283	61398	08288	00708	21816	39615	03102	02834	04116
68256	51225	92645	77747	33104	81206	00112	53445	04212	58476
38744	81018	41909	70458	72459	66136	97266	26490	10877	45022
44375	19619	35750	59924	82429	90288	61064	26489	87001	84273
57780	97609	52482	12783	88768	12323	64967	22970	11204	37576
68327	00067	17487	49149	25894	23639	86557	04139	10756	76285
55888	82253	67464	91628	88764	43598	45481	00331	15900	97699
84910	44827	31173	44247	56573	91759	79931	26644	27048	53704
35654	53638	00563	57230	07395	10813	99194	81592	96834	21374
46381	60071	20835	43110	31842	02855	73446	24456	24268	85291
11212	06034	77313	66896	47902	63483	09924	83635	30013	61791
49703	07226	73337	49223	73312	09534	64005	79267	76590	26066
05482	30340	24606	99042	16536	14267	84084	16198	94852	44305
92947	65090	47455	90675	89921	13036	92867	04786	76776	18675
51806	61445	32437	01129	03644	70024	07629	55805	85616	59569
16383	30577	91319	67998	72423	81307	75192	80443	09651	30068
30893	85406	42369	71836	74479	68273	78133	34506	68711	58725

(*Continued*)

TABLE A1 *Random Digits (Continued)*

59790	11682	63156	10443	99033	76460	36814	36917	37232	66218
06271	74980	46094	21881	43525	16516	26393	89082	24343	57546
93325	61834	40763	81178	17507	90432	50973	35591	36930	03184
46690	08927	32962	24882	83156	58597	88267	32479	80440	41668
82041	88942	57572	34539	43812	58483	43779	42718	46798	49079
14306	04003	91186	70093	62700	99408	72236	52722	37531	24590
63471	77583	80056	59027	37031	05819	90836	19530	07138	36431
68467	17634	84211	31776	92996	75644	82043	84157	10877	12536
94308	57895	08121	07088	65080	51928	74237	00449	86625	06626
52218	32502	82195	43867	79935	34620	37386	00243	46353	44499
46586	08309	52702	85464	06670	18796	74713	81632	34056	56461
07869	80471	69139	82408	33989	44250	79597	15182	14956	70423
46719	60281	88638	26909	32415	31864	53708	60219	44482	40004
74687	71227	59716	80619	56816	73807	94150	21991	22901	74351
42731	50249	11685	54034	12710	35159	00214	19440	61539	25717
71740	29429	86822	01187	96497	25823	18415	06087	05886	11205
96746	05938	11828	47727	02522	33147	92846	15010	96725	67903
27564	81744	51909	36192	45263	33212	71808	24753	72644	74441
21895	29683	26533	14740	94286	90342	24674	52762	22051	31743
01492	40778	05988	65760	13468	31132	37106	02723	40202	15824
55846	19271	22846	80425	00235	34292	72181	24910	25245	81239
14615	75196	40313	50783	66585	39010	76796	31385	26785	66830
77848	15755	91938	81915	65312	86956	26195	61525	97406	67988
87167	03106	52876	31670	23850	13257	77510	42393	53782	32412
73018	56511	89388	73133	12074	62538	57215	23476	92150	14737
29247	67792	10593	22772	03407	24319	19525	24672	21182	10765
17412	09161	34905	44524	20124	85151	25952	81930	43536	39705
68805	19830	87973	99691	25096	41497	57562	35553	77057	06161
40551	36740	61851	76158	35441	66188	87728	66375	98049	84604
90379	06314	21897	42800	63963	44258	14381	90884	66620	14538
09466	65311	95514	51559	29960	07521	42180	86677	94240	59783
15821	25078	19388	93798	50820	88254	20504	74158	35756	42100

(*Continued*)

TABLE A1 *Random Digits (Continued)*

10328	60890	05204	30069	79630	31572	63273	13703	52954	72793
49727	08160	81650	71690	56327	06729	22495	49756	43333	34533
71118	41798	34541	76432	40522	51521	74382	06305	11956	30611
53253	23100	03743	48999	37736	92186	19108	69017	21661	17175
12206	24205	32372	46438	67981	53226	24943	68659	91924	69555

TABLE A2 *Cumulative Standardized Normal Distribution*

$A(z)$ is the integral of the standardized normal distribution from $-\infty$ to z (in other words, the area under the curve to the left of z). It gives the probability of a normal random variable not being more than z standard deviations above its mean. Values of z of particular importance:

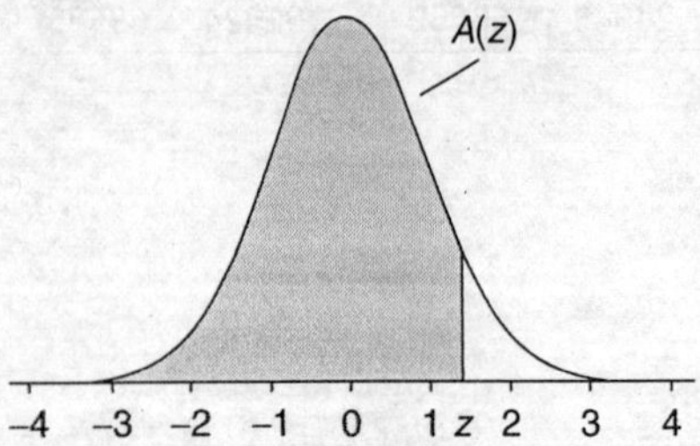

z	$A(z)$	
1.645	0.9500	Lower limit of right 5% tail
1.960	0.9750	Lower limit of right 2.5% tail
2.326	0.9900	Lower limit of right 1% tail
2.576	0.9950	Lower limit of right 0.5% tail
3.090	0.9990	Lower limit of right 0.1% tail
3.291	0.9995	Lower limit of right 0.05% tail

z	0.00	0.01	0.02	0.03	0.04	0.05	0.06	0.07	0.08	0.09
0.0	0.5000	0.5040	0.5080	0.5120	0.5160	0.5199	0.5239	0.5279	0.5319	0.5359
0.1	0.5398	0.5438	0.5478	0.5517	0.5557	0.5596	0.5636	0.5675	0.5714	0.5753
0.2	0.5793	0.5832	0.5871	0.5910	0.5948	0.5987	0.6026	0.6064	0.6103	0.6141
0.3	0.6179	0.6217	0.6255	0.6293	0.6331	0.6368	0.6406	0.6443	0.6480	0.6517
0.4	0.6554	0.6591	0.6628	0.6664	0.6700	0.6736	0.6772	0.6808	0.6844	0.6879
0.5	0.6915	0.6950	0.6985	0.7019	0.7054	0.7088	0.7123	0.7157	0.7190	0.7224
0.6	0.7257	0.7291	0.7324	0.7357	0.7389	0.7422	0.7454	0.7486	0.7517	0.7549
0.7	0.7580	0.7611	0.7642	0.7673	0.7704	0.7734	0.7764	0.7794	0.7823	0.7852
0.8	0.7881	0.7910	0.7939	0.7967	0.7995	0.8023	0.8051	0.8078	0.8106	0.8133
0.9	0.8159	0.8186	0.8212	0.8238	0.8264	0.8289	0.8315	0.8340	0.8365	0.8389
1.0	0.8413	0.8438	0.8461	0.8485	0.8508	0.8531	0.8554	0.8577	0.8599	0.8621
1.1	0.8643	0.8665	0.8686	0.8708	0.8729	0.8749	0.8770	0.8790	0.8810	0.8830
1.2	0.8849	0.8869	0.8888	0.8907	0.8925	0.8944	0.8962	0.8980	0.8997	0.9015
1.3	0.9032	0.9049	0.9066	0.9082	0.9099	0.9115	0.9131	0.9147	0.9162	0.9177
1.4	0.9192	0.9207	0.9222	0.9236	0.9251	0.9265	0.9279	0.9292	0.9306	0.9319
1.5	0.9332	0.9345	0.9357	0.9370	0.9382	0.9394	0.9406	0.9418	0.9429	0.9441
1.6	0.9452	0.9463	0.9474	0.9484	0.9495	0.9505	0.9515	0.9525	0.9535	0.9545
1.7	0.9554	0.9564	0.9573	0.9582	0.9591	0.9599	0.9608	0.9616	0.9625	0.9633
1.8	0.9641	0.9649	0.9656	0.9664	0.9671	0.9678	0.9686	0.9693	0.9699	0.9706
1.9	0.9713	0.9719	0.9726	0.9732	0.9738	0.9744	0.9750	0.9756	0.9761	0.9767
2.0	0.9772	0.9778	0.9783	0.9788	0.9793	0.9798	0.9803	0.9808	0.9812	0.9817
2.1	0.9821	0.9826	0.9830	0.9834	0.9838	0.9842	0.9846	0.9850	0.9854	0.9857

(*Continued*)

TABLE A2 *Cumulative Standardized Normal Distribution (Continued)*

z	0.00	0.01	0.02	0.03	0.04	0.05	0.06	0.07	0.08	0.09
2.2	0.9861	0.9864	0.9868	0.9871	0.9875	0.9878	0.9881	0.9884	0.9887	0.9890
2.3	0.9893	0.9896	0.9898	0.9901	0.9904	0.9906	0.9909	0.9911	0.9913	0.9916
2.4	0.9918	0.9920	0.9922	0.9925	0.9927	0.9929	0.9931	0.9932	0.9934	0.9936
2.5	0.9938	0.9940	0.9941	0.9943	0.9945	0.9946	0.9948	0.9949	0.9951	0.9952
2.6	0.9953	0.9955	0.9956	0.9957	0.9959	0.9960	0.9961	0.9962	0.9963	0.9964
2.7	0.9965	0.9966	0.9967	0.9968	0.9969	0.9970	0.9971	0.9972	0.9973	0.9974
2.8	0.9974	0.9975	0.9976	0.9977	0.9977	0.9978	0.9979	0.9979	0.9980	0.9981
2.9	0.9981	0.9982	0.9982	0.9983	0.9984	0.9984	0.9985	0.995	0.9986	0.9986
3.0	0.9987	0.9987	0.9987	0.9988	0.9988	0.9989	0.9989	0.9989	0.9990	0.9990
3.1	0.9990	0.9991	0.9991	0.9991	0.9992	0.9992	0.9992	0.9992	0.9993	0.9993
3.2	0.9993	0.9993	0.9994	0.9994	0.9994	0.9994	0.9994	0.9995	0.9995	0.9995
3.3	0.9995	0.9995	0.9995	0.9996	0.9996	0.9996	0.9996	0.9996	0.9996	0.9997
3.4	0.9997	0.9997	0.9997	0.9997	0.9997	0.9997	0.9997	0.9997	0.9997	0.9998
3.5	0.9998	0.9998	0.9998	0.9998	0.9998	0.9998	0.9998	0.9998	0.9998	0.9998
3.6	0.9998	0.9998	0.9999							

TABLE A3 *The Normal Distribution*

The table gives the proportion of the total area under the curve which lies beyond any given z value (that is, the shaded area in the diagram). It is therefore appropriate for a one-tailed (directional) test. For a two-tailed (non-directional) test, the proportions must be doubled..

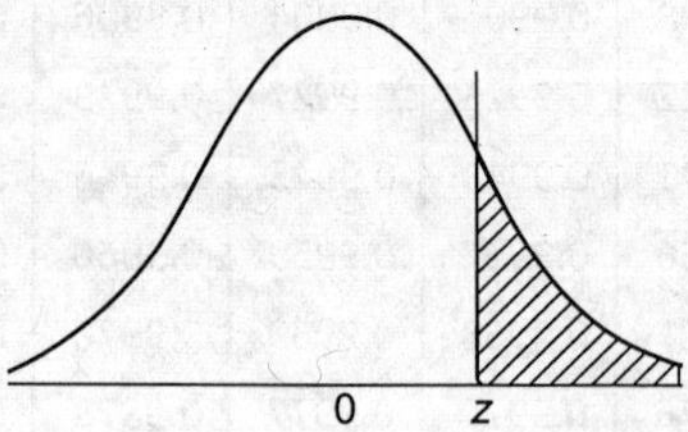

The figures down the left-hand side give values of z to the first decimal place, and those across the top give the second decimal place.

z	0.00	0.01	0.02	0.03	0.04	0.05	0.06	0.07	0.08	0.09
0.0	0.5000	0.4960	0.4920	0.4880	0.4840	0.4801	0.4761	0.4721	0.4681	0.4641
0.1	0.4602	0.4562	0.4522	0.4483	0.4443	0.4404	0.4364	0.4325	0.4286	0.4247
0.2	0.4207	0.4168	0.4129	0.4090	0.4052	0.4013	0.3974	0.3936	0.3897	0.3859
0.3	0.3821	0.3783	0.3745	0.3707	0.3669	0.3632	0.3594	0.3557	0.3520	0.3483
0.4	0.3446	0.3409	0.3372	0.3336	0.3300	0.3264	0.3228	0.3192	0.3156	0.3121
0.5	0.3085	0.3050	0.3015	0.2981	0.2946	0.2912	0.2877	0.2843	0.2810	0.2776
0.6	0.2743	0.2709	0.2676	0.2643	0.2611	0.2578	0.2546	0.2514	0.2483	0.2451
0.7	0.2420	0.2389	0.2358	0.2327	0.2296	0.2266	0.2236	0.2206	0.2177	0.2148
0.8	0.2119	0.2090	0.2061	0.2033	0.2005	0.1977	0.1949	0.1922	0.1894	0.1867
0.9	0.1841	0.1814	0.1788	0.1762	0.1736	0.1711	0.1685	0.1660	0.1635	0.1611
1.0	0.1587	0.1562	0.1539	0.1515	0.1492	0.1469	0.1446	0.1423	0.1401	0.1379
1.1	0.1357	0.1335	0.1314	0.1292	0.1271	0.1251	0.1230	0.1210	0.1190	0.1170
1.2	0.1151	0.1131	0.1112	0.1093	0.1075	0.1056	0.1038	0.1020	0.1003	0.0985
1.3	0.0968	0.0951	0.0934	0.0918	0.0901	0.885	0.0869	0.0853	0.0838	0.0823
1.4	0.0808	0.0793	0.0778	0.0764	0.0749	0.735	0.0721	0.0708	0.0694	0.0681
1.5	0.0668	0.0655	0.0643	0.0630	0.0618	0.0606	0.0594	0.0582	0.0571	0.0559
1.6	0.0548	0.0537	0.0526	0.0156	0.0505	0.0495	0.0485	0.0475	0.0465	0.0455
1.7	0.0446	0.0436	0.0427	0.0418	0.0409	0.0401	0.0392	0.0384	0.0375	0.0367
1.8	0.0359	0.0351	0.0344	0.0336	0.0329	0.0322	0.0314	0.0307	0.0301	0.0294
1.9	0.0287	0.0281	0.0274	0.0268	0.0262	0.0256	0.0250	0.0244	0.0239	0.0233
2.0	0.0228	0.0222	0.0217	0.0212	0.0207	0.0202	0.0197	0.0192	0.0188	0.0183
2.1	0.0179	0.0174	0.0170	0.0166	0.0162	0.0158	0.0154	0.0150	0.0146	0.0143
2.2	0.0139	0.0136	0.0132	0.0129	0.0125	0.0122	0.0119	0.0116	0.0113	0.0110

(Continued)

TABLE A3 *The Normal Distribution (Continued)*

z	0.00	0.01	0.02	0.03	0.04	0.05	0.06	0.07	0.08	0.09
2.3	0.0107	0.0104	0.0102	0.0099	0.0096	0.0094	0.0091	0.0089	0.0087	0.0084
2.4	0.0082	0.0080	0.0078	0.0075	0.0073	0.0071	0.0069	0.0068	0.0066	0.0064
2.5	0.0062	0.0060	0.0059	0.0057	0.0055	0.0054	0.0052	0.0051	0.0049	0.0048
2.6	0.0047	0.0045	0.0044	0.0043	0.0041	0.0040	0.0039	0.0038	0.0037	0.0036
2.7	0.0035	0.0034	0.0033	0.0032	0.0031	0.0030	0.0029	0.0028	0.0027	0.0026
2.8	0.0026	0.0025	0.0024	0.0023	0.0023	0.0022	0.0021	0.0021	0.0020	0.0019
2.9	0.0019	0.0018	0.0018	0.0017	0.0016	0.0016	0.0015	0.0015	0.0014	0.0014
3.0	0.0013	0.0013	0.0013	0.0012	0.0012	0.0011	0.0011	0.0011	0.0010	0.0010
3.1	0.0010	0.0009	0.0009	0.0009	0.0008	0.0008	0.0008	0.0008	0.0007	0.0007
3.2	0.0007	0.0007	0.0006	0.0006	0.0006	0.0006	0.0006	0.0005	0.0005	0.0005
3.3	0.0005	0.0005	0.0005	0.0004	0.0004	0.0004	0.0004	0.0004	0.0004	0.0003
3.4	0.0003	0.0003	0.0003	0.0003	0.0003	0.0003	0.0003	0.0003	0.0003	0.0002
3.5	0.0002	0.0002	0.0002	0.0002	0.0002	0.0002	0.0002	0.0002	0.0002	0.0002

TABLE A4 *The t-distribution*

The table gives critical values of *t* for significance at various levels, in a two-tailed/non-directional or a one-tailed/directional test, for different numbers of degrees of freedom. These critical values are the values beyond which lies that proportion of the area under the curve which corresponds to the significance level.

	Significance Level: Two-tailed/non-directional				
	0.20	0.10	0.05	0.02	0.01
	Significance Level: One-tailed/directional				
Degrees of Freedom	0.10	0.05	0.025	0.01	0.005
1	3.078	6.314	12.71	31.82	63.66
2	1.886	2.920	4.303	6.965	9.925
3	1.638	2.353	3.182	4.541	5.841
4	1.533	2.132	2.776	3.747	4.604
5	1.476	2.015	2.571	3.365	4.032
6	1.440	1.943	2.447	3.143	3.707
7	1.415	1.895	2.365	2.998	3.499
8	1.397	1.860	2.306	2.896	3.355
9	1.383	1.833	2.262	2.821	3.250
10	1.372	1.812	2.228	2.764	3.169
11	1.363	1.796	2.201	2.718	3.106
12	1.356	1.782	2.179	2.681	3.055
13	1.350	1.771	2.160	2.650	3.012
14	1.345	1.761	2.145	2.624	2.977
15	1.341	1.753	2.131	2.602	2.947
16	1.337	1.746	2.120	2.583	2.921
17	1.333	1.740	2.110	2.567	2.898
18	1.330	1.734	2.101	2.552	2.878
19	1.328	1.729	2.093	2.539	2.861
20	1.325	1.725	2.086	2.528	2.845
21	1.323	1.721	2.080	2.518	2.831
22	1.321	1.717	2.074	2.508	2.819
23	1.319	1.714	2.069	2.500	2.807

(*Continued*)

TABLE A4 *The t-distribution (Continued)*

	Significance Level: Two-tailed/non-directional				
	0.20	**0.10**	**0.05**	**0.02**	**0.01**
	Significance Level: One-tailed/directional				
Degrees of Freedom	**0.10**	**0.05**	**0.025**	**0.01**	**0.005**
24	1.318	1.711	2.064	2.492	2.797
25	1.316	1.708	2.060	2.485	2.787
26	1.315	1.706	2.056	2.479	2.779
27	1.314	1.703	2.052	2.473	2.771
28	1.313	1.701	2.048	2.467	2.763
29	1.311	1.699	2.045	2.462	2.756
30	1.310	1.697	2.042	2.457	2.750
40	1.303	1.684	2.021	2.423	2.704
60	1.296	1.671	2.000	2.390	2.660
120	1.289	1.658	1.980	2.358	2.617
∞	1.282	1.645	1.960	2.326	2.576

TABLE A5 *The F Distribution*

The table gives the critical values of F for different numbers of degrees of freedom (df) in the numerator and in the denominator of the expression for F. For each entry, two values are given. The upper value is the critical value for the $p \leq 0.05$ level in a one-tailed/directional test, and for the $p \leq 0.10$ level in a two-tailed/non-directional test. The lower value is the critical value for the $p \leq 0.01$ level in a one-tailed/directional test and for the $p \leq 0.02$ level in a two-tailed/non-directional test.

df in Denominator	df in Numerator															
	1	2	3	4	5	6	7	8	9	10	12	15	20	30	50	∞
1	161 4052	200 5000	216 5403	225 5625	230 5764	234 5859	237 5928	239 5981	241 6022	242 6056	244 6106	246 6157	248 6209	250 6261	252 6303	254 6366
2	18.5 98.5	19.0 99.0	19.2 99.2	19.2 99.2	19.3 99.3	19.3 99.3	19.4 99.4	19.4 99.4	19.4 99.4	19.4 99.4	19.4 99.4	19.4 99.4	19.4 99.4	19.5 99.5	19.5 99.5	19.5 99.5
3	10.1 34.1	9.55 30.8	9.28 29.5	9.12 28.7	9.01 28.2	8.94 27.9	8.89 27.7	8.85 27.5	8.81 27.3	8.79 27.2	8.74 27.1	8.70 26.9	8.66 26.7	8.62 26.5	8.58 26.4	8.53 26.1
4	7.71 21.2	6.94 18.0	6.59 16.7	6.39 16.0	6.26 15.5	6.16 15.2	6.09 15.0	6.04 14.8	6.00 14.7	5.96 14.5	5.91 14.4	5.86 14.2	5.80 14.0	5.75 13.8	5.70 13.7	5.63 13.5
5	6.61 16.3	5.79 13.3	5.41 12.1	5.19 11.4	5.05 11.0	4.95 10.7	4.88 10.5	4.82 10.3	4.77 10.2	4.74 10.1	4.68 9.89	4.62 9.72	4.56 9.55	4.50 9.38	4.44 9.24	4.36 9.02
6	5.99 13.7	5.14 10.9	4.76 9.78	4.53 9.15	4.39 8.75	4.28 8.47	4.21 8.26	4.15 8.10	4.10 7.98	4.06 7.87	4.00 7.72	3.94 7.56	3.87 7.40	3.81 7.23	3.75 7.09	3.67 6.88
7	5.59 12.2	4.74 9.55	4.35 8.45	4.12 7.85	3.97 7.46	3.87 7.19	3.79 6.99	3.73 6.84	3.68 6.72	3.64 6.62	3.57 6.47	3.51 6.31	3.44 6.16	3.38 5.99	3.32 5.86	3.23 5.65
8	5.32 11.3	4.46 8.65	4.07 7.59	3.84 7.01	3.69 6.63	3.58 6.37	3.50 6.18	3.44 6.03	3.39 5.91	3.35 5.81	3.28 5.67	3.22 5.52	3.15 5.36	3.08 5.20	3.02 5.07	2.93 4.86
9	5.12 10.6	4.26 8.02	3.86 6.99	3.63 6.42	3.48 6.06	3.37 5.80	3.29 5.61	3.23 5.47	3.18 5.35	3.14 5.26	3.07 5.11	3.01 4.96	2.94 4.81	2.86 4.65	2.80 4.52	2.71 4.31
10	4.96 10.0	4.10 7.56	3.71 6.55	3.48 5.99	3.33 5.64	3.22 5.39	3.14 5.20	3.07 5.06	3.02 4.94	2.98 4.85	2.91 4.71	2.85 4.56	2.77 4.41	2.70 4.25	2.64 4.12	2.54 3.91

11	4.84 9.65	3.98 7.21	3.59 6.22	3.36 5.67	3.20 5.32	3.09 5.07	3.01 4.89	2.95 4.74	2.90 4.63	2.85 4.54	2.79 4.40	2.72 4.25	2.65 4.10	2.57 3.94	2.51 3.81	2.40 3.60
12	4.75 9.33	3.89 6.93	3.49 5.95	3.26 5.41	3.11 5.06	3.00 4.82	2.91 4.64	2.85 4.50	2.80 4.39	2.75 4.30	2.69 4.16	2.62 4.01	2.54 3.86	2.47 3.70	2.40 3.57	2.30 3.36
13	4.67 9.07	3.81 6.70	3.41 5.74	3.18 5.21	3.03 4.86	2.92 4.62	2.83 4.44	2.77 4.30	2.71 4.19	2.67 4.10	2.60 3.96	2.53 3.82	2.46 3.66	2.38 3.51	2.31 3.38	2.21 3.17
14	4.60 8.86	3.74 6.51	3.34 5.56	3.11 5.04	2.96 4.69	2.85 4.46	2.76 4.28	2.70 4.14	2.65 4.03	2.60 3.94	2.53 3.80	2.46 3.66	2.39 3.51	2.31 3.35	2.24 3.22	2.13 3.00
15	4.54 8.68	3.68 6.36	3.29 5.42	3.06 4.89	2.90 4.56	2.79 4.32	2.71 4.14	2.64 4.00	2.59 3.89	2.54 3.80	2.48 3.67	2.40 3.52	2.33 3.37	2.25 3.21	2.18 3.08	2.07 2.87
16	4.49 8.53	3.63 6.23	3.24 5.29	3.01 4.77	2.85 4.44	2.74 4.20	2.66 4.03	2.59 3.89	2.54 3.78	2.49 3.69	2.42 3.55	2.35 3.41	2.28 3.26	2.19 3.10	2.12 3.97	2.01 2.75
17	4.45 8.40	3.59 6.11	3.20 5.18	2.96 4.67	2.81 4.34	2.70 4.10	2.61 3.93	2.55 3.79	2.49 3.68	2.45 3.59	2.38 3.46	2.31 3.31	2.23 3.16	2.15 3.00	2.08 2.87	1.96 2.65
18	4.41 8.29	3.55 6.01	3.16 5.09	2.93 4.58	2.77 4.25	2.66 4.01	2.58 3.84	2.51 3.71	2.46 3.60	2.41 3.51	2.34 3.23	2.27 3.23	2.19 3.08	2.11 2.92	2.04 2.78	1.92 2.57
19	4.38 8.18	3.52 5.93	3.13 5.01	2.90 4.50	2.74 4.17	2.63 3.94	2.54 3.77	2.48 3.63	2.42 3.52	2.38 3.43	2.31 3.30	2.23 3.15	2.16 3.00	2.07 2.84	2.00 2.71	1.88 2.49
20	4.35 8.10	3.49 5.85	3.10 4.94	2.87 4.43	2.71 4.10	2.60 3.87	2.51 3.70	2.45 3.56	2.39 3.46	2.35 3.37	2.28 3.23	2.20 3.09	2.12 2.94	2.04 2.78	1.97 2.64	1.84 2.42
25	4.24 7.77	3.39 5.57	2.99 4.68	2.76 4.18	2.60 3.85	2.49 3.63	2.40 3.46	2.34 3.32	2.28 3.22	2.24 3.13	2.16 2.99	2.09 2.85	2.01 2.70	1.92 2.54	1.84 2.40	1.71 2.17
30	4.17 7.56	3.32 5.39	2.92 4.51	2.69 4.02	2.53 3.70	2.42 3.47	2.33 3.30	2.27 3.17	2.21 3.07	2.16 2.98	2.09 2.84	2.01 2.70	1.93 2.55	1.84 2.39	1.76 2.25	1.62 2.01
35	4.12 7.42	3.27 5.27	2.87 4.40	2.64 3.91	2.49 3.59	2.37 3.37	2.29 3.20	2.22 3.07	2.16 2.96	2.11 2.88	2.04 2.74	1.96 2.60	1.88 2.44	1.79 2.28	1.70 2.14	1.56 1.89
40	4.08 7.31	3.23 5.18	2.84 4.31	2.61 3.83	2.45 3.51	2.34 3.29	2.25 3.12	2.18 2.99	2.12 2.89	2.08 2.80	2.00 2.66	1.92 2.52	1.84 2.37	1.74 2.20	1.66 2.06	1.51 1.80

(*Continued*)

TABLE A5 *The F Distribution (Continued)*

df in Denominator	df in Numerator															
	1	**2**	**3**	**4**	**5**	**6**	**7**	**8**	**9**	**10**	**12**	**15**	**20**	**30**	**50**	**∞**
45	4.06	3.20	2.81	2.58	2.42	2.31	2.22	2.15	2.10	2.05	1.97	1.89	1.81	1.71	1.63	1.47
	7.23	5.11	4.25	3.77	3.45	3.23	3.07	2.94	2.83	2.74	2.61	2.46	2.31	2.14	2.00	1.74
50	4.03	3.18	2.79	2.56	2.40	2.29	2.20	2.13	2.07	2.03	1.95	1.87	1.78	1.69	1.60	1.44
	7.17	5.06	4.20	3.72	3.41	3.19	3.02	2.89	2.78	2.70	2.56	2.42	2.27	2.10	1.95	1.68
60	4.00	3.15	2.76	2.53	2.37	2.25	2.17	2.10	2.04	1.99	1.92	1.84	1.75	1.65	1.56	1.39
	7.08	4.98	4.13	3.65	3.34	3.12	2.95	2.82	2.72	2.63	2.50	2.35	2.20	2.03	1.88	1.60
80	3.96	3.11	2.72	2.49	2.33	2.21	2.13	2.06	2.00	1.95	1.88	1.79	1.70	1.60	1.51	1.32
	6.96	4.88	4.04	3.56	3.26	3.04	2.87	2.74	2.64	2.55	2.42	2.27	2.12	1.94	1.79	1.49
100	3.94	3.09	2.70	2.46	2.31	2.19	2.10	2.03	1.97	1.93	1.85	1.77	1.68	1.57	1.48	1.28
	6.90	4.82	3.98	3.51	3.21	2.99	2.82	2.69	2.59	2.50	2.37	2.22	2.07	1.89	1.74	1.43
120	3.92	3.07	2.68	2.45	2.29	2.18	2.09	2.02	1.96	1.91	1.83	1.75	1.66	1.55	1.46	1.25
	6.85	4.79	3.95	3.48	3.17	2.96	2.79	2.66	2.56	2.47	2.34	2.19	2.03	1.86	1.70	1.38
∞	3.84	3.00	2.60	2.37	2.21	2.10	2.01	1.94	1.88	1.83	1.75	1.67	1.57	1.46	1.35	1.00
	6.63	4.61	3.78	3.32	3.02	2.80	2.64	2.51	2.41	2.32	2.18	2.04	1.88	1.70	1.52	1.00

TABLE A6 *The Chi-square Distribution*

The table gives the critical values of χ^2 in a two-tailed/non-directional test, for different numbers of degrees of freedom (df). For significance, the calculated value must be *greater than or equal to* the critical value.

	Significance level					
df	**0.20**	**0.10**	**0.05**	**0.025**	**0.01**	**0.001**
1	1.64	2.71	3.84	5.02	6.64	10.83
2	3.22	4.61	5.99	7.38	9.21	13.82
3	4.64	6.25	7.82	9.35	11.34	16.27
4	5.99	7.78	9.49	11.14	13.28	18.47
5	7.29	9.24	11.07	12.83	15.09	20.52
6	8.56	10.64	12.59	14.45	16.81	22.46
7	9.80	12.02	14.07	16.01	18.48	24.32
8	11.03	13.36	15.51	17.53	20.09	26.12
9	12.24	14.68	16.92	19.02	21.67	27.88
10	13.44	15.99	18.31	20.48	23.21	29.59
11	14.63	17.28	19.68	21.92	24.72	31.26
12	15.81	18.55	21.03	23.34	26.22	32.91
13	16.98	19.81	22.36	24.74	27.69	34.53
14	18.15	21.06	23.68	26.12	29.14	36.12
15	19.31	22.31	25.00	27.49	30.58	37.70
16	20.47	23.54	26.30	28.85	32.00	39.25
17	21.61	24.77	27.59	30.19	33.41	40.79
18	22.76	25.99	28.87	31.53	34.81	42.31
19	23.90	27.20	30.14	32.85	36.19	43.82
20	25.04	28.41	31.41	34.17	37.57	45.31
21	26.17	29.62	32.67	35.48	38.93	46.80
22	27.30	30.81	33.92	36.78	40.29	48.27
23	28.43	32.01	35.17	38.08	41.64	49.73
24	29.55	33.20	36.42	39.36	42.98	51.18
25	30.68	34.38	37.65	40.65	44.31	52.62
26	31.79	35.56	38.89	41.92	45.64	54.05
27	32.91	36.74	40.11	43.19	46.96	55.48
28	34.03	37.92	41.34	44.46	48.28	56.89
29	35.14	39.09	42.56	45.72	49.59	58.30
30	36.25	40.26	43.77	46.98	50.89	59.70

(*Continued*)

TABLE A6 *The Chi-square Distribution (Continued)*

	Significance level					
df	**0.20**	**0.10**	**0.05**	**0.025**	**0.01**	**0.001**
40	47.27	51.81	55.76	59.34	63.69	73.40
50	58.16	63.17	67.50	71.42	76.15	86.66
60	68.97	74.40	79.08	83.30	88.38	99.61
70	79.71	85.53	90.53	95.02	100.4	112.3

TABLE A7 *The Pearson Product–Moment Correlation Coefficient*

The table gives the critical values of the pearson product–moment correlation coefficient, r, for different numbers of pairs of observations, N. For significance, the calculated value of r must be *greater than or equal to* the critical value.

	Significance Level: Two-tailed/non-directional			
	0.20	**0.10**	**0.05**	**0.01**
	Significance Level: One-tailed/directional			
N	**0.10**	**0.05**	**0.025**	**0.005**
3	0.951	0.988	0.997	1.000
4	0.800	0.900	0.950	0.990
5	0.687	0.805	0.878	0.959
6	0.608	0.729	0.811	0.917
7	0.551	0.669	0.754	0.875
8	0.507	0.621	0.707	0.834
9	0.472	0.582	0.666	0.798
10	0.443	0.549	0.632	0.765
11	0.419	0.521	0.602	0.735
12	0.398	0.497	0.576	0.708
13	0.380	0.476	0.553	0.684
14	0.365	0.458	0.532	0.661
15	0.351	0.441	0.514	0.641
16	0.338	0.426	0.497	0.623
17	0.327	0.412	0.482	0.606
18	0.317	0.400	0.468	0.590
19	0.308	0.389	0.456	0.575
20	0.299	0.378	0.444	0.561
21	0.291	0.369	0.433	0.549
22	0.284	0.360	0.423	0.537
23	0.277	0.352	0.413	0.526
24	0.271	0.344	0.404	0.515
25	0.265	0.337	0.396	0.505
26	0.260	0.330	0.388	0.496
27	0.255	0.323	0.381	0.487
28	0.250	0.317	0.374	0.479

(*Continued*)

TABLE A7 *The Pearson Product–Moment Correlation Coefficient (Continued)*

	Significance Level: Two-tailed/non-directional			
	0.20	**0.10**	**0.05**	**0.01**
	Significance Level: One-tailed/directional			
N	**0.10**	**0.05**	**0.025**	**0.005**
29	0.245	0.311	0.367	0.471
30	0.241	0.306	0.361	0.463
40	0.207	0.264	0.312	0.403
50	0.184	0.235	0.279	0.361
60	0.168	0.214	0.254	0.330
70	0.155	0.198	0.235	0.306
80	0.145	0.185	0.220	0.286
90	0.136	0.174	0.207	0.270
100	0.129	0.165	0.197	0.256
200	0.091	0.117	0.139	0.182

TABLE A8 *The Spearman Rank Correlation Coefficient*

The table gives the critical values of the spearman rank correlation coefficient, ρ, for different numbers of pairs of observations, N.

	Significance Level: Two-tailed/non-directional			
	0.20	**0.10**	**0.05**	**0.01**
	Significance Level: One-tailed/directional			
N	**0.10**	**0.05**	**0.25**	**0.005**
5	0.800	0.900	1.000	–
6	0.657	0.829	0.886	1.000
7	0.571	0.714	0.786	0.929
8	0.524	0.643	0.738	0.881
9	0.483	0.600	0.700	0.833
10	0.455	0.564	0.648	0.794
11	0.427	0.536	0.618	0.755
12	0.406	0.503	0.587	0.727
13	0.385	0.484	0.560	0.703
14	0.367	0.464	0.538	0.679
15	0.354	0.446	0.521	0.654
16	0.341	0.429	0.503	0.635
17	0.328	0.414	0.488	0.618
18	0.317	0.401	0.472	0.600
19	0.309	0.391	0.460	0.584
20	0.299	0.380	0.447	0.570
21	0.292	0.370	0.436	0.556
22	0.284	0.361	0.425	0.544
23	0.278	0.353	0.416	0.532
24	0.271	0.344	0.407	0.521
25	0.265	0.337	0.398	0.511
26	0.259	0.331	0.390	0.501
27	0.255	0.324	0.383	0.492
28	0.250	0.318	0.375	0.483
29	0.245	0.312	0.368	0.475
30	0.240	0.306	0.362	0.467
35	0.222	0.283	0.335	0.433

(*Continued*)

TABLE A8 *The Spearman Rank Correlation Coefficient (Continued)*

	Significance Level: Two-tailed/non-directional			
	0.20	**0.10**	**0.05**	**0.01**
	Significance Level: One-tailed/directional			
N	**0.10**	**0.05**	**0.25**	**0.005**
40	0.207	0.264	0.313	0.405
45	0.194	0.248	0.294	0.382
50	0.184	0.235	0.279	0.363
55	0.175	0.224	0.266	0.346
60	0.168	0.214	0.255	0.331

TABLE A9 *The Sign Test*

The table gives critical values of x (the number of cases with the less frequent sign) for different values of N (the number of non-tied pairs of scores). For significance, the computed value of x must be *smaller than or equal to* the critical value.

	Significance Level: Two-tailed/non-directional		
	0.10	**0.05**	**0.02**
	Significance Level: One-tailed/directional		
N	**0.05**	**0.025**	**0.01**
5	0	–	–
6	0	0	–
6	0	0	0
8	1	0	0
9	1	1	0
10	1	1	0
11	2	1	1
12	2	2	1
13	3	2	1
14	3	2	2
15	3	3	2
16	4	3	2
17	4	4	3
18	5	4	3
19	5	4	4
20	5	5	4
21	6	5	4
22	6	5	5
23	7	6	5
24	7	6	5
25	7	7	6

TABLE A10 *The Wilcoxon Signed-ranks Test*

The table gives critical values of W for different values of N (the number of non-tied pairs of scores). For significance, the calculated value must be *smaller than or equal to* the critical value.

	Significance Level: Two-tailed/non-directional	
	0.05	**0.01**
	Significance Level: One-tailed/directional	
N	**0.025**	**0.005**
6	0	–
7	2	–
8	3	0
9	5	1
10	8	3
11	10	5
12	13	7
13	17	9
14	21	12
15	25	15
16	29	19
17	34	23
18	40	27
19	46	32
20	52	37
21	58	42
22	65	48
23	73	54
24	81	61
25	89	68

TABLE A11 *The Mann–Whitney U-test*

The first table gives the critical values for significance at the $p \leq 0.05$ level in a two-tailed/non-directional test, and for the $p \leq 0.025$ level in a one-tailed/directional test. The second table gives the critical values for the $p \leq 0.01$ level in a two-tailed/non-directional test, and for the $p \leq 0.005$ level in a one-tailed/directional test. For significance, the calculated value of U must be *smaller than or equal to* the critical value. N_1 and N_2 are the number of observations in the smaller and larger group, respectively.

	N_2															
N_1	5	6	7	8	9	10	11	12	13	14	15	16	17	18	19	20
$p \leq 0.05$ (two-tailed), $p \leq 0.025$ (one-tailed)																
5	2	3	5	6	7	8	9	10	11	12	13	14	15	17	19	20
6		5	6	8	10	11	13	14	16	17	19	21	22	24	25	27
7			8	10	12	14	16	18	20	22	24	26	28	30	32	34
8				13	15	17	19	22	24	26	29	31	34	36	38	41
9					17	20	23	26	28	31	34	37	39	42	45	48
10						23	26	29	33	36	39	42	45	48	52	55
11							30	33	37	40	44	47	51	55	58	62
12								37	41	45	49	53	57	61	65	69
13									45	50	54	59	63	67	72	76
14										55	59	64	69	74	78	83
15											64	70	75	80	85	90
16												75	81	86	92	98
17													87	93	99	105
18														99	106	112
19															113	119
20																127
$p \leq 0.01$ (two-tailed), $p \leq 0.005$ (one-tailed)																
5	0	1	1	2	3	4	5	6	7	7	8	9	10	11	12	13
6		2	3	4	5	6	7	9	10	11	12	13	15	16	17	18
7			4	6	7	9	10	12	13	15	16	18	19	21	22	24
8				7	9	11	13	15	17	18	20	22	24	26	28	30
9					11	13	16	18	20	22	24	27	29	31	33	36
10						16	18	21	24	26	29	31	34	37	39	42
11							21	24	27	30	33	36	39	42	45	48
12								27	31	34	37	41	44	47	51	54
13									34	38	42	45	49	53	57	60

(*Continued*)

TABLE A11 *The Mann–Whitney U-test (Continued)*

	N_2															
N_1	**5**	**6**	**7**	**8**	**9**	**10**	**11**	**12**	**13**	**14**	**15**	**16**	**17**	**18**	**19**	**20**
14										42	46	50	54	58	63	67
15											51	55	60	64	69	73
16												60	65	70	74	79
17													70	75	81	86
18														81	87	92
19															93	99
20																105

Glossary

Abstract concepts The concepts that are not readily observable and whose meanings are more distant from specific time, space, and referent group.

Abstract review A brief summary of a research article, thesis, review, conference proceedings, or any in-depth analysis of a particular subject or discipline.

Accessible population The aggregate of cases that conform to designated criteria and are accessible for a study.

Action research A practical form of research, which aims at a specific problem and situation with little or no control over independent variables and depends mainly on observation and behavioural data; constant monitoring and evaluation are carried out and the findings of the research are applied immediately and monitored further.

Anonymity A strong guarantee of privacy.

Applied research Scientific investigation conducted not only for the purpose of acquiring and expanding knowledge but most specifically to find a solution to a problem that requires an impending solution in practice. It is focused on nursing interventions, procedures, processes, and methods of patient care.

Associative hypothesis A relationship between variables that occurs or exists in a natural setting without manipulation.

Assumption A basic principle accepted as true based on logic or reason but without proof or verification.

Attrition The loss of participants over the course of a study, which can create bias by changing the composition of the sample initially drawn (particularly if more participants are lost from one group than another) and can threaten the study's internal validity.

Basic research The type of research considered to be pure research; it is conducted primarily for the purpose of obtaining new knowledge without any intent to apply this knowledge and is useful in formulating and refining concepts and theories.

Beneficence An ethical principle that seeks to prevent harm and exploitation of, and maximize benefits for, study participants.

Bibliography A list that includes all sources consulted during research for background or further reading.

Boolean searching The most common method of searching, which is also called as keyword searching. Words such as AND, OR, and NOT are used while searching through a database.

Bracketing In phenomenological enquiries, the process of identifying and holding in abeyance any preconceived beliefs and opinions about the phenomena under study.

Bricolage The tendency in qualitative research to derive a complex array of data from a variety of sources using a variety of methods.

Card catalogue An alphabetical file of authors, subjects, and titles for materials acquired by a library.

Categorical variable An attribute with values that function as labels rather than as numbers but can be coded with numbers; it is also referred to as a *nominal variable.*

Causal hypothesis The cause and effect relationship between two or more dependent and independent variables in an experimental or interventional setting, wherein the independent variable is manipulated by the researcher to examine its effect on the dependent variable.

Causal hypothesis-testing research An approach that addresses causal relationships among variables in an attempt to predict something.

Cluster sampling A form of sampling in which large groups (clusters) are selected first with successive sub-sampling of smaller units or the process of randomly selecting intact groups, not individuals, within the defined population sharing similar characteristics.

Code A symbolic abbreviation used to classify data.

Coding The process of categorizing and indexing data to facilitate data analysis and retrieval.

Coefficient of variation (C.V.) Standard deviation expressed as a percentage of the arithmetic mean; $C.V. = (SD \times 100)/\text{Mean}$.

Cohort study A kind of trend study that focuses on a specific sub-population (which is often an age-related subgroup) from which different samples are selected at different points in time, for example, the cohort of patients who are admitted in 2000 and 2010.

Communication of research findings Developing and disseminating report through presentations and publications.

Complex hypothesis A statement that reflects the relationship between more than two variables.

Concept An abstract idea of an object and a word picture that strikes in our mind and is formed by generalizing an object from particular characteristics.

Conceptual framework A framework that depicts the relationship between concepts and links concepts selected from various theories, from previous research results, and from researcher's own experiences.

Conceptual map The way of using diagrams for expressing the interrelationships of concepts and statements that contribute totally or partially, directly or indirectly, and in sequence or cumulatively to cause or produce an outcome of the study.

Conceptual model A symbolic or visual representation of highly abstract cluster of concepts under study; it is also known as a schematic model or flowchart and diagrammatically depicts the concepts and their relationships by using boxes, arrows, and other symbols.

Confidentiality Managing of private data in research in such a way that only the researcher knows the subjects' identities and can link them with their responses.

Conformability The consistency and repeatability of decision-making about the processes of data collection and data analysis. One approach to ensure conformability is audit trail, which is an ongoing documentation regarding the researcher's decision about the data analysis and collection process. Changes in methodological approach with the rationale need to be noted in a diary or in memos.

Confounding variables The variables that cannot be controlled.

Consent form A written agreement signed by a study participant and a researcher concerning the terms and conditions of voluntary participation in a study.

Constant comparative method Data are compared with other data continuously as they are acquired during research.

Construct A cluster of concepts or a newly invented concept that represents an index of behaviour, events, or other phenomena.

Construct validity The degree to which an instrument measures the construct under investigation.

Content analysis The process of understanding, interpreting, and conceptualizing the meanings in qualitative data. The researcher does this by first breaking down the data into units that are meaningful and then developing a categorization scheme (based on the ideas found in the data). The process of breaking down and labelling large amounts of data to identify the category to which they belong is called coding or data reduction.

Content validity The degree to which the items in an instrument adequately represent the universe of content for the concept being measured or the degree to which an instrument has an appropriate sample of items for the construct being measured and adequately covers the construct's domain.

Content validity index (CVI) The attribute calculated by asking the experts to evaluate individual items on the given measure as well as the overall instrument.

Continuous variable An attribute that has numeric values such as 1, 2, and 3 and the relative magnitude of the values is significant. This is also referred as an ordered or a monotonic variable.

Control group The group not exposed to the experimental treatment in a study in which the sample is randomly selected.

Convenience sampling The method of selecting the most readily available persons as participants in a study; it is also termed as accidental sampling.

Correlational analysis The analysis used to find the *direction* (positive or negative) and *magnitude* (strength) of the relationship between two variables; it is also called a *bivariate correlation*.

Correlational research A research study that examines the relationship between and among variables to explain the nature of relationships without any active intervention by the researcher.

Covariance A measure of how much two random variables change together.

Credibility A criterion for evaluating data quality in qualitative studies, referring to confidence in the truth of the data.

Criterion validity The degree to which the instrument determines a subject's response at the present time or predicts subject's response in the future.

Critical appraisal skill The process by which a reader can evaluate a piece of written material and assess whether it possesses validity (i.e., is it close to the truth) and applicability (i.e., is it clinically useful).

Critical reading skill An active, intellectually engaging process in which the reader participates in an inner dialogue with the writer.

Critical theory A theory that believes in the creative nature of the knowledge and in the existence of multiple realities to change the world by empowering the subject's enquiry to enact social change.

Data The information collected during a study.

Data analysis The step-by-step process of dissecting, scrutinizing, cleaning, and transforming raw data into clear information, which can answer the research questions presented as study hypotheses, suggest conclusions, and support decision-making.

Data categorization The process of organizing or arranging data and dividing them into several homogeneous groups or classes on the basis of common characteristics.

Data collection Systematic gathering of information relevant to the research study.

Data compilation The process of arranging data in a meaningful order.

Data editing The process of checking the data for accuracy, usefulness, and adequacy.

Debriefing The complete disclosure of the study purpose and results at the end of a study.

Deception The deliberate withholding of information to study participants usually to reduce potential biases.

Deductive approach A logical process from the complexities or whole observed situation to arrive at a particular or certain single idea.

Deductive reasoning A process of reasoning that moves thinking from stated general principles to specific elements.

Degree of freedom (df) The number of observations that are free to vary in a set of observations.

Delimitations The boundaries of the study for the researcher. It aids the researcher as a guide and shows the path—horizontal and vertical—in the study.

Dependent variable A variable that is the outcome or response due to the effect of the independent variable and which the researcher wants to predict or explain.

Descriptive research A research study in which a particular situation or event that already exists is described systematically.

Design The blueprint for conducting a study.

Directional hypothesis The expected direction of the relationship between variables.

Effect size The actual size of the effect the researcher is looking for; it may be the effect of an independent variable on the dependant variable.

Element The object about which or from which information is collected.

Empirical concepts The concepts that can be observed directly, have their meanings, and can be measured but limit the comprehensiveness of research findings. These are also called *descriptive concepts*.

Empirics Scientific knowledge derived through testing the theories and models by objective or quantitative approach.

Ethical committee A group of individuals from diverse backgrounds who support health care institutions by providing ethics consultation and developing and/or revising select policies pertaining to clinical ethics.

Ethical principles The basis for nurse's decisions on consideration of consequences and of universal moral principles when making clinical judgements and refers to the principles of respect for persons, beneficence, and justice, which are relevant to the conduct of research.

Ethics Moral knowledge that does what ought to be and what is good or right; it is a set of moral and social standards, which includes both *prohibitions against* and *prescriptions for* specific kinds of behaviour in research.

Ethics in nursing research The act of moral principles that the researcher has to follow in the conduct of nursing research to ensure the rights and welfare of participants.

Ethnographic research A method of conducting enquiry of a life process by studying individuals, artefacts, or documents in their natural settings and includes both anthropology and historical forms of research.

Ethnography A branch of human enquiry that describes and interprets a cultural or social group or system.

Evidence-based practice A practice that involves making clinical decisions on the basis of best available evidence, with an emphasis on evidence from disciplined research.

Experimental group The subjects who receive the experimental treatment or intervention.

Experimental research A study in which the researcher manipulates and controls one or more variables and observes the effect of manipulation on the other variables.

External validity The degree to which the study results can be generalized to settings or samples other than the one studied.

Extraneous variable A factor that is not a part of the study but may affect the measurement of the study variable or a variable other than the independent variable that could cause a change in the dependent variable, such as gender, ethnicity, social class, genetics, intelligence, and age.

Face validity The extent to which a measuring instrument looks as though it is measuring what it purports to measure.

Factor-isolating theories The type of theories used for observing, describing, and naming the concepts.

Factor-relating theories The theories showing the relationship among the factors or the concepts.

Fidelity Faithfulness towards one's duties and obligations and keeping one's promises.

Focus groups Measurement strategy where groups are assembled to obtain the participants' perceptions in focused areas in settings that are permissive and non-threatening in a qualitative study.

Framework A set of principles and ideas that can be used to make decisions and judgements when given a meaning to them.

General objectives The outcome of a researcher's expectation at the end of the study.

Generalization The process of applying the research findings obtained by testing the selected samples to the population of a particular setting.

Global concepts The broad concepts that have many interrelated, diverse, and empirical manifestations. These concepts are also called *domain concepts*.

Graph A visual representation of data by a continuous curve on a squared (graph) paper.

Grand theories The theories that address the phenomena of concern and models, from which hypothesis can be derived; they are also termed as *macro theories*.

Grounded theory research An inductive technique that emerged from the discipline of sociology; an important research method for the study of nursing theories of phenomena relevant to nurses.

Halo effect The tendency of the investigator to be influenced by one characteristic while judging another unrelated characteristic.

Hawthorne effect The effect on the dependent variable resulting from subjects' awareness that they are participants under study.

Heterogeneous sample A sample in which subjects have a broad range of values being studied, which increases the representativeness of the sample and the ability to generalize from the accessible population to the target population.

Historical research A research study that provides a narrative description or analysis of events that occurred in the past.

Homogeneous sample A sample in which subjects' score on selected measurement methods in a study are similar, resulting in a limited distribution of scores.

Hypothesis A testable or expected relationship between two or more than two variables, which are measurable or potentially measurable.

Independent variable A stimulus or activity that is manipulated or varied by the researcher to create an effect on the dependent variable.

Index A systematic list of book titles or author's names, giving cross-references and the location of each book; catalogue.

Inductive approach A logical process wherein a generalization is drawn from several observations and specific instances or the process of reasoning from particular to a whole group of ideas, phenomena, or situations.

Inductive reasoning A process of reasoning that moves thinking from specific elements to general principles, in which particular instances are observed and then combined into a larger whole or general statement.

Inference The process of explaining the findings in depth and drawing a conclusion about the situation or issue being investigated.

Inferential statistics The type of statistics that permits inferences on whether relationships observed in a sample are likely to occur in the larger population.

Information-seeking skill The process by which a reader scans literature manually or using computerized methods to identify a set of potentially useful articles and books.

Informed consent The ethical principle that requires a researcher to inform the subjects, and to ensure that they understand, the reason for the proposed intervention or study and its benefits and risks such that they are in a position to make rational decision about participating in the study; subjects agree to the intervention by signing a consent form.

Internal validity The degree to which it can be inferred that the experimental treatment rather than uncontrolled extraneous factors is responsible for the observed effects.

Inter-quartile range The difference between the upper and lower quartile, hence covering the middle 50 per cent of the observations in the group.

Interval indicator The type of indicator in which the specific distance is identified between each level of variable and includes all the characteristics of nominal and ordinal scales of measurement; the units of measurement are constant and equal, and zero point is not true but rather arbitrary.

Intervening variables Intangible attributes that are very difficult to control or condition.

Intervention The treatment or independent variable that is manipulated during the conduct of a study to produce an effect on the dependent or outcome variable.

Intuition A truth that the mind grasps immediately without any proof, testing, or experimentation.

Justice The promotion of equity or fairness in every situation a nurse encounters in the care of the client.

Key informants The individuals who have special knowledge, status, or communication skills and are willing to teach the ethnographer about the phenomenon. A major part of information is obtained from the key informants. Secondary informants are used by the researcher to confirm or refute the information provided by the key informants, to widen the database as theory is developed, or to search for negative cases.

Level of significance The probability of rejecting a null hypothesis when it is true and is represented by the Greek letter alpha (α); the symbol of probability level is p.

Limitations The restriction of the study due to theoretical or methodological reasons, which may decrease the credibility and generalizability of the research findings.

Lines graph A way to summarize how two pieces of information are related and how they vary depending on one another. It allows comparison of multiple sets of data over time in the same graph.

Literature review A critical summary of research on a topic of interest, often prepared to generate a picture of what is known and not known about a particular problem.

Logical reasoning A problem-solving method that uses experience, intellectual faculties, and thought process with inductive and deductive reasoning.

Longitudinal design A research design used to examine changes in the same subjects over an extended time period.

Manipulation A treatment or intervention introduced by the researcher in an experimental or quasi-experimental study to assess its impact on the dependent variable.

Matching Pairing of subjects of one group with subjects of another group based on their similarity in one or more dimensions to enhance the overall comparability of groups.

Mean The sum of all the observations (values) in a group divided by the total number of observations (values) in that group.

Measurement A process of assigning numbers to objects, situations, or events according to some rules.

Measurement error The difference between what exists in reality and what is measured by a research instrument.

MEDLINE A comprehensive database for health literature managed by National Library of Medicine, USA.

Meta-analysis A technique for quantitatively combining and statistically analysing the results of multiple studies on a common given topic.

Meta-paradigms The paradigms that define the domain of interest and questions to be addressed and identify appropriate theories, methods, and instruments to be utilized; they serve as the framework within which more models and theories can be developed.

Meta-synthesis The non-statistical technique used to integrate, evaluate, and interpret the findings of multiple qualitative research studies.

Methodological limitations The limitations that result from some of the methodological factors such as un-repetitive sample, weak design, single setting, limited control over extraneous variables, and poor implementation of treatments protocol.

Middle range concepts The concepts that are more refined than global concepts and are derived from global concepts.

Middle range theories The theories that examine the facts and identify a few key variables; propositions are clearly formulated and tested hypothesis can be derived through inductive or deductive approach.

Model A symbolic representation of some phenomena, which may be concrete or abstract, in structural, pictorial, or mathematical form that provides a more concrete analogy for thinking about the various concepts and how they actually operate.

Narrative review An overview of the research findings on a particular topic, including critical summary of the content, written by experts after examining the published work.

Naturalist philosophy The philosophy that stays on the fundamental pattern of human thought, behaviour, and experiences.

Nesting An advanced search strategy that allows combining multiple search terms by using Boolean operators and wildcards.

Nominal indicator The indicator that classifies variables into subcategories that are mutually exclusive and exhaustive, do not vary in degree, and cannot be ranked or ordered.

Non-directional hypothesis The relationship between two or more variables that does not specify the anticipated direction and nature of relationship.

Non-experimental research Studies that are more descriptive or exploratory in nature. The main focus is to describe how phenomena exist in nature without manipulation.

Non-maleficence One of the ethical principles whose meaning is to do no harm.

Normal curve The graphical representation of a normal distribution.

Normal distribution A theoretical frequency distribution.

Normal probability curve The probability curve when the total area under it is *equal to unity.*

Null hypothesis A hypothesis stating no relationship between the variables under study.

Nursing research A systematic approach designed to examine phenomena important to nursing and nurses.

Nursing theory The body of knowledge to define or explain various aspects of nursing.

Operational definition Description of variables or concepts measured or manipulated in a study, which links the concept to the real world and identifies empirical referents (indicators) of the concept that can be observed and measured.

Ordinal indicators The variables that can be ranked in addition to being mutually exclusive and exhaustive but cannot quantify in degree and are not of equal interval or an absolute zero.

Outcome research Research designed to document the effectiveness of health care services and the end results of patient care.

Paradigm A core cluster of concepts or constructs.

Parameters The measures of population.

Phenomenology The subjective reality of an event, as perceived by the study population; it is the study of a phenomenon.

Phenomenological research Descriptive qualitative methodology developed from phenomenological philosophy for the purpose of describing experiences as they are lived by the study participants.

Pie diagram A circular diagram—a circle (pie) divided by the radii into components.

Pilot study Smaller version of a proposed study conducted to develop and refine the methodology, instruments, or data collection process to be used in the larger study.

Plagiarism A type of scientific misconduct with appropriation of another person's ideas, processes, results, or words without giving appropriate credit, including those obtained through confidential review of others' research proposals and manuscripts, stealing intellectual property, or taking credit for another individual's work.

Population The entire aggregation of cases that meets a specified set of criteria.

Positivist philosophy The philosophy that believes anyone worth knowing can be known objectively, that is, measured or quantified and typically represented numerically and verified by independent observers.

Practice theories The theories that are very limited in their scope such as descriptive, explanatory, and predictive theories.

Pre-paradigms The constructs when in a developing stage and not reached a dominant phase.

Primary source Original materials or research reports that provide first-hand records of events, experiments, creative works, or statistics conducted by the researcher.

Print database resources Indexes, card catalogues, and abstract reviews.

Propositions The linkages or relationships that spell out how concepts are interrelated.

Prospective research A research design that starts with a presumed cause and then goes forward in time to presumed effect.

Psychometrics A theory underlying the principles of measurement and the application of the theory in the development of measuring tools.

Purposive sampling A non-probability sampling method in which the researcher selects participants based on personal judgement and according to preselected criteria relevant to a particular research question.

Qualitative research A systematic, subjective, and methodological approach used to describe life experiences and give them meaning.

Quantitative research A formal, objective, and systematic process that involves conceptualizing, planning, implementing, and communicating the findings, which are used to describe variables, test relationships between them, and examine cause-and-effect relationships among variables.

Quasi-experimental research A research design in which the researcher initiates an experimental treatment but some characteristic of true experiment, either control or randomization, is lacking.

Questionnaire A printed self-report form designed to collect information from the respondents mostly in written form.

Quota sampling A type of non-probability method of sampling in which researcher decides while designing the study the number people with pre-specified characteristics to be included as participants.

Random assignment The assignment of subjects to treatment or control groups in a random manner, which is also termed as randomization.

Random sampling The technique in which every member of the population has an equal probability of being included in the study.

Range The interval between the highest and lowest values of the observations (highest – lowest).

Ratio indicator The highest level of measurement that allows comparison between variable values; it has all the properties of nominal, ordinal, and interval scales plus an absolute or a true zero value.

Reference list A list that includes the books, articles, web pages, and so on that are cited in the text of the document.

Referencing A standardized way of acknowledging the sources of information and ideas that are used in a study.

Reflectivity An interactive process that a researcher goes through to uncover the underlying factors that may influence the study's findings.

REFWORKS A web-based bibliography and database manager that allows to create one's own personal database by importing references from text files or online databases and other various sources.

Reliability The degree of consistency or dependability with which an instrument measures the attribute it is designed to measure or the ability of the instrument to create reproducible results, because without the ability to reproduce results no truth can be known.

Representative sample The sample whose key characteristics closely approximate those of the population.

Research critiques A careful appraisal of the strengths and weaknesses of a research study or report.

Research ethics A set of principles or guidelines that will assist the researcher in making difficult research decisions and in deciding which goals are most important in reconciling conflicting values.

Research hypothesis The existence of relationship between two or more variables.

Research problem A question that a researcher wants to answer or a problem that a researcher wants to solve.

Research report A means of communicating key aspects of a study to the research consumer and also the vehicle through which the nurse researcher disseminates crucial information about the investigation.

Research utilization A process of communicating and using research generated knowledge in order to make an impact on or a change in the existing practices in health care system.

Research utilization continuum The starting point of a research to the emergence of new knowledge and ideas and the utilization of research.

Research variables The variables observed or measured in natural settings as they exist, without manipulating or imposing the effect of intervention or treatment.

Retrospective research A type of research in which a phenomenon existing in the present is linked to phenomena that occurred in the past, before the study was initiated.

Rigour Striving for excellence in research.

Sample A subset of the population that is selected for a study.

Sample size The number of participants needed to achieve statistical conclusion validity.

Sampling The process of selecting a portion of the population to represent the entire population.

Sampling bias The systematic over-representation or under-representation of sample.

Sampling error The fluctuations of the value of a statistic from one sample to another drawn from the same population. It is sometimes referred to as chance or standard error.

Sampling frames The potential participants who meet the definition of the population and are accessible to the researcher.

Saturation The collection of data in a qualitative study to the point where a sense of closure is attained because new data yield redundant information.

Scatter plots The graphical presentation of the relationship between two *continuous variables*, including its direction and magnitude. They are also called *scatter diagrams* or *scattergrams.*

Secondary source The description or summary by somebody other than the original researcher or second-hand records of events, experiments, creative works, or statistics.

Simple hypothesis A statement that reflects the relationship between two variables.

Situation-producing theories The theories that prescribe the activities necessary to attain a defined goal; these are also known as prescription theories.

Situation-relating theories The theories that just depict the proximity in relationship in a given situation; they are also termed as situation-depicting theories.

Snowball sampling The selection of participants through referrals from earlier participants. It is also called as network sampling.

Solomon four-group design An experimental design that uses a before–after design for one pair of experimental and control groups and an after only design for another pair.

Specific objectives The factors influencing the various aspects of the statement of the problems.

Stability The extent to which similar results or responses are obtained on two or more separate occasions of an instrument.

Standard normal curve When the mean is 'zero' and the standard deviation is 'one'.

Standard score The number of standard deviations from the mean; it is also called the 'sigma' or '*z*-score'.

Statistical unit The individual subject or object upon whom or which information is collected.

Statistics Measures of the samples.

Stop words The commonly used words that will automatically stop a computer keyword search because they occur too frequently in records.

Strata Mutually exclusive segments of population based on specific characteristics.

Stratified random sampling A type of sample selection where the subjects are randomly selected from two or more strata of the population independently.

Study framework The relationship between variables or concepts and links variables or concepts selected from the research problem.

Systematic error A measurement error that is not random but occurs consistently in the same direction.

Systematic reviews Rigorous and well-defined approach for reviewing the literature in a specific subject area.

Systematic sampling The process of selecting every small k^{th} individual from an ordered list of all members of a population, using a randomly selected starting point.

Target population The aggregate of cases about which a researcher would like to generalize.

Tertiary source A description of study prepared by synthesizing and explaining the research work from secondary sources.

Theoretical concepts The concepts that are not readily observable and whose meanings are derived from the theory in which they are embedded.

Theoretical definition The concept that is defined in relation to other concepts as defined in the particular theory.

Theoretical framework A collection of interrelated concepts based on one existing theory; it provides a context for examining the problem and is a frame of reference as a base for observations, definitions of concepts, interpretation, and generalization; it defines overall design of a research study.

Theoretical limitations The limitations that restrict the ability of research findings to generalize due to the use of specific theoretical concept in study, or limiting the study of variables through operational definitions.

Theory An abstract generalization that is developed from concepts and reveals the relationship between the concepts, which are in the form of propositional statements and are connected in a logical system of thought.

Thesaurus A directory of assigned subject headings.

Theses or dissertations Documents that describe completely the steps followed in carrying out a research investigation.

Transferability The extent to which findings relate to other settings or groups.

Triangulation It refers to combining different methods, theories, data sources (including data collected from different sites or at different times), or investigators to converge on a single construct. The idea is that looking at a single question through multiple 'glasses' will give a more complete understanding of the issue being studied. Triangulation provides an opportunity to increase the strength and consistency of evidence provided by the use of both qualitative and quantitative research methods.

Truncation A way to find different forms of words in a Boolean or keyword search.

Type I error The error that occurs when the researcher concludes that the samples tested are from different populations when, in fact, the samples are from the same population.

Type II error The error that occurs when the researcher concludes that no significant differences exist between the samples examined when, in fact, a difference exists.

Universal assumptions Beliefs that are assumed to be true by a large part of society, but testing such assumption is not always possible.

Unstructured interview An oral self-report in which the researcher asks a respondent questions without having a predetermined plan regarding the content or flow of information to be gathered.

Unwarranted assumptions The assumptions stated without any supportive evidence.

Validity The degree to which an instrument measures what it is intended to measure or the truthfulness of the measure in an instrument in assessing the phenomenon of interest in a given sample or population.

Variables The qualities, properties, or characteristics of persons, things, or situations that change or vary and are manipulated or measured in research.

Veracity The quality of telling the truth; it incorporates the concept that individuals should always be told the truth.

Verbal research report A format of reporting the research studies or presenting the research study by the researcher in research conferences or professional conferences.

Warranted assumptions The assumptions stated along with evidence to support.

Written research report A scholarly work of a researcher done for disseminating the research findings through the research articles or research abstracts in research journals or various professional nursing journals.

***z*-Score** The distance of a particular observation (value) from the mean in terms of standard deviations.

Index